Statistics in Endocrinology

*Proceedings of a Workshop Conference held at
Endicott House, Dedham, Massachusetts, December 4–7, 1967*

THE MIT PRESS
Cambridge, Massachusetts, and London, England

Statistics
in
Endocrinology

Edited by Janet W. McArthur
and Theodore Colton

Contents

Supplement: Competitive Protein-Binding Assays

I. Theoretical Aspects

II. Statistical Aspects

Preface

The Workshop Conference on Statistics in Endocrinology was organized for the purpose of acquainting endocrine investigators with modern experimental design and statistical analysis. Although most endocrinologists have had the benefit of an elementary course in statistics, only rarely have they been grounded sufficiently in mathematical principles to make full use of the statistical armamentarium. In consequence, many experimenters operate within unnecessary constraints, unaware of the variety and power of the instruments created by their ally, the statistician. Yet, with the artful use of statistical tools the endocrinologist not only can increase the economy and validity of his experiments but can add a dimension of elegance.

The Conference had a long gestation period. Its moment of conception can be dated accurately as August 19, 1964, when a few American experimenters were privileged to attend a half-day symposium on the mathematical analysis of data in experimental endocrinology held at the Second International Congress of Endocrinology in London. Despite the limitation of time the symposium was outstandingly successful, and upon our return some of us began to explore means whereby we could share this experience with a wider circle of investigators. It seemed that a longer meeting, with greater opportunity for interchange between experimenter and statistician, was needed.

When we began to consider what to include in the program, we started in true statistical fashion by conducting a survey. A checklist questionnaire of possible topics was sent to a group of some sixty endocrinologists. If not a random sample of experimenters, it constituted one representing a wide variety of research interests. Thirty-nine replies were received and were utilized in evolving the content of the Workshop. In addition to completing the checklist the respondents offered many valuable suggestions. One was that the statistical analyses be illustrated with endocrine data insofar as practicable. Another was that the subject of competitive protein-binding assays be considered in a mathematical and statistical context. Two supplementary sessions were accordingly arranged and, although this portion of the Conference constituted a digression from the original plan, the presentations fitted in with the overall theme.

The Conference was supported by grants from the Endocrinology Study Section and the Special Mathematics Study Section of the National Institutes of Health. Supplementary funds were generously donated by CIBA Pharmaceutical Company, Ortho Research Foundation, Syntex Research, and Wyeth Laboratories.

We are deeply grateful to those who contributed to this volume, not only with their formal presentations, but by their responsiveness in the discussions. We wish also to acknowledge our indebtedness to the members of the Organizing Committee: Chester I. Bliss, William G. Cochran, Roy O. Greep, Sidney H. Ingbar, Hilton A. Salhanick, Armen H. Tashjian, Jr., and Jane Worcester.

Especial gratitude is due Mrs. Elim M. O'Shaughnessy, Director of Endicott House, and her staff for the perfection of the physical arrangements for the Conference and Miss Rita J. Nickerson for untiring assistance in the conduct of the meeting. Mrs. Charlotte Casler gave invaluable help in the preparations for the Workshop, and she, together with Mrs. Lydia Du Pertuis and Mrs. Elizabeth Palmer, typed the manuscript. To them and to Drs. Andrew G. Frantz and Edward W. Webster, who gave expert assistance to the editors in the preparation of the proceedings, we wish to express our warm thanks.

Janet W. McArthur, M.D., Sc.D. (hon.)
*Associate Clinical Professor of
Obstetrics and Gynecology,
Harvard Medical School*

Theodore Colton, Sc.D.
*Associate Professor of Biostatistics,
Harvard Medical School*

Boston, Massachusetts
July 1969

List of Contributors

PETER ARMITAGE, PH.D.
Professor of Medical Statistics
London School of Hygiene
and Tropical Medicine
London, England

SOLOMON A. BERSON, M.D.
Professor and Chairman of Medicine
Mt. Sinai School of Medicine
New York, New York
Senior Medical Investigator
Veterans Administration
Bronx, New York

CHESTER I. BLISS, PH.D.
Research Associate
Yale University
New Haven, Connecticut
Biometrician
Connecticut Agricultural Experiment
Station
New Haven, Connecticut

BYRON WILLIAM BROWN, JR., PH.D.
Professor of Biostatistics
Stanford University
Stanford, California

WILLIAM G. COCHRAN, M.A.
Professor of Statistics
Harvard University
Cambridge, Massachusetts

JEROME CORNFIELD, B.S.
Research Professor in Biostatistics
University of Pittsburgh
Pittsburgh, Pennsylvania

C. PHILIP COX, M.A.
Professor of Statistics
Iowa State University
Ames, Iowa

WILFRID J. DIXON, PH.D.
Professor of Biomathematics
Health Sciences Computing Facility
University of California
Los Angeles, California

CHARLES W. DUNNETT, D.SC.
Statistician
Lederle Laboratories Division
American Cyanamid Company
Pearl River, New York

MURRAY EDEN, PH.D.
Professor of Electrical Engineering
Massachusetts Institute of Technology
Cambridge, Massachusetts
Lecturer in Preventive Medicine
Harvard Medical School
Boston, Massachusetts

ROGER EKINS, PH.D.
Reader in Medical Nucleonics
University of London
London, England
Institute of Nuclear Medicine
Middlesex Hospital Medical School
London, England

C. W. EMMENS, D.SC., PH.D.
Professor of Veterinary Physiology
University of Sydney
Sydney, Australia

SALLY B. FAND, M.D.
Associate Professor of Pathology
Wayne State University
School of Medicine
Detroit, Michigan
Chief, Special Histochemistry
Veterans Administration Hospital
Allen Park, Michigan

DAVID J. FINNEY, SC.D., F.R.S., F.R.S.E.
Professor of Statistics
University of Edinburgh
Edinburgh, Scotland

JOHN P. GILBERT, PH.D.
Staff Statistician
Harvard Computing Center
Cambridge, Massachusetts

EDWARD M. KAPLAN, M.S.
Staff Analyst
Harvard Computing Center
Cambridge, Massachusetts

RICHARD B. MCHUGH, PH.D.
Professor and Director of Biometry
Health Sciences Center
University of Minnesota
Minneapolis, Minnesota

CURTIS L. MEINERT, PH.D.
Associate Professor of Epidemiology
  and Biostatistics
Institute of International Medicine
University of Maryland
Baltimore, Maryland

G. B. NEWMAN, M.A.
Lecturer in Mathematics
Institute of Nuclear Medicine
Middlesex Hospital Medical School
London, England

J. L. H. O'RIORDAN, B.M.
Senior Lecturer in Medicine
Middlesex Hospital Medical School
London, England

P. L. RAYFORD, B.S.
Research Technician
Endocrinology Branch
National Cancer Institute
Bethesda, Maryland

RICHARD D. REMINGTON, PH.D.
Associate Dean
University of Texas School of
  Public Health
Houston, Texas

DAVID RODBARD, M.D.
Research Associate
National Institute of Child Health
  and Human Development
Bethesda, Maryland

GRIFF T. ROSS, M.D., PH.D.
Head, Endocrinology Service
Assistant Chief,
Endocrinology Branch
National Cancer Institute
Bethesda, Maryland

I. RICHARD SAVAGE, PH.D.
Visiting Professor of Statistics
Yale University
New Haven, Connecticut
Professor of Statistics
Florida State University
Tallahassee, Florida

HARRY SMITH, JR., PH.D.
Professor of Biostatistics
University of North Carolina
Chapel Hill, North Carolina

RICHARD P. SPENCER, M.D., PH.D.
Professor of Nuclear Medicine
  (Radiology)
Yale University School of Medicine
New Haven, Connecticut

JAMES F. TAIT, PH.D., F.R.S.
Senior Scientist
Worcester Foundation for
  Experimental Biology
Shrewsbury, Massachusetts

ROSALYN S. YALOW, PH.D.
Research Professor of Medicine
Mt. Sinai School of Medicine
New York, New York
Chief, Radioimmunoassay
  Reference Laboratory
Veterans Administration Hospital
Bronx, New York

List of Participants

ALEXANDER ALBERT, PH.D., M.D.
Mayo Clinic
Rochester, Minnesota

GEORGE ALLEN, M.A.
Ortho Research Foundation
Raritan, New Jersey

WAYNE BACON, PH.D.
Ohio Agricultural Research and
Development Center
Wooster, Ohio

DEREK BANGHAM, B.S., M.B.
National Institute for Medical
Research
London, England

DELPHINE B. BARTOSIK, M.D.
Worcester Foundation for
Experimental Biology
Shrewsbury, Massachusetts

GABRIEL BIALY, PH.D.
Worcester Foundation for
Experimental Biology
Shrewsbury, Massachusetts

MARION K. BIRMINGHAM, PH.D.
Allan Memorial Institute of
Psychiatry
Montreal, Canada

RUDI BORTH, PH.D.
University of Toronto School of
Medicine
Toronto, Canada

CLAUDE DESJARDINS, PH.D.
Jackson Laboratory
Bar Harbor, Maine

CLAUDE FORTIER, PH.D.
Faculté de Médecine
Université Laval
Quebec, Canada

ROGER GUILLEMIN, PH.D., M.D.
Baylor University Medical School
Houston, Texas

ERLIO GURPIDE, PH.D.
College of Physicians and Surgeons of
Columbia University
New York, New York

ARTHUR L. HERBST, M.D.
Harvard Medical School
Boston, Massachusetts

JEROME M. HERSHMAN, M.D.
Veterans Administration Hospital
Birmingham, Alabama

PHILIP HIRSCH, PH.D.
University of North Carolina
Medical School
Chapel Hill, North Carolina

C. M. KNEBEL, PH.D.
Wyeth Laboratories
Philadelphia, Pennsylvania

SHELDON KUGLER, M.S.
Syntex Laboratories
Palo Alto, California

WILLIAM B. LANGAN, PH.D.
Villanova University
Villanova, Pennsylvania

E. TRAVIS LITTLEDIKE, D.V.M., PH.D.
Iowa State University
Ames, Iowa

ALBERT C. LOWENSTEIN, B.A.
Wyeth Laboratories
Philadelphia, Pennsylvania

LLOYD MILLER, PH.D.
U.S. Pharmacopeia
New York, New York

ARNOLD MOSES, M.D.
Veterans Administration Hospital
Syracuse, New York

FREDERICK MOSTELLER, PH.D.
Harvard University
Cambridge, Massachusetts

MARJORIE MUSSETT, B.SC.
National Institute for Medical
  Research
London, England

KATHLEEN B. O'KEEFE, PH.D.
University of Washington
Pacific Northwest Research
  Foundation
Seattle, Washington

WILLIAM H. PEARLMAN, PH.D.
Harvard Medical School
Boston, Massachusetts

SAMUEL REFETOFF, M.D.
Harvard Medical School
Boston, Massachusetts

GILBERT A. RINARD, PH.D.
Case Western Reserve University
Cleveland, Ohio

JACOB ROBBINS, M.D.
National Institute of Arthritis and
  Metabolic Diseases
Bethesda, Maryland

ELIJAH B. ROMANOFF, PH.D.
Worcester Foundation for
  Experimental Biology
Shrewsbury, Massachusetts

ALLEN ROOT, M.D.
University of Pennsylvania School of
  Medicine
Philadelphia, Pennsylvania

EUGENIA ROSEMBERG, M.D.
Medical Research Institute of
  Worcester
Worcester, Massachusetts

MARIE L. D. SCHÖNBAUM, M.SC.
University of Toronto
Toronto, Canada

ROMUALD STUPNICKI, PH.D.
Worcester Foundation for
  Experimental Biology
Shrewsbury, Massachusetts

HANNA D. SYLWESTROWICZ, M.S.
CIBA Pharmaceutical Company
Summit, New Jersey

WILLIAM TAYLOR, PH.D.
Mayo Clinic
Rochester, Minnesota

KOJI YOSHINAGA, PH.D.
Worcester Foundation for
  Experimental Biology
Shrewsbury, Massachusetts

Statistics in Endocrinology

CHAPTER ONE

Experimental Design

PETER ARMITAGE AND
RICHARD D. REMINGTON

1. Basic principles

Introduction

Whether one is an endocrinologist experimenting with animals, a practicing physician, or a statistician charged with the analysis of experimental data, the design of one's experiments is of central importance. Logically and chronologically, the design of an experiment precedes its analysis, and to a large extent the design determines the validity of the analysis: many investigations are so ill designed as to be beyond salvation, however ingenious the analysis. Furthermore, it is a useful beginning point, since the general principles we shall discuss require little in the way of mathematical justification.

We shall use examples from endocrinological work, but basically we shall be talking about principles that are equally applicable in most branches of biology. This is not to deny that endocrinology may give rise to special problems of experimental design.

In many fields of science it is often extremely difficult to get the same answer twice. Particularly in quantitative observations on some scale of measurement, variation is often present, variation that is not wholly controllable by the investigator. In the physical sciences such variation may arise mainly from measurement errors or from failure to control the environment. In the biological sciences variations from one organism to another or in the physiological state of a single organism are likely to be at least as important. One of the central tasks of statistical science is to provide methods of handling data of this type. We are concerned with experiments in which (a) the observations are subject to this sort of variation and (b) the purpose is to compare the effects of various treatments on some sort of experimental material. This covers many, perhaps most, biological experiments but excludes investigations in which no comparisons are made. This is an important group of exclusions. In physics, for example, one might wish to measure some absolute quantity, such as the speed of light, as accurately as possible; in medicine one might wish to discover some characteristics of a certain species, such as the distribution of the survival time after exposure to a toxic agent or the mean urinary concentration of a certain steroid. Investigations of this sort may well involve considerable interference with nature, as they do in the determination of survival times, but conceptually they are more like surveys than comparative experiments. Statistical considerations are certainly present, but one is usually concerned at least as much about the relevance of the experiment: whether there is a systematic bias in the method, or whether the animals are typical of those in general use, and so on.

Even when interest centers on the effect of one particular treatment — say the injection of a certain substance into rats or the administration of a certain drug to human patients — the experimenter or the physician will often deem it advisable to include a control group treated in some relevant way. A noncomparative experiment thus becomes comparative. In any such experiment there will be certain experimental units to which alternative treatments could be allotted. They may be towns, people, animals, different periods of observations on the same organism, bacteria, or pieces of inert matter. In each case the question arises: "How should one allot the rival treatments to the different experimental units?" This question will underlie most of our discussion.

It may be useful at this stage to mention two largely nonmathematical books that deal with this subject, one by Cox (1958) and one (a shorter book) by Finney (1955). The work of Cochran and Cox (1957) is a comprehensive handbook, and a number of other books, such as those of Federer (1955) and Finney (1960), deal at great length with the mathematical theory. Fisher's classic book, *The Design of Experiments* (1935), is perhaps best read after one has gained some preliminary knowledge of the subject. Mention of this book may serve to remind us that the whole idea that the design of comparative experiments is a part of statistical theory and methodology deserving systematic study is due to the late R. A. Fisher. Most of what we have to say will be an attempted exposition of the basic principles that he enunciated during the 1920's and 1930's and that still underlie most of the current work on experimental design. Their application to clinical experiments, which was largely promoted by Hill (1962) in the 1940's and 1950's involved rather simple designs, although it has raised a number of difficult practical and ethical issues.

Randomization

One of the most important of Fisher's precepts was that the effect of extraneous variables should be controlled by the device of randomization. If two or more treatments of groups of experimental units are to be compared, one would like the groups to be as similar as possible in the various factors that might influence the level of response. Some of these factors can be recognized in advance. One could then try to match the individuals in the various groups: for example, in an animal experiment, by selecting groups of animals of about the same weight and about the same age and, in a clinical comparison, by selecting groups of patients in whom the various degrees of severity of their illness are similarly distributed. But there remains a basic problem: how can one ensure that the groups do not differ in some unmatched characteristic that may well affect the result of the experiment?

Fisher's solution was to allot the individuals to groups randomly, that is, by some chance mechanism like the toss of a coin or the spin of a roulette wheel. Such an overt use of gambling apparatus may be a little unseemly, and the allocation can conveniently and more discreetly be done from tables of random numbers or random permutations. Randomization may be thought of as a way of dealing with all the unrecognized factors that may influence response, once the recognizable factors, if any, have been allowed for by some sort of systematic balancing. It does not ensure that groups are absolutely alike in all relevant aspects; nothing can do that. It does ensure that they are all unlikely to differ on the average by more than a moderate amount in any given characteristic, and it enables the statistician to assess the extent to which an observed difference in response to different treatments can be explained by the hazards of random allocation.

Randomization in animal experiments is, no doubt, a nuisance. Animals have to be numbered, tables consulted, and care taken over the allocation. Yet in comparison with other aspects of most experiments it is relatively inexpensive in time, effort, and cost. Furthermore, it is difficult to imagine any other procedure as free from potential hazards. Emmens (1948) points out that the haphazard selection of animals from a cage may lead to a systematic difference in weight between the animals chosen first and those chosen later. The animals are also likely to differ in behavior (for example, in tameness) and quite possibly in a number of other features related to the response to treatment. Clinical comparisons similarly are fraught with artifacts. The reasons for the clinician's use of one treatment rather than another are so frequently related to the condition of the patient that comparisons of the effectiveness of different treatments are rarely of any value unless the groups of patients have been formed by random allocation.

Randomization, of course, will not necessarily remove all potential biases in the comparison. In an animal experiment the investigator may carefully select two groups of animals at random and then place the cages containing animals due for treatment A at one end of the room and those for treatment B at the other end. A well-chosen draft would wreck the experiment. The positions in the room and not only the animals should have been randomized. In clinical comparisons there is a special danger that different standards of assessment may be used for different treatments, particularly when the patient or the doctor knows which treatment is being applied on any one occasion. The well-known devices of single- and double-blind administrations of therapies are designed to overcome this problem, although of course they are not always both feasible and desirable.

Replication

A second basic principle is that of replication, or the use of more than one experimental unit with a given treatment. There are a number of different points to bear in mind here. One point relates to the analysis that will follow the completion of the experiment. In that analysis it will be important not only to measure the apparent relative effects of the different treatments but also to assess the extent to which these comparisons might have been affected by the inescapable random variation. To do this one must measure the random variation, and one can most easily do so by having a number of experimental units treated in the same way and seeing how they differ in their response. As we shall see, some experimental designs do not require this simple type of replication, but replication of some sort must certainly be present.

A second point about replication is that, the greater the number of units to which each treatment is applied, the more precise the comparison of treatment effects. This is intuitively obvious, and it follows theoretically from the fact that the sampling variance of a mean, a proportion, or almost any other quantity that is likely to be relevant in a comparison is inversely proportional to the number of observations.

A further reason for replication is to extend the range of applicability of the results. Any experiment permits only limited generalization. A contrast revealed by a particular experiment and shown by a statistical analysis to be reasonably precise when random variation is allowed for is not necessarily valid under conditions other than those of the experiment or for experimental units different in kind from those used. The nature of these units will be difficult to define rigorously unless they have been selected at random from some large population, and that is not usually the case. It will often, therefore, be illuminating to use a variety of experimental environments, various strains of animal, different techniques, and so forth. The relevant comparisons can then be made separately within each subdivision of the experiment, and their consistency can be examined. For example, a clinical trial to compare certain medical treatments may be run in a number of hospitals, so that minor variations in therapy are represented in the experiment.

All these points bear on the frequently asked question of how big an experiment should be, and from this point of view the most important criterion is that of precision. If the experimenter can decide how precise a comparison he wants, and if some measure of the degree of random variation is available, the statistician can provide him with a figure. If the random variation is initially of unknown extent, it may be possible to measure it during the early stages of an experiment. The difficulty usually is that the experimenter is not at all certain how precise an answer he wants. In a context of technology it may be possible to work this out by hard-headed economics. Experimentation costs money, but an improvement in, say, the yield of crops saves money; somewhere a balance can be struck. If, on the other hand, it is a matter of measuring, say, the ACTH in the sera of scorbutic guinea pigs, one must surely rely on more arbitrary assessments of the precision required. The experimenter may well find that his original target implied an impossibly large number of observations, in which case he will have to lower his sights.

Reduction of random variation

The third basic principle is the use of techniques of experimental design for the reduction of random variation, or what Fisher often called the "local control of variability."

We have discussed so far the simplest example of an experimental design, the *simple randomization* design, in which experimental units are allotted at random to the groups receiving the various treatments. In such an experiment the precision of a comparison depends not only on the number of replicates, which we have just discussed, but also on the basic random variability in response between units treated in the same way. We should like, in fact, to perform the experiment on units that are as homogeneous as possible in their responses. The investigator will often try to work with such homogeneous material by using, for instance, inbred strains of animals or, in a clinical trial, by carefully restricting the clinical condition of the patients. We must remember, though, that the more successful he is in this aim the less successful he will be in one of the aims of replication, which is to cover a variety of experimental conditions.

A solution to this dilemma lies in the use of a *randomized block* design. Suppose we can arrange the experimental units in groups (or, as we shall say, blocks) such that members of the same block are on the whole likely to behave more similarly than members of different blocks. For example, in some circumstances littermates may be more alike in their response than members of different litters (whether for genetic or environmental reasons). If, say, five treatments are to be compared, one could take litters of five animals and allocate treatments at random to the individual animals in each litter so that each treatment occurred once in each litter (Table 1). Each litter would provide a small experiment, and

TABLE 1   A Randomized Block Design

Litter	Animal				
	1	2	3	4	5
1	D	C	A	E	B
2	C	B	A	E	D
3	D	B	C	A	E
4	C	E	A	D	B
5	B	A	E	C	D
6	E	C	D	B	A
7	D	B	A	C	E
8	B	E	A	C	D
9	E	A	B	C	D
10	C	B	D	E	A

in the whole experiment the comparison of treatments would be affected only by the random variation *within* a litter, not by the extra variation between litters.

If the blocks are sufficiently large, it may be possible to arrange that each treatment occurs two or more times within a block. Each block then provides its own internal replication, and it becomes possible in the analysis to see whether the relative treatment effects vary appreciably from one block to another. This may be particularly useful if the blocks are really interesting in their own right — if, for instance, they differentiate between animals of different strains or weights rather than of different litters.

Another common example of blocking occurs in experiments in which an individual animal can be used on more than one occasion, with a different treatment on each occasion. It is generally found that repeated observations of the same individual are more alike than observations of different individuals. The individual animal now forms the block, and treatments may be allocated at random to the successive occasions on which an animal is observed. In particular, in clinical comparisons it is often possible to arrange that each patient receives the rival treatments on successive occasions, the order of administration being determined randomly.

We have mentioned the possibility that the effect of an extraneous variable such as the weight of an animal may be controlled by the formation of blocks consisting of animals of similar weights. Leech and Paterson (1952), for instance, investigating the effects of thyroxine and thiouracil on the tubercular reactions of guinea pigs, wished to divide thirty-six animals into nine treatment groups. They formed four blocks according to weight and allocated the nine treatments at random within each block.

They do not appear, however, to have taken this arrangement into account in the analysis. If a blocking system is effective, it should certainly be exploited in the analysis; otherwise the investigator takes an unduly modest view of the precision of his experiment.

An alternative approach to the control of the variation in response due to some identifiable variable such as weight is to use a simple, randomized experiment, without blocking, and then to allow for the effect of this variable in the analysis. The improvement in precision is much the same as that in a randomized block experiment; the choice is largely whether one wants the extra complications in the design or in the analysis. The basic statistical method for this situation is the analysis of covariance (see Chapter 7), although modifications may be required in some circumstances.

2. Factorial experiments

Introduction

The purpose of this section is to examine one category of design, the factorial design, which illustrates the basic principles. Historically, factorial designs were developed to deal with experiments in agronomy and agricultural science, but their usefulness and appropriateness are now realized by workers in nearly every category of experimental science. In endocrinology they are particularly useful in unsnarling the multiple complicated sources of experimental variability that seem to characterize this field.

The view of factorial experiments we shall take is a general one: we shall consider factorial arrangements of experimental units and treatments. A factorial experiment, then, is an experiment that permits the simultaneous assessment of the effects of several factors. For many years it was considered a maxim of sound experimentation that all factors but one should be held constant, to permit evaluation of the influence of that single factor. That view was outmoded years ago when Fisher, Yates, and other workers showed us how to plan factorial experiments and to analyze the resulting data.

Some examples of experimental factors relevant to endocrinological research are hormone preparation in an experiment for comparing the milk-ejecting potency of oxytocin and deaminooxytocin, hormone dosage or concentration, sex of an experimental animal, right versus left side of an animal treated with a topical preparation, days in an experiment for determining day-to-day fluctuation in adrenocortical activity, and subjects in an experiment for assessing the importance of intersubject variation. Each of these factors occurs at several levels; for example,

hormone preparation has as its levels oxytocin and deaminooxytocin, sex
has the levels male and female, and subjects has several levels, each level
corresponding to a particular subject.

The 2^2 factorial: main effects and interaction

To illustrate some basic concepts of factorial experimentation we shall
abstract a portion of a design used by Althabe et al. (1966) in a study
made to assess the milk-ejecting potencies of oxytocin and deaminooxytocin in lactating women. Although the full design is rather complicated, we are here interested in only one portion of it, in which each of
the two compounds is used at a high and a low dose level, and the
response variable is the rise in intramammary pressure. The experiment
thus contains two factors (compound and dose), each occurring at two
levels, and is called a 2^2 factorial. The basic design is shown in Table 2.

TABLE 2   A 2^2 Factorial Experiment*

Hormone compound	Dose	
	Low	High
Oxytocin	$\bar{y}_{11}$	$\bar{y}_{12}$
Deaminooxytocin	$\bar{y}_{21}$	$\bar{y}_{22}$

* Abstracted from Althabe et al. (1966).

The mean rises in intramammary pressure are indicated by $\bar{y}$ with appropriate subscripts, the first subscript giving the level of the first factor
(compound) and the second giving the level of the second factor (dose).
For example, $\bar{y}_{12}$ is the mean rise in intramammary pressure following
administration of oxytocin at high dose. We shall assume that each mean
is based on the same number of observations, say r. Thus the basic
compound by dose layout with a single observation in each cell may be
regarded as being repeated, or replicated, r times; we say there are r
replicates.

The simple effect of compound at low dose might be measured by
$\bar{y}_{21} - \bar{y}_{11}$, the average amount by which response to deaminooxytocin
exceeds that to oxytocin when both are at low dose. Similarly, the simple
effect of compound at high dose is measured by $\bar{y}_{22} - \bar{y}_{12}$. The overall,
main effect of compound is the sum of these simple effects:

$$\bar{y}_{21} - \bar{y}_{11} + \bar{y}_{22} - \bar{y}_{12} \tag{1}$$

This quantity is often multiplied by the factor $1/2$, but since this
refinement is of more import in analysis than design, we shall omit it.

Again, the simple effects of dose at the two levels of compound are, respectively,

$$\bar{y}_{12} - \bar{y}_{11} \quad \text{and} \quad \bar{y}_{22} - \bar{y}_{21}$$

and the main effect of dose is their sum,

$$\bar{y}_{12} - \bar{y}_{11} + \bar{y}_{22} - \bar{y}_{21} \tag{2}$$

An important question for investigation in factorial experimentation concerns the constancy of the two simple effects. That is, are the simple effects of compound constant at the two dose levels? More generally, we ask whether the effect of the first factor is constant at the two levels of the second. Of course, this question is asked relative to the populations from which the observations have been drawn. Sampling fluctuations will affect the observed values. The question we have asked may be re-phrased to read, "Is there any *interaction* between compound and dose?" If simple effects are not constant, then interaction is present. A natural measure of interaction is the difference between the two simple effects of compound at high and low dose, or

$$(\bar{y}_{22} - \bar{y}_{12}) - (\bar{y}_{21} - \bar{y}_{11})$$

or, the parentheses removed,

$$\bar{y}_{22} - \bar{y}_{12} - \bar{y}_{21} + \bar{y}_{11} \tag{3}$$

Alternatively we might ask whether or not the simple effects of dose are constant across the two levels of compound and measure lack of constancy by

$$(\bar{y}_{22} - \bar{y}_{21}) - (\bar{y}_{12} - \bar{y}_{11})$$

which becomes

$$\bar{y}_{22} - \bar{y}_{21} - \bar{y}_{12} + \bar{y}_{11}$$

and which is an expression identical in value with Equation 3, the earlier expression for interaction. Thus the interaction is symmetric and measures the lack of constancy of one factor across the levels of another.

Interaction depends strongly upon the scale of measurement. This is easy to see numerically. Suppose we consider a single replicate of a 2^2 factorial experiment and have observations as shown in Table 3, first part. Here the main effects are as follows.

Row effect: $16 - 4 + 76 - 64 = 24$
Column effect: $64 - 4 + 76 - 16 = 120$

The interaction is $76 - 64 - 16 + 4 = 0$.

TABLE 3   A Single Replicate of a
Hypothetical 2^2 Factorial Experiment

Levels of row factor	Levels of column factor	
	1	2
	Raw data:	
1	4	64
2	16	76
	Data after square-root transformation:	
1	2.0	8.0
2	4.0	8.7

Suppose, however, we used a different scale of measurement on which observations were taken to be the square roots of the original measurements. The second part of Table 3 shows the data on the transformed scale. Now the interaction is $8.7 - 8.0 - 4.0 + 2.0 = 1.3$. A simple change in scale has produced an interaction where none was present before.

Higher factorials

We are often interested in experiments involving larger numbers of factors than those given in the preceding paragraphs, or larger numbers of levels per factor, or both. If we have three factors, each at two levels, a single replicate will consist of eight observations, one at each level of each factor. The resulting experiment is called a 2^3 factorial. Three main effects corresponding to each of the three factors A, B, and C can be estimated. Three two-factor interactions, those of A with B, A with C, and B with C, can be estimated, but a three-factor interaction of A, B, and C is also estimable. This higher-order interaction measures the lack of constancy of a two-factor interaction, say that of A and B, across the levels of the third factor, C.

It is reasonable that larger numbers of factors, each at two levels, might be employed. With four such factors we have a 2^4 factorial. In general, an experiment with k factors, each at two levels, is called a 2^k factorial. Again, the number 2^k is the number of observations necessary to form one complete replicate.

If there are two factors, each at three levels, nine observations are needed per replicate, and the resulting experiment is a 3^2 factorial. In general, an experiment with k factors, each at p levels, is a p^k factorial. It is not necessary that all factors have an equal number of levels. If there are three factors, the first two at two levels and the third at three levels, the result is a $2 \times 2 \times 3$ factorial. Again, there are twelve observations per replicate.

The following are several endocrinological examples of experiments with higher factorials. Meckler and Collins (1965) investigated the relative adrenal weights of adult offspring from all possible mating combinations of four strains of mice. The design was a $4 \times 4 \times 2 \times 2$ factorial with the following factors: dam's strain at four levels, sire's strain at four levels, sex of offspring, and laterality (right versus left adrenal). Pollard and Martin (1967) investigated the inhibiting of estradiol and estrone by dimethylstilbestrol in a mouse vaginal tetrazolium assay. This was a $6 \times 2 \times 2$ factorial with time of administration of DMS at six levels (0, 1, 2, 4, 8, and 16 minutes after the estrogens), hormone at two levels (estradiol and estrone), and a repetition of the entire experiment at two different times. Mackinnon et al. (1963) in a study of the influence of rapid altitude change on adrenocortical activity used a three-factor experiment to study variations in palmar sweat index. The factors were subjects, times of day, and days, producing a $7 \times 19 \times 4$ experiment. Feuer and Broadhurst (1962) examined the effect of thyrotropic hormone on defecation scores in rats selectively bred for emotional elimination. They used a 2^3 factorial arrangment with treatment (hormone or saline control), strain (reactive or nonreactive), and sex as factors.

Analysis of factorial experiments

The details of analysis of factorial experiments are considered in Chapter 2. The usual analytical scheme involves analysis of variance, which can be used either to test the statistical significance of main effects and interactions or to construct confidence intervals. Under appropriate assumptions (see pp. 44–47) test statistics will follow the F distribution, and interval estimators will often be based on the t distribution. The choice of an appropriate error term from the analysis of variance depends upon both the experimental design and the nature of the factors under study. In particular, one must decide whether the levels of a particular factor may be considered a sample of levels from some large population (which is ordinarily the case, as, for example, when the experimental subject is the factor), or whether the included levels are the only relevant ones (as when a treatment is being compared with a control). For more complete discussions see Cornfield and Tukey (1956), Bennett and Franklin (1954, Chapter 7), and Cox (1958).

Crossed and nested factors

Up to this point we have considered only cases in which experimental factors are crossed, that is, situations such that every level of a given factor could occur jointly with every level of the other factors. For instance, in the 2^2 example each level of the row factor (oxytocin and deaminooxytocin) occurred at each level of the column (dose) factor. Some factorial designs involve factors that are nested rather than crossed; that is, the levels of one factor occur within particular levels of another factor. An example will clarify the situation. Munford (1963) investigated the histological structure of mammary glands of rats and mice during pregnancy, lactation, and involution. Animals were sacrificed at three-day intervals during these stages. Thus, considering the two factors time of sacrifice (or, alternatively, stage in the lactational cycle) and rat, we see that the rat factor is nested within the time factor. A particular rat can be studied only at one time; in other words, even a rat has only one life to give for its experiment. Thus, the main effect for rat-to-rat variation can be studied only within the particular times. A pooled, rat main effect is formed by adding across the levels of the time factor. In this study there are the additional nestings of glands within rats, slides within glands, sections within slides, fields within sections, and alveoli within fields, producing a seven-factor, fully nested design. Such designs are sometimes called *hierarchical* designs.

Glover (1956) examined the effect of scrotal insulation on fructose concentration in the semen of the ram. The experiment included two crossed factors: treatment (scrotal insulation or none) by time period (before, during, or after treatment), producing a 2 × 3 factorial design. Within each of these factors another factor was nested: rams within treatment and weeks within time period.

Incomplete designs

It is obvious that to form even a single replicate of an experiment with three or more factors many experimental units will be needed. For instance, one replicate of a three-factor experiment with each factor at five levels will require a hundred and twenty-five units. For this reason investigators and statisticians have sought designs that permit at least the assessment of main effects of several factors, but at a reduction in the number of units required. Factorial designs in which not all combinations of factor levels are present in the experiment are called *incomplete factorials*.

Perhaps the most familiar incomplete factorial is the *Latin square*. This is a design that permits assessment of the main effects of three factors with only the number of units required by a two-factor experiment. The design requires that each of the factors have the same number of levels. Furthermore, in such an experiment no assessment of interaction is available, and the design probably should be avoided if there is reason to believe that large interaction effects are present. Table 4 shows a 5 × 5 Latin square; the factors are rows, columns, and Latin letters, and each factor has five levels. The essential, defining property of the Latin

TABLE 4 Some Latin-Square Designs

A 5 × 5 Latin square					A 5 × 5 Greco-Latin square					A 6 × 6 Latin square for carryover effects					
A	E	C	D	B	Cγ	Dε	Eβ	Aδ	Bα	A	B	F	C	E	D
C	B	E	A	D	Dδ	Eα	Aγ	Bε	Cβ	B	C	A	D	F	E
D	C	A	B	E	Eε	Aβ	Bδ	Cα	Dγ	C	D	B	E	A	F
E	D	B	C	A	Bβ	Cδ	Dα	Eγ	Aε	D	E	C	F	B	A
B	A	D	E	C	Aα	Bγ	Cε	Dβ	Eδ	E	F	D	A	C	B
										F	A	E	B	D	C

square is that each of the letters A through E occurs once and only once in each row and each column. Notice that only twenty-five experimental units are required, compared with the hundred and twenty-five for a full replicate of a 5^3 factorial.

As is true of many experimental designs, an early use of the Latin square was for agronomic field trials comparing the yields of several varieties of a grain, such as barley. In our example letters A to E represent the varieties, and the square is a field or land area. The varieties are planted in experimental plots arranged geometrically in the field, as in the 5 × 5 Latin square in Table 4. If there are fertility or meteorologic gradients in a horizontal or vertical direction across the field, the defining property of the Latin square guarantees that the varieties are planted in a balanced pattern and that no variety is either enhanced or inhibited by such gradients.

Bradley and Clarke (1956) used a 5 × 5 Latin square in a study of the response of rabbit mammary glands to intraductally injected prolactin preparations. The response variable was weight of gland per unit area, the row factor was the individual rabbit, and the column factor was the anterior or posterior portions of a pair of injected abdominal nipples on the rabbit. Each nipple pair was divided into anterior and posterior injection sites, except for the posterior nipple pair, which received injections only in the anterior portion. The Latin-letter factor was the injected dose of prolactin.

There are many different Latin squares of a given size. In designing an experiment of this type it is good practice to select a square at random from all possible squares of the appropriate size or at least to select from some very large group of such squares. Fisher and Yates (1963) describe the selection process in detail.

The Latin-square principle can be extended to permit assessment of the main effects of four factors in a two-factor array. The resulting design is called a *Greco-Latin square*. Table 4 shows a 5 × 5 Greco-Latin square. Notice that the Latin letters form a Latin square when considered alone, as do the Greek letters. Furthermore, every two letters consisting of one Latin and one Greek letter occur together once and only once in the square. These are the defining characteristics of the Greco-Latin square.

Certain special Latin-square designs can be useful in some situations. For example, in the administration of a succession of treatments to the same subject a problem of carryover from one treatment to the next may arise. Williams (1949) found a way to deal with this difficulty, and Cox (1958, Section 13.3) discusses the appropriate designs. A Latin square in which rows denote subjects, columns denote time periods, and Latin letters denote treatments is used. The square is so constructed that every treatment follows every other treatment except itself the same number of times. An example of such a square is given by Cox (1958, p. 273) and is shown in Table 4. For an odd number of treatments the situation is a bit more complicated, requiring pairs of squares and guaranteeing that in each pair every treatment follows every other treatment exactly twice.

Another use of the Latin square is in *crossover designs*. The simplest crossover experiment divides subjects at random into two groups for administration of treatment and control preparations. Group 1 gets treatment during the first time period, and the control during the second; group 2 has the sequence reversed.

Emmens (1957) investigated the effect of estrogen and proestrogen in ovariectomized mice. The basic response variable was the presence or absence of a positive vaginal smear, although transformations and modifications of this variable were also used. Mice were randomly subdivided into eight groups of twenty-four animals each, four doses each of estrogen and proestrogen were used, and the mice were tested every two weeks. Table 5 shows the design. Notice that groups I to IV received estrogen first and proestrogen second, and groups V to VIII the reverse. Notice, too, that not only is the full array an 8 × 8 Latin square but it is composed of four 4 × 4 Latin subsquares.

Further modifications of Latin-square designs are available. For example, a series of randomly selected squares of given size can be used. Another modification arises when it is impossible to use as many levels of the column factor as are available for the row and letter factors; here a modification known as the *Youden square* can be used. Cox (1958, Section 11.3) gives a description of this design.

Incomplete blocks

As indicated, blocking is a device that is often used to control extraneous variation by grouping experimental units into relatively homogeneous sets or blocks. The notions of blocking and factorial design can be combined. If, for example, each block consists of four units, then the

TABLE 5   A Latin-Square Crossover Design*

Group	Time period†							
	1	2	3	4	5	6	7	8
I	E_2	E_4	E_3	E_1	P_1	P_3	P_4	P_2
II	E_4	E_3	E_1	E_2	P_4	P_2	P_1	P_3
III	E_1	E_2	E_4	E_3	P_2	P_1	P_3	P_4
IV	E_3	E_1	E_2	E_4	P_3	P_4	P_2	P_1
V	P_1	P_3	P_2	P_4	E_4	E_2	E_3	E_1
VI	P_2	P_1	P_4	P_3	E_3	E_4	E_1	E_2
VII	P_3	P_4	P_1	P_2	E_1	E_3	E_2	E_4
VIII	P_4	P_2	P_3	P_1	P_2	P_1	P_4	P_3

* Emmens (1957).

† E_1, E_2, E_3, and E_4 are 4 doses of estrogen; P_1, P_2, P_3, and P_4 are 4 doses of proestrogen.

four treatment combinations of a 2^2 factorial experiment like that in Table 2 can be applied at random to the units within each block of a randomized block design. The resulting elimination of block differences allows a more precise assessment of main effects and interaction.

Occasionally it will be impractical to use blocks of size sufficient to accommodate a full replicate. This will be particularly true in the case of higher factorials. In this situation blocks consisting of less than a full replicate are used, and the experiment is called a *randomized incomplete-block* experiment, provided treatments have been assigned within the blocks at random, as they should be. Incomplete-block experiments have the property that some main effects or interactions will be mixed up or *confounded* with interblock differences. An expression that estimates a certain effect will also estimate block-to-block variation.

To show how this works we again use the 2^2 factorial example. Suppose blocks will accommodate only two units, and we divide the total available blocks randomly into two groups, each containing the same number of blocks. In one group of blocks we apply the treatment combinations "22" and "11" at random to the two units in each block, and in the other group we apply the treatment combinations "12" and "21" (the numerals ij mean that factor 1 is at level i, factor 2 at level j, so that 21 indicates level 2 of the first factor and level 1 of the second).

Table 6 shows the two block types. Recall that the main effects for the factors are

Factor 1: $\bar{y}_{21} - \bar{y}_{11} + \bar{y}_{22} - \bar{y}_{12}$
Factor 2: $\bar{y}_{12} - \bar{y}_{11} + \bar{y}_{22} - \bar{y}_{21}$

Notice that these effects include the combination 22 with a plus sign and the combination 11 with a minus sign, permitting the effect of a given

TABLE 6   A 2^2 Factorial Experiment
in Two Incomplete Blocks

Block, type I	Block, type II
22	21
11	12

block of type I to cancel out. Similarly, the effects of blocks of the second type cancel out, since the responses to the treatment combinations 12 and 21 occur with opposite signs in each main effect. We say the main effects are not *confounded* with blocks.

However, the interaction effect

$$\bar{y}_{22} - \bar{y}_{12} - \bar{y}_{21} + \bar{y}_{11}$$

shows no such cancellation. In fact, responses on all units in type I blocks are added, while responses in type II blocks are subtracted. Thus, the expression that measures interaction also compares the two block types. Interaction is confounded with blocks. In designing an incomplete-block experiment, particularly when more than two factors are involved, we often decide to confound one or more high-order interactions with blocks.

Split-unit designs

In some situations reasons of economy and the nature of the experimental material may make it advisable to define two or more levels of experimental units. Large experimental units, often consisting of, say, a whole animal, might be assigned to one factorial array, while subdivisions of an animal might be assigned to another array. This would arise, for example, when patches of skin were used as subunits. The animal would then be a unit, or plot, and a particular skin area would be a subunit. The error variance for factors applied to the large units would be based upon variation between large units, and that for factors applied to subunits would be based upon variation between subunits. Error variation between the large units is likely to be greater than the corresponding variation between subunits — a property to keep in mind in designing a split-plot experiment.

In the study made by Bradley and Clarke (1956), discussed earlier, in which the response of rabbit mammary glands to prolactin injection was measured, the 5 × 5 Latin square was subdivided into a split-plot structure. Recall that anterior and posterior segments of abdominal nipple pairs were the experimental units. These can quite naturally be divided into split units: that is, right and left nipples. Doses of standard and test prolactin assumed to be approximately equipotent were randomly allocated to a right or left nipple site. The full design is shown in Table 7.

TABLE 7   A Split-Plot Latin-Square Design for Determining Response of Rabbit Mammary Gland to Prolactin*

| Injection site | Rabbit† | | | | | | | | | |
| | 1 | | 2 | | 3 | | 4 | | 5 | |
	R	L	R	L	R	L	R	L	R	L
1	S50	T75	T300	S200	S100	T150	T210	S140	T600	S400
2	T150	S100	S400	T600	T300	S200	S50	T75	T210	S140
3	S140	T210	S50	T75	S400	T600	S200	T300	T150	S100
4	T600	S400	T210	S140	S50	T75	T150	S100	S200	T300
5	S200	T300	S100	T150	T210	S140	S400	T600	T75	S50

* Bradley and Clarke (1956).

† Table entries refer to doses of standard and test preparations; for example S50 means "50 µg of standard."

Summary

It is possible only to scratch the surface of the field of factorial experimentation in this chapter. The area is large, rich, and varied. Although factorial designs are not panaceas, they do permit orderly, simultaneous assessments of main effects and interactions of several factors. Furthermore, they are flexible enough to permit structures appropriate to the realities of most experimental situations, provided the structure is determined prior to the collection of data. However, the experimenter should beware of including extra factors simply because an experimental configuration that will accommodate them can be found. If extraneous factors strongly interact with factors of primary interest, our evaluation of the important factors can be seriously and adversely affected. Furthermore, as the number of factors increases, so does the difficulty of organizing and managing the experimental situation. With these caveats factorial arrangements are useful and can contribute much to the design of endocrinological experiments.

3. Other designs

Sequential designs

So far we have considered experimental situations in which all the main features of the investigation, except the results themselves, could be laid down in advance: the general design, the choice of treatments and of conditions under which they would be used, and the number of observations. In many situations the investigator cannot proceed in this way. There may be so many imponderables, so much uncertainty about the experimental material and its likely response, that no rational choice among the various possibilities can be made. The natural procedure is then to proceed sequentially, that is, to allow the progressive accumulation of experimental results to determine the pattern of future observations. It is, of course, the procedure in most long-term programs of scientific research, and we are merely saying here that it will often be advisable also in the short-term ones.

Sometimes the major uncertainty is the choice of treatment comparisons. Here one can often progress quite well by a series of designs of a standard type, the choice of treatment comparisons in each being determined by the results of the previous experiments. Claringbold and Lamond (1957), for example, studied the optimal conditions for the biological assay of gonadotropins by a series of four experiments, of which two were factorials and the others the rather similar simplex designs (Claringbold, 1955c) appropriate for comparing mixtures of treatments. Working in a different field, Ellis et al. (1964) investigated the optimal conditions for the electrical stimulation of the bladder in dogs by using a series of factorial designs.

It is perhaps surprising that in biological research the techniques for exploring response surfaces, developed largely by Box and his colleagues (Cochran and Cox, 1957, Chapter 8A), have not been more often utilized. In many situations the mean response y is a function of a number of controllable variables, $x_1, x_2, \ldots$, etc., and one wishes to know as much as possible about the "surface" relating y to the x's near a supposed maximum. Some relevant questions are the following. What is the maximal y? For what values of x does it occur? What are the contours of constant response near the maximum? The writers recently examined some results from experiments in which a certain measure of activity in rats was determined for various combinations of doses of dexamphetamine and chlordiazepoxide. The surface is described quite well by a second-degree equation for which the contours are ellipses. These were in fact fitted by the technique known as multiple regression, after all the data had been collected (see Chapter 10), but one could imagine a similar situation, in which the surface had to be explored by a trial-and-error procedure in which the chosen combination of doses in successive stages would gradually climb up the surface until the summit was straddled. Box's results provide one with a strategy for this sequential program of experiments. One problem may be that in many biological systems the effect of random variation in the results of a small experiment (such as might constitute one stage of this approach) will be so great as to provide little evidence of the local shape of the surface, in which case one's mountaineering would be very ineffective indeed.

Sequential designs of a rather different sort have been much used in clinical trials. The problem here is not the choice of relevant treatments (although no doubt more attention could be given to the optimal choice of dose) so much as the decision when to stop the trial. Clinical trials are, of course, a very special branch of medical experimentation because of the ethical issues involved. Ethical considerations will often prevent a randomized trial from being started. They may similarly impel a clinical investigator to terminate a trial that initially seemed justified, because at some stage the evidence in favor of one treatment is so strong that it seems wrong to withhold its use any longer from any of the patients in the trial.

What sort of considerations should one bring to bear on the question whether a trial should be stopped at any particular stage? It seems unlikely that any one theoretical approach will be appropriate for all clinical situations. As regards the ethical problem, for instance, we can distinguish among situations presenting various levels of ethical difficulty.

In a first category are comparisons in which the problem hardly exists, either because the clinical condition being treated is very mild or because the comparison concerns treatments for episodes in a chronic disease in which a less than optimal treatment given at any one stage can be replaced later with a better treatment. Here the aim will usually be to make a comparison of adequate precision, and this will often lead to a nonsequential design. However, it has often been pointed out that if there is a finite number of patients to be treated — and we can think, perhaps, of the number of patients who possibly receive any of the rival treatments before each is replaced with yet a better choice — then one can devise a sequential design that in a certain sense will optimize one's expectations of the good done to the whole group of patients (Colton, 1963; Anscombe, 1963). Thus far there has been very little application of these theoretical results. It seems possible that the main moral to be drawn is that clinical trials in such situations should be almost as large as one could conceive of making them. Practical considerations of time, cost, and enthusiasm, in fact, are likely to be the limiting factors.

In a second category are situations in which any treatment should be dropped from the trial if in some sense there is quite strong evidence that it is worse than a rival treatment. Armitage (1960) describes a number of sequential designs that derive from this approach, and several examples of the use of these designs exist in the endocrinological literature. For example, Watkinson (1958) demonstrated the effectiveness of hydrocortisone administered by rectal drip for patients with ulcerative colitis. Different approaches to the question of what constitutes "strong evidence" lead to somewhat different designs, but the results are qualitatively rather similar.

In a third category are situations in which we should be willing to abandon a treatment if it is only moderately worse than another. If, for example, a new drug is compared with a standard treatment of recognized efficacy, there might be little point in continuing with a randomized trial long enough to be able to prove beyond much doubt that the new drug is really worse than the standard. One will want to do this if the new drug is apparently better, but if the evidence is running against the new drug, it should probably be dropped pretty quickly.

In a fourth category, which may be very rare, one could place comparisons rather like those in the third category, but in which the response is exceedingly severe, involving, say, life and death. Here one may feel it proper to start a randomized trial, being genuinely unconvinced of a superiority either way, and indeed hoping that the new drug will be an improvement over the standard one. One may feel, though, in situations of such severity that the trial should be abandoned if at any stage there is the slightest suspicion of an advantage in using the standard, even if this means stopping after two observations.

Quite apart from this variety of attitudes, we must remember the importance of adverse effects, to which it may be almost as important to pay attention as it would be to therapeutic effects, and which may certainly lead to the early termination of a trial. Circumstances are thus so diverse that it would be wrong to impose on all of them the same rigid form of sequential design. Two particularly regrettable tendencies are to apply stopping rules appropriate for the second category when the situation is really in the first and to use designs for which the maximal number of observations possible is far too small. In either case the consequence is that trials have often included so few observations that no comparison of any useful degree of precision could be made.

Unbalanced designs

The types of design discussed in the earlier sections all possess high degrees of symmetry. In the simple randomization design, it is true, different numbers of experimental units may be allotted to different treatment groups. In the more complex designs the numbers either are equal or must be distributed proportionately over the blocks or other factors of interest. There are many advantages in this sort of balance. The statistical analysis is very much facilitated, and the contrasts between treatments can be measured by simple summarizing statistics with, at the most, minor adjustments. Furthermore, a given number of experimental units will usually yield comparisons of greatest precision when they are distributed equally among the treatments.

Sometimes, however, there are practical reasons that prevent the investigator from using a standard design. There may be severe restrictions on the combinations of factors that can appear together, or the experimenter may have incomplete control over the choice of factors. Mandl and Zuckerman (1950), for instance, studied the number of follicles in the ovaries of rats. Ovariectomy was performed at various stages of the estrous cycle, these stages being determined by vaginal smear. The distribution of rats from different litters according to the stage of the cycle is shown in Table 8. The authors do not say whether the lack of balance was unavoidable.

TABLE 8 Distribution of Rats According to Stage of Estrous Cycle*

Litter	Early diestrus	Diestrus	Late diestrus	Early estrus	Estrus	Late estrus
1	0	3	0	0	0	0
2	0	1	1	1	0	1
3	1	0	0	1	0	0
4	2	0	1	0	0	0
5	1	0	1	1	1	0
6	0	1	0	0	2	0
7	1	4	0	0	0	0
8	0	0	0	1	2	1
9	2	1	2	0	1	2

* Data of Mandl and Zuckerman (1950).

Until recently it would have seemed impossible to analyze such experiments at all adequately, and makeshift methods of analysis would have been applied. The electronic computer now makes the analysis relatively simple. Pearce (1965, Chapters 5 and 6) has discussed special methods available for unbalanced block designs. In more general situations, in which many factors are involved, the analysis can be effected by means of a multiple-regression program, perhaps used several times on the same data with different sets of variables. Although this chapter avoids detailed discussion of the statistical analysis of experimental designs, it is worth noting that the basic method of analysis for standard designs, the analysis of variance, is a convenient way of expressing the results of an application of the methods of least squares and that multiple regression is another formulation of these methods (see, for example, pp. 180–183).

A similar point arises when we consider the analysis of designs in which the basic observations are quantal: for example, the positive or negative reaction of tissue to a certain stimulus. In theory, the usual assumptions underlying the analysis of variance are invalid. A solution by the general approach of maximum likelihood can, however, be obtained by applying the probit or logistic transforms with several independent variables, and here again general computer programs may be used.

Finally, a small degree of imbalance often occurs when there are a few missing readings in an experiment that would otherwise have followed a standard design. There are well-known devices for correcting for these deficiencies before applying standard forms of analysis. The investigator should always beware of missing readings, however. The tendency to be missing, whatever the cause, may be related to the size of the response that would otherwise be observed. For instance, animals that are eaten by their neighbors may be those that would have given unusually high or low responses to some treatment. In such case the available observations give a somewhat biased picture of the whole set of data. If only one or two observations are missing, this bias would probably have little effect. The results of experiments with more than a very small proportion of missing data should usually be put to one side and the experiments repeated, if possible, with additional precautions.

DISCUSSION

HIRSCH   Would you comment on a difficulty that strict, formal randomization often presents to experimenters, namely impracticability? For example, suppose we want to examine the effect of an endocrinectomy hourly over a six-hour period. The operation takes four or five hours. As a matter of convenience, the operations on the animals to be examined at six hours are performed first, those for the five hours next, etc. The selection of animals for operation and the order of chemical analyses are determined by randomization, but the operations are scheduled according to the hours. Other investigators have similar problems.

ARMITAGE   As I understand the position, the observations over the longer time intervals are started earlier, so that all the observations end at about the same time. This means that when one is examining the effect of time interval, one may also be partly examining the effect of starting time. If there are environmental changes that differentially affect responses started at different points of the experiment, they may to some extent get mixed up with the effect of the length of the time interval. If convenience is of overriding importance, and one cannot randomize the starting times for the various time intervals, then one is confronted with this dilemma. One may, of course, have good reason for believing that the risk is small.

HIRSCH   A risk is involved. However, may not the risk be overshadowed by the necessity of having the experiment proceed smoothly? We have undertaken complicated experiments with adherence to strict randomization but have lost all its advantages as a result of poor execution.

FINNEY   During a number of years of association with biological experiments I have tried to become more and more sympathetic to the needs of experimenters. I believe strongly that the statistician must try to understand exactly the experimenter's aims and in his planning of a design and analysis try to answer the right questions. The one thing on which my opinions have steadily hardened is randomization. Randomization is one of the essential features of most experiments. The investigator who declines to randomize is digging a hole for himself, and he cannot expect the statistician to provide the ladder that will help him out. He is entitled to say, "As an experimenter in this field, I know that randomizing for this particular factor does not matter." If he can stand by that assertion, then I, as statistician, have nothing to say. I find difficulty in believing that a civilization able to put rockets exactly on a selected point of the moon needs to find randomizing of an animal experiment too difficult and too complicated.

I was struck by the example in Table 8. I am not entirely sure what this experiment was, but I thought it contained a danger that was not mentioned. If the investigator is seeking to compare treatments applied to animals at different stages of the estrous cycle, I envisage him as giving a drug and then, at sacrifice of the animal, determining the stage of the cycle and hoping to discuss differential effects of the drug at different stages of the estrous cycle. Should one, perhaps, examine the risk that the stage of a cycle is itself related to the block structure? Why were there three animals in the first litter that were all in the same stage of the cycle, and yet there were four animals in the second litter in completely different stages? If there is any fear that something about the first litter makes its animals linger a little longer at one point of the cycle than do those in the second litter, one might have block differences tied up with assessments of treatment effects. Such an idea may be nonsense. The statistician should not be ashamed of occasionally asking silly questions, for the answers may produce a healthy critical examination of implicit assumptions.

ALBERT   I was heartened by Professor Finney's statement that one should consider each case on its merits. Consider the bioassay for follicle-stimulating hormone by the augmentation reaction. This is a very good assay as judged by λ (index of precision), Finney's g, and the 95% confidence interval. Let us assay the same pair of hormone materials on an unrandomized basis and with strict formal randomization. What power does randomization give to the assay? Does it really make it any better?

ARMITAGE   I should argue that it confers some element of guarantee that the contrasts measured in the biological assay — between treatments and between doses of the same treatment — are really produced by the factors one thinks they are produced by, and not by some quite extraneous effect, such as differences between one group of animals and another, differences in environmental factors, and differences in ways of measuring things from one day to another.

ALBERT   The reason I asked the question is that we have, in fact, done this. We were trained in formal randomization, but when we realized how good this bioassay for follicle-stimulating hormone was, our randomization became, at best, informal. No laboratory that I know of in this field carries out this assay with formal randomization.

ARMITAGE   You may be in a very fortunate position, because many people do not have the ability to check their results against other work in which randomization has been carried out. Furthermore, you may suddenly run into difficulties. There may be factors creeping into your work that were not previously present and that may affect the situation without your realizing it.

ALBERT   We have been doing this for some years. We maintain external checks, and nothing has crept in.

BORTH   With regard to Dr. Albert's experiment, in which the omission of randomization resulted in no worse precision, I have two comments. First, if one does not randomize and runs the risk of having animals more alike within dose groups than between them, then a false appearance of high precision may result. Second, randomization, on theoretical grounds, provides insurance against the effects of unassessed sources of variation. If none are there, randomization makes no difference.

EMMENS   I am tempted to ask Dr. Albert how he does not randomize.

ALBERT   Thank you, Dr. Emmens. I purposely withheld some information. We are dealing with animals that are, in effect, already randomized. The Sprague-Dawley rat is highly inbred and exhibits remarkable uniformity in its sensitivity to gonadotropin.

EMMENS   How do you decide which six animals to put on the dose level? Are the animals enumerated in any sort of way? Are they listed? Or are they just a collection of animals from a box?

ALBERT   We put one hundred animals in a large box and then serially distribute one rat per cage for each of twenty-five cages, until each cage houses four rats. The end points for comparison are the index of precision, Finney's *g*, and the relative potency. We compare these with the same values obtained in other laboratories or within our own laboratory. We cannot see any difference, no matter how we allocate the animals. Biologically, it is hard to visualize what effect a few grams' difference in weight of the rat, or a difference in speed of a rat, could have on the sensitivity of the rat ovary to exogenous follicle-stimulating hormone. Considering the haphazard supply of rats thirty years ago, randomization was vitally necessary then. Today we have supplies of rats of reagent-grade purity, as it were.

ARMITAGE Effectively, this is a form of systematic allocation. It is rather like systematic sampling versus random sampling. One has a population of animals arranged in a rather haphazard, but perhaps not entirely random, order. Even if there is some tendency to pull out tame animals first, one is allowing for most of the effect of this by a systematic, almost blocking, effect by arranging that every tenth one will be put into this cage, every tenth one into that, and so on. It is a general finding that systematic sampling of that sort has very much the same effect as random sampling, perhaps even to the extent of increasing the precision by effectively doing a bit of blocking as well.

BLISS Some years ago Youden indicated that in certain situations selection of material in a systematic order was equivalent to random selection. For example, consider a study on the bilirubin content of the blood of medical students, a measurement which presumably lacks any external sign. The subjects were those at hand, all healthy young men. To have picked names at random from a list of all medical students would not have been any more reliable, I believe, than to have picked the seven or eight who were conveniently near when these tests on bilirubin levels were conducted.

ARMITAGE Was this a comparative experiment? On the seven or eight that were around, were they doing an experiment to compare different treatments, or were they measuring the mean bilirubin level?

BLISS They were studying the variation between and within individuals, to determine a normal level within the limitations of a sample of eight. I think the same situation might hold if they were trying an experiment on each.

ARMITAGE I think we must distinguish between the random selection of experimental units from a population and the random allocation of available experimental units to different treatments. If one wanted to get an authoritative statement about the mean bilirubin content or the effect of treatment on bilirubin content and wanted one's answer to refer to that particular population of students, then one ought to have selected the students at random. This is what I would call a part of sample survey rather than of experimental design methodology.

If one is not concerned with the particular group of students but merely wants to have some opportunity of getting a fair assessment of the effect of treatments A versus B on available experimental material, then perhaps one can dispense with the initial random selection and say, "Here are eight students. These provide our experimental material, which we shall proceed to allocate randomly to treatments."

What should we randomize? I suppose one factor would be occasions. With as few as eight we should probably have a crossover design, in which some subjects start on A and go on to B, while others start on B and go on to A, and in which this is determined at random. If there are such features as the order in which, or, indeed, the position in the room in which, the person is inoculated or anything that may affect the response, then these ought to be randomized within the experiment.

SMITH   One must be careful of being too complacent after randomizing the allocation of treatments to experimental units. Randomization is done mainly to minimize or negate the effects of unknown variables on the estimates of treatment effects. When an experiment is complete, it is wise to check other known sources of variability. Although these may have been ignored in the design of the experiment and randomization utilized effectually to eliminate them from consideration, one can examine residuals from the model to determine whether, in fact, other sources of variability had any effect. In my opinion there is insufficient emphasis in the statistical literature on the importance of checking the assumptions made in statistical analyses. Sometimes the examination of residuals will indeed indicate that randomization was poor. I repeat the warning: randomization, although a necessary procedure, does *not* guarantee that all the estimates of the parameters in a model will be unbiased. This must always be checked.

MCHUGH   To what extent was randomization used in the examples cited?

REMINGTON   It is not always possible to determine from a published report the extent to which randomization was carried out. However, Dr. Cox and Dr. Emmens, who were involved in certain of the original experiments, are fortunately present and can furnish additional information.

COX   With regard to Table 7 this, in my view, is a good example of the collaboration we were able to achieve between Bradley, who is an

Australian endocrinologist, and Clarke, who is a statistician. In fact, we did exactly what Professors Armitage and Remington have suggested. We allowed for known, recognizable sources of variability, such as rabbits, which provided the columns, and the longitudinal positions of injection sites on the animal, which provided the rows. We randomized for left and right, on the assumption of no consistent left or right effect. Unlike Dr. Albert, therefore, we randomized in the area of ignorance. As I remember it, the experiment turned out to be very satisfactory. Bradley seemed enthusiastic and cooperative about randomization because, I think, he appreciated the reason for it.

EMMENS Bradley worked in my laboratory for two years. In this kind of mouse experiment the mice live in boxes in small communites of four or six or a dozen, or whatever number you may choose. What we do in a large experiment (there were twenty-four mice per group and eight groups) is to randomize the mice into boxes, and thereafter we randomize the mice by boxes in dose groups. I feel that this is quite justified when six different boxes and six different parts of the animal house will be going into each dose group. When a Latin-square design is used, our selection of the particular Latin square is at random. We do one further thing that, I think, is essential in this kind of work: we make the order of injection of the animals also at random. It takes half a day to administer the injections, the site being intravaginal. In case there is an effect, the operator does not know the solution he is using. He takes a series of numbered vials, and he injects the animals in the course of a morning. The man who looks at the vaginal smears does not know what he is looking at. All observations are decoded later. Occasionally the answer to a test of this sort is complete nonsense. Then one realizes that somewhere something has gone astray or somebody has mixed things up. Randomization and "blind" procedures carry the risk of an occasional complete waste of time because somewhere an error has been made.

BLISS Note that when the design in Table 6 is amplified by repeating it in the reverse order, it becomes the standard crossover design for the assay of insulin in rabbits. The assay is thereby simplified by a reduction in the number of determinations from each rabbit to two on successive days (see pp. 206–209 and U.S. Pharmacopeia, 1965).

FINNEY I want to suggest the need for caution in the analysis of the experiment of Table 5. The standard Latin-square analysis may be inappropriate because of a possible heterogeneity of variance arising from the comparisons between the first four times and the second four times. Probably this was taken into account. The experiment has two levels of classification, a 2×2 Latin square for estrogen versus proestrogen and, within each element of the 2 × 2 square, a 4 × 4 Latin square. I am not sure how the analysis should go.

EMMENS   The form of this experiment was determined by a number of factors. It was not one that I would have preferred to use. It had to be in a form in which it gathered some information on the way. There was heterogeneity, not within each of the estrogen or proestrogen squares, but over all. However, it wasn't serious. This was taken into account in the analysis.

ROSS   I am surprised that no mention has yet been made of what seems to me to be a significant point. This concerns the intended use of the data. This is important, especially to those of us who are charged with responsibility for assays for clinical diagnostic purposes. In our laboratory at Bethesda we utilize a mouse uterus weight assay in which nothing is randomized. As a matter of fact, we studiously try to avoid anything random, since the people on whom we depend for the performance of this assay might become confused. The assay is used for following the response to treatment and for diagnosing remission of disease in women with tumors that produce a hormone like human chorionic gonadotropin, excreted in the urine. The hormone is extracted from the urine and assayed by a method so crude that only values differing by a factor greater than 10 are regarded as different. Despite this imprecision, in sixty-seven diagnoses of remission based upon this assay there has been only one instance of exacerbation of disease among patients followed for periods of three to fourteen years. This gives a predictive value in excess of 90% for information obtained by a method which, according to the standards here recommended, is grossly inadequate. Is it in error to assume that the intended use of the information should influence the sophistication of the design?

ARMITAGE   I should like to make a general point before I discuss your remarks. I think we must be careful not to assert that any nonrandomized experiment necessarily gives a foolish result. One may, in fact, get a perfectly satisfactory or correct result with very high precision from a nonrandomized experiment, a result that perhaps transgresses, not only randomization, but various other general principles one may lay down. What I think is important is that in many circumstances, perhaps in most, one can never really be sure that this is so. If one fails to take out life insurance, one does not necessarily expect to die next week, but that may happen. Now, it may be either that one is in a very fortunate position and need not worry about the sort of difficulties we are discussing or that, if problems do arise through nonrandomization or any other features one may regard as defects, the consequences are relatively small in comparison with the general imprecision of the results. Dr. Ross suggested that the precision is rather low. This would have led one to expect rather poor prediction, yet, as he says, the procedure has very good predictive value which, I suppose, indicates that differences between individuals with good and bad prognoses are much greater than the errors of estimation. Many people with similar problems would not be so fortunate, so I doubt whether your experience is a safe guide for other workers.

CHAPTER TWO

Analysis of Variance

W. G. COCHRAN AND C. I. BLISS*

1. Introduction

The primary objectives of this chapter are to describe some of the effects of failures in the assumptions that are made in the standard analyses of variance and to give advice on methods of coping with these failures. As a preliminary some examples of the three commonest types of analysis — the one-way, two-way, and Latin-square classifications — will be presented so as to provide a brief review of the technique.

The analysis of variance is a flexible tool with many uses. The writer once heard Fisher describe the analysis-of-variance table as simply a convenient way of doing the bookkeeping for the calculations needed in the preliminary stages of interpreting the results of an experiment.

In the analysis-of-variance table we start with the total sum of squares of deviations of the observations from their mean, $\sum (y - \bar{y})^2$. This quantity is broken down into a number of component sums of squares, SS, one for each of the classifications, plus a residual, or remainder, sum of squares. There is a corresponding breakdown of the total degrees of freedom, $N - 1$, into degrees of freedom, DF, for each of the component sums of squares. When each sum of squares is divided by its degrees of freedom, a column of mean squares, MS, is produced. The most useful outcomes of this calculation are the following:

1. The residual mean square is an unbiased estimate of the error variance per observation in the experiment. Its square root, the standard deviation per observation, is required for computing the standard errors of differences between the treatment means and for testing the significance of these differences.

2. The treatments mean square is a measure of the amount of variation that exists between the treatment means. The ratio of the treatments mean square to the error mean square, usually denoted by F, furnishes a test of the null hypothesis that there are no real differences among the effects of the treatments.

3. Often the investigator chooses the treatments so that the experiment will supply answers to a number of separate and distinct questions.

* The final draft of Sections 1 to 9 was prepared by W. G. Cochran; that of Sections 10 to 15, by C. I. Bliss.

In such case the treatments sum of squares can itself be subdivided into a number of parts, each related to one of the questions. Rules for doing this, with illustrations, are presented in Section 5 and applied in Sections 10 and 11.

4. The other classifications in the experiment — for example, animals and dates of testing in a Latin square — are usually employed in the hope that they will remove major sources of variation and thus increase the precision of the comparisons of treatment means. The ratio of the mean square for any such classification to the error mean square indicates the extent to which the classification has been successful in this respect.

2. One-way classification

One-way classifications are used in experiments in which the experimental animals or other units have been arranged by randomization (see pp. 4–6) in groups of size n, each group receiving a different treatment. Suppose that there are k treatments. The symbol y_i stands for an individual response, where i denotes the treatment (i goes from 1 to k). In this one-way classification the treatments are the classes.

The assumptions made as a background to the analysis of variance are usually expressed as follows:

$$y_{ij} = \mu + \alpha_i + e_{ij} \qquad \begin{matrix} i = 1, \ldots k \\ j = 1, \ldots n \end{matrix} \qquad (1)$$

The symbol μ represents the mean response over the whole experiment, and α_i represents the effect of the ith treatment. The term e_i stands for the combined effect of all other sources of variation that make one animal differ in response from other animals receiving the same treatment. Thus, e_i represents the contribution of experimental errors. If we can envisage a repetition of the experiment under similar conditions, the terms μ and α_i remain unchanged, but the e_i vary from one repetition to another. In the standard analysis of variance the e_i are assumed to follow a normal distribution with mean 0 and variance σ^2 and to be independent of one another.

The analysis-of-variance table depends on an algebraic relation that holds among sums of squares, with a corresponding relation among degrees of freedom. Let $\bar{y}_t$ denote the average of the n observations for a treatment and $\bar{y}$ the overall mean. Then,

$$\text{SS:} \qquad \sum (y - \bar{y})^2 = n \sum (\bar{y}_t - \bar{y})^2 + \sum (y - \bar{y}_t)^2 \qquad (2)$$

$$\text{DF:} \qquad \underset{\text{total}}{kn - 1} = \underset{\text{treatments}}{k - 1} + \underset{\text{residual = error}}{k(n - 1)}$$

Let us consider first the residual sum of squares. From Equation 1 it follows that

$$y_i - \bar{y}_t = e_i - \bar{e}_t$$

since the symbols μ and α_i cancel out. Hence, within a given treatment we have $\sum (y - \bar{y}_t)^2 = \sum (e_i - \bar{e}_t)^2$. If we divided by $n - 1$, we would get the usual estimate of σ^2 for a sample of size n. Thus, $\sum (y - \bar{y}_t)^2$ estimates $(n - 1)\sigma^2$. When we add over the k treatments, we get a pooled estimate of $k(n - 1)\sigma^2$, so that on dividing by $k(n - 1)$ the residual mean square is an unbiased estimate of σ^2; it is appropriately called the error mean square.

Now let us consider the treatments mean square. Its average value over repetitions of the experiment may be shown to be

$$\frac{n \sum (\alpha_i - \bar{\alpha})^2}{k - 1} + \sigma^2 \tag{3}$$

This relation is quite informative. If all the α_i are equal (no differences in the effects of the treatments), the treatments mean square, like the

TABLE 1 One-Way Classification for Experiment on Uterine Weights of Immature Rats Four Days after Stilbestrol*

Data, totals, and means:

$$y = \log \text{weight} - 1.4$$
$$x = \log \text{dose}$$

x:	0.30	0.45	0.60	0.75	0.90	
y:	−0.038	0.083	0.219	0.261	0.308	
	0.100	0.138	0.270	0.306	0.396	
	0.122	0.197	0.181	0.206	0.406	
	0.139	0.197	0.237	0.341	0.456	
	0.149	0.232	0.150	0.354	0.386	
	0.214	0.251	0.183	0.390	0.337	
	0.144	0.173	0.223	0.309	0.354	
Total T_t:	0.830	1.271	1.463	2.167	2.643	$8.374 = T$
Mean $\bar{y}_t$:	0.119	0.182	0.209	0.310	0.378	$0.239 = \bar{y}$

Calculations:

$\sum y^2 = 2.4059$, $C_m = T^2/nk = 8.374^2/35 = 2.0035$

Total SS $= \sum (y - \bar{y})^2 = \sum y^2 - C_m = 0.4024$

Between-doses SS $= \dfrac{\sum T_t^2}{n} - C_m = \dfrac{(0.830^2 + \cdots + 2.643^2)}{7} - 2.0035 = 0.3002$

Analysis of variance:

Term	DF	SS	MS	F
Between doses	$4 = k - 1$	0.3002	0.0750	22.0 ($P < 0.01$)
Residual = error	$30 = k(n - 1)$	0.1022	0.00341	
Total	$34 = kn - 1$	0.4024		

* Data of Lee et al. (1942).

error mean square, is an unbiased estimate of σ^2, so that the ratio $F = $ (treatments MS)/(error MS) should be about 1, apart from sampling fluctuations. As the α_i diverge from one another, the treatments mean square tends to become large because of the first term in Equation 3, causing F to become large.   •

Table 1 gives a numerical example. The data are the log uterine weights of immature rats after injection with five different doses of stilbestrol. In the analysis-of-variance calculations in the table, Equation 2 for the sums of squares is expressed in a form that is quicker for calculations. First we compute the correction for the mean, $C_m = T^2/kn$, where T is the grand total. Then we rewrite Equation 2 as

$$\underset{\text{total SS}}{\sum y^2 - C_m} \;\; \underset{=}{=} \;\; \underset{\text{treatments SS}}{\sum T_t^2/n - C_m} \;\; \underset{+}{+} \;\; \underset{\text{error SS}}{\text{(found by subtraction)}}$$

TABLE 2   One-Way Classification (Unequal Sample Sizes) for Experiment on Comb Growth of Capons Injected for Five Days with Androsterone*

Data and calculations:

$$y = \log [\text{length} + \text{height (mm)}]$$
$$x = 1 + \log \text{dose}$$

n_t:	10	10	8	9	9	$46 = N = \sum n_t$
$n_t x$:	4.00	7.00	8.00	10.62	11.70	$41.32 = \sum n_t x$
x:	0.40	0.70	1.00	1.18	1.30	
y:	0.30	0.48	0.48	0.70	0.81	
	0.30	0.54	0.60	0.78	0.93	
	0.30	0.54	0.78	0.81	0.93	
	0.40	0.60	0.81	0.85	0.98	
	0.48	0.65	0.81	0.90	1.00	
	0.54	0.65	0.82	0.90	1.00	
	0.54	0.65	0.85	0.94	1.02	
	0.60	0.70	0.85	1.00	1.02	
	0.60	0.78		1.04	1.04	
	0.74	0.81				
T_t:	4.80	6.40	6.00	7.92	8.73	$33.85 \quad = T$
T_t^2/n_t:	2.3040	4.0960	4.5000	6.9696	8.4681	$26.3377 = \sum T_t^2/n_t$
			$C_m = T^2/N = 33.85^2/46 = 24.9092$			

Analysis of variance:

Term	DF	SS	MS	F
Doses	4	$\sum T_t^2/n_t - C_m = 1.4285$	0.3571	25.76 $(P < 0.01)$
Error	41	By subtraction $= 0.5684$	0.01386	
Total:	45	$\sum y^2 - C_m = 1.9969$		

* Data of Emmens (1939b).

Having found the total sum of squares and the treatments sum of squares, we obtain the error sum of squares by subtraction. In the analysis of variance the F value of 22.0 with 4 and 30 DF is highly significant. Actually, in this experiment the value of F is of only mild interest. The objective is to express the uterine weight as a function of the log dose, so we proceed to fit this response curve or, in technical terms, to examine the regression of the treatment means on log dose. Methods of doing this are presented in Section 10.

Other data to be used in Section 10 come from Table 2, an example of a one-way-classification experiment with unequal sample sizes in the classes. The only change required in the calculations is that in finding the treatments sum of squares. The square T_t^2 of any treatment total is divided by the sample size n_t for that treatment, the quotient being written down, as shown in the table. The error sum of squares and the degrees of freedom are again found by subtraction in the analysis-of-variance table.

3. Two-way classification

Two-way classifications are used in experiments in which the units, say animals, are grouped into replications, and each treatment is applied to a different member within any replication, the member being selected by some randomization process (see pp. 4–9). Usually the purpose in forming replications is to increase the precision of the comparisons among treatments. In a replication one tries to group units expected to show similar responses. For instance, if responses may be expected to be somewhat different in male and female animals and in old and young animals, one would try to have one replication composed of young males, another of young females, and so on.

If i denotes the treatment (i goes from 1 to k) and j the replication or group (j goes from 1 to n), the model is

$$y_{ij} = \mu + \alpha_i + \beta_j + e_{ij} \tag{4}$$

There are two key assumptions, as follows.

1. Treatment and group effects are *additive*. This implies that the difference between the effects of two treatments is, apart from experimental errors, the same in all groups. There is no natural reason why additivity should obtain. In the first paper in which an analysis of variance appeared in print (Fisher and Mackenzie, 1923) the section introducing this tool was entitled "Analysis of Variation on the Sum Basis." In the experiment the crop was potatoes, the treatments were fertilizers, and the groups were different potato varieties. The authors write: "In order to make clear the method of the analysis of variation,

we will first carry through the process on the assumption that the yield to be expected from a given variety grown with a given manurial treatment is the sum of two quantities, one depending on the variety and the other on the manure. This assumption is evidently an unsatisfactory one." The authors claimed that a product formula, in which the *ratio* of the yields of two treatments was assumed constant from group to group, would be more reasonable. The effects of nonadditivity and methods of handling it are discussed in Sections 6 and 9.

2. As in the one-way classification, the residuals e_{ij} are assumed normally and independently distributed with means 0 and variance σ^2, that is, NID(0, σ^2).

In terms of the observed responses the additive relationship y may be expressed as follows:

$$y = \underset{\text{mean}}{\bar{y}} + \underset{\text{treatment}}{(\bar{y}_t - \bar{y})} + \underset{\text{group}}{(\bar{y}_g - \bar{y})} + \underset{\text{residual = error}}{(y - \bar{y}_t - \bar{y}_g + \bar{y})} \qquad (5)$$

where $\bar{y}_t$ denotes, as before, the average of the n observations for a treatment, $\bar{y}_g$ denotes the average of the k observations in a group or replicate, and $\bar{y}$ denotes the overall mean. Any individual response is expressed as the sum of elements due to the overall mean, the treatment to which it has been subjected, the group in which it lies, and a residual, or error, term. If the additive model, Equation 4, holds, it is easily shown that the residual term above equals $e_{ij} - \bar{e}_t - \bar{e}_g + \bar{e}$ and hence is composed entirely of genuine "error" components. If the model does not hold, the computed residuals are inflated by nonadditivity.

Table 3 describes an experiment of this type, in which the groups are breeds of chicks. The treatments are again increasing doses of stilbestrol, the response being the log of the relative oviduct weight. The table gives the elements from Equation 5. On a desk machine these elements are rather tedious to find and write down, but since electronic computers can easily print all the individual residuals, printouts of residual elements are becoming a routine matter. Inspection of the residual elements for signs of gross errors, nonadditivity, and anything else that looks suspicious is recommended, as will be discussed in Section 6.

With k treatments and n groups the usual method of computing the sums of squares in the analysis of variance of $\sum (y - \bar{y})^2$ is as follows, where C_m is equal to T^2/kn, as before.

$$\text{SS:} \quad \sum \sum y^2 - C_m = (\sum T_t^2/n - C_m) + (\sum T_g^2/k - C_m)$$

$$+ \text{ (found by subtraction)} \quad (6)$$

$$\text{DF:} \quad \underset{\text{total}}{kn - 1} = \underset{\text{doses}}{(k - 1)} + \underset{\text{breeds}}{(n - 1)} + \underset{\text{error}}{(k - 1)(n - 1)}$$

TABLE 3   Two-Way Classification for Experiment on Oviduct
Response of Four Breeds of Chicks to Stilbestrol*

Data, totals, means, and deviations:

$y = \log [100 \text{ oviduct wt. (mg)/body wt. (g)}]$

Breed	Dose, μg 50	100	200	400	Breed total T_g	Breed mean $\bar{y}_g$	$\bar{y}_g - \bar{y}$
WL	0.74	0.85	1.16	1.43	4.18	1.045	−0.030
WR	0.76	0.94	1.20	1.38	4.28	1.070	−0.005
RI	0.68	0.92	1.24	1.48	4.32	1.080	0.005
Hy	0.64	1.01	1.32	1.45	4.42	1.105	0.030
Treat. total T_t:	2.82	3.72	4.92	5.74	17.20 = T		0.000
Treat. mean $\bar{y}_t$:	0.705	0.930	1.230	1.435	1.075 = $\bar{y}$		
$\bar{y}_t - \bar{y}$:	−0.370	−0.145	0.155	0.360	0.000		

Deviation elements:

Breed	Dose, μg 50	100	200	400	Dose, μg 50	100	200	400
	Element $\bar{y}$ for mean				Element $\bar{y}_t - \bar{y}$ for dose			
WL	1.075	1.075	1.075	1.075	−0.370	−0.145	0.155	0.360
WR	1.075	1.075	1.075	1.075	−0.370	−0.145	0.155	0.360
RI	1.075	1.075	1.075	1.075	−0.370	−0.145	0.155	0.360
Hy	1.075	1.075	1.075	1.075	−0.370	−0.145	0.155	0.360
	Element $\bar{y}_g - \bar{y}$ for breeds				Residual $y - \bar{y}_t - \bar{y}_g + \bar{y}$			
WL	−0.030	−0.030	−0.030	−0.030	0.065	−0.050	−0.040	0.025
WR	−0.005	−0.005	−0.005	−0.005	0.060	0.015	−0.025	−0.050
RI	0.005	0.005	0.005	0.005	−0.030	−0.015	0.005	0.040
Hy	0.030	0.030	0.030	0.030	−0.095	0.050	0.060	−0.015

Analysis of variance:

Term	DF	SS	MS	F
Breeds	3	0.0074	0.0025	0.7
Doses	3	1.2462	0.4154	110.0 ($P < 0.01$)
Error	9	0.0340	0.00378	
Total:	15	1.2876		
C_m:	1	18.4900		

* Data of Dorfman and Dorfman (1948).

Alternatively, since we have calculated the elements for doses, breeds,
and residuals, the sums of squares for doses, breeds, and error can be
found by computing the sums of squares of the elements in the

appropriate tables. This calculation may help in understanding both the additive model and the additive sum-of-squares relationship that underlie an analysis of variance. There is no indication of differences in response among breeds ($F = 0.7$), but there are large differences among doses, as might be expected.

4. The Latin square

The Latin square is a plan that enables one to group units, say animals, simultaneously in two different ways, so that the treatments are balanced with respect to two potential sources of variability (see pp. 14–16). In the numerical example Table 4, which compares the effects of four doses of insulin on the blood sugar of four rabbits, the first grouping was the individual rabbit, each rabbit serving as his own control, and the second grouping was days, each rabbit being injected with a different dose on four different days.

If i represents the treatment (dose), j the row (date), and k the column (rabbit), the additive model is carried one step further,

$$y_{ijk} = \mu + \alpha_i + \beta_j + \gamma_k + e_{ijk} \tag{7}$$

the e_{ijk} being $\mathrm{NID}(0, \sigma^2)$. For our data the additive relation is written as follows:

$$y = \bar{y} + \underbrace{(\bar{y}_t - \bar{y})}_{\text{treatment}} + \underbrace{(\bar{y}_r - \bar{y})}_{\text{row}} + \underbrace{(\bar{y}_c - \bar{y})}_{\text{column}}$$

$$+ \underbrace{(y - \bar{y}_t - \bar{y}_c - \bar{y}_r + 2\bar{y})}_{\text{residual} = \text{error}}$$

The elements corresponding to the terms on the right-hand side of this equation are shown in Table 4. In a natural extension of the corresponding result, Equation 6, for the two-way classification, the breakdown of $\sum (y - \bar{y})^2$ in an $n \times n$ Latin square is as follows:

$$\underbrace{\sum y^2 - C_m}_{\text{total}} = \underbrace{\left(\sum T_t^2/n - C_m\right)}_{\text{treatments}} + \underbrace{\left(\sum T_r^2/n - C_m\right)}_{\text{rows}}$$

$$+ \underbrace{\left(\sum T_c^2/n - C_m\right)}_{\text{columns}}$$

$$+ \text{residual (found by subtraction)}$$

Each sum of squares on the right-hand side can also be found by squaring and adding the elements in the corresponding table of elements. The degrees of freedom for error are $(n - 1)(n - 2)$. In the analysis of variance the mean squares both for dates and for rabbits are substantially greater than the error mean square, indicating that both groupings helped to increase precision, and the doses mean square is large.

TABLE 4 Latin Square for Experiment on Effects of Four Doses of Insulin on Blood Sugar of Rabbits*

Data, totals, and means:

$y = $ mg/(100 cm^3 blood sugar) 50 min after injection.

A, B, C, and D denote the four doses of insulin.

Initial variates y_{ijk}

Day of month	Dose and y (rabbit no.)				Row T_r	$\bar{y}_r$	Treatment Dose†	T_t	$\bar{y}_t$
	1	2	3	4					
23	B 24	C 46	D 34	A 48	152	38	A S$_1$	224	56
25	D 33	A 58	B 57	C 60	208	52	B S$_2$	160	40
26	A 57	D 26	C 60	B 45	188	47	C U$_1$	212	53
27	C 46	B 34	A 61	D 47	188	47	D U$_2$	140	35
T_c:	160	164	212	200	736 = T			736	
$\bar{y}_c$:	40	41	53	50		46 = $\bar{y}$			46

Deviation elements:

Day of month	Rabbit no.				Row total	Treat. total		Rabbit no.				Row tot.	Treat. total
	1	2	3	4				1	2	3	4		
	Row element $\bar{y}_r - \bar{y}$							Column element $\bar{y}_c - \bar{y}$					
23	−8	−8	−8	−8	−32	A 0		−6	−5	7	4	0	A 0
25	6	6	6	6	24	B 0		−6	−5	7	4	0	B 0
26	1	1	1	1	4	C 0		−6	−5	7	4	0	C 0
27	1	1	1	1	4	D 0		−6	−5	7	4	0	D 0
Col. total:	0	0	0	0	0			0	−24	−20	28	16	0	0
	Treatment element $\bar{y}_t - \bar{y}$							Residual $y - \bar{y}_t - \bar{y}_r - \bar{y}_c + 2\bar{y}$					
23	−6	7	−11	10	0	A 40		−2	6	0	−4	0	A 0
25	−11	10	−6	7	0	B −24		−2	1	4	−3	0	B 0
26	10	−11	7	−6	0	C 28		6	−5	−1	0	0	C 0
27	7	−6	10	−11	0	D −44		−2	−2	−3	7	0	D 0
Col. total:	0	0	0	0	0			0	0	0	0	0	0

Analysis of variance:

Term	DF	SS	MS	F
Dates (rows)	3	408	136.0	3.81
Rabbits (columns)	3	504	168.0	4.71
Doses	3	1,224	408.0	11.43 ($P < 0.01$)
Error	6	214	35.7	
Total:	15	2,350		
C_m:	1	33,856		

* Data of Young and Romans (1948).

† S, standard preparation; U, unknown preparation; subscripts 1 and 2 denote low and high dose respectively.

5. Comparisons among the treatment means

The analysis of variance provides the value s^2 of the experimental error mean square with its degrees of freedom. From s^2 we obtain s, the standard deviation per observation. When we examine and compare the treatment means in more detail, a few additional rules are useful.

If $\bar{y}_i$ denotes a typical treatment mean, most of the quantities of interest in a summary of the results of an experiment are of the form $\sum c_i \bar{y}_i$, where the c_i are numerical constants whose sum is zero. For example, in the difference between two means, $\bar{y}_1 - \bar{y}_2$, we have $c_1 = 1$ and $c_2 = -1$. If treatments 1 and 2 are of one kind and treatments 3, 4, and 5 are of another kind, one might be interested in a comparison of the average performances of each kind of treatment. This is the quantity

$$L = \frac{\bar{y}_1 + \bar{y}_2}{2} - \frac{\bar{y}_3 + \bar{y}_4 + \bar{y}_5}{3} \tag{8}$$

Here $c_1 = c_2 = 1/2$ and $c_3 = c_4 = c_5 = -1/3$. A quantity $L = \sum c_i \bar{y}_i$ with $\sum c_i = 0$ is called a *comparison*, or *contrast*, among the treatment means.

Rule 1. In a standard design (one-way with equal sample sizes, two-way, or Latin square) the estimated standard error of L is

$$s_L = \frac{s}{\sqrt{n}} \sqrt{\sum c_i^2}$$

where n is the sample size for each treatment mean. The degrees of freedom are those in s. In the example above, Equation 8, with four replications, or groups,

$$s_L = \frac{s}{\sqrt{4}} \sqrt{\left(\frac{1}{4} + \frac{1}{4} + \frac{1}{9} + \frac{1}{9} + \frac{1}{9} \right)} = \frac{s}{2} \sqrt{\frac{5}{6}} = 0.456s$$

Rule 2. The quantity $nL^2 / \sum c_i^2$ is a component of the treatments sum of squares, with 1 DF. The remainder,

treatments SS $- nL^2 / \sum c_i^2$

is also a component of the treatments sum of squares, with $k - 2$ DF. The mean square for each component may be tested by an F test, the degrees of freedom being 1 and f for the first component and $k - 2$ and f for the second, where f is the number of error degrees of freedom in the analysis of variance.

Two examples will be given. In the first we suppose the treatments to consist of three agents that are qualitatively similar and a fourth treatment that is a control (no agent). If $\bar{\bar{y}}_3 = (\bar{y}_1 + \bar{y}_2 + \bar{y}_3)/3$ represents the mean of the three agents, the comparison

$$L = \bar{\bar{y}}_3 - \bar{y}_4$$

estimates their *average* effect. Here $\sum c_i^2 = 4/3$; so $3nL^2/4$ is a part of the treatments sum of squares with 1 DF. The remaining part has 2 DF; as might be anticipated, it may be shown to satisfy the following identity:

$$\text{treatments SS} - 3nL^2/4 = n \sum_{i=1}^{3} (\bar{y}_i - \bar{\bar{y}}_3)^2$$

Thus the remaining part measures differences in effect among the three agents. If the agents are all effective to about the same degree, we may expect to find a significant F for the first component but a nonsignificant F for the second (2 DF) component.

The second example is similar; it occurs when the treatments represent different amounts x_i of some agent. If the relation between $\bar{y}_i$ and x_i appears linear when the two are plotted, we may fit a linear regression of $\bar{y}_i$ on x_i. By the usual formula, the regression coefficient is

$$b = \frac{\sum (\bar{y}_i - \bar{y})(x_i - \bar{x})}{\sum (x_i - \bar{x})^2} = \frac{\sum \bar{y}_i(x_i - \bar{x})}{\sum (x_i - \bar{x})^2}$$

since, as may be shown, the term in $\bar{y}$ is 0. Clearly, b is also a comparison among the $\bar{y}_i$, with $c_i = (x_i - \bar{x})/\sum (x_i - \bar{x})^2$ and $\sum c_i^2 = 1/\sum (x_i - \bar{x})^2$. Hence, by Rule 2, the relation

$$nb^2 \sum (x_i - \bar{x})^2 = n[\sum (\bar{y}_i - \bar{y})(x_i - \bar{x})]^2/\sum (x_i - \bar{x})^2$$

is a component of the treatments sum of squares, with 1 DF, representing the slope of the regression of $\bar{y}_i$ on x_i.

Now, if the treatment means lay *exactly* on this line, we should have

$$\bar{y}_i = \bar{y} + b(x_i - \bar{x})$$

so that

$$\text{treatments SS} = n \sum (\bar{y}_i - \bar{y})^2 = nb^2 \sum (x_i - \bar{x})^2$$
$$= \text{slope SS (1 DF)}$$

Hence, the *remainder* of the treatments sum of squares, with $k - 2$ DF, must measure the extent to which the treatment means $\bar{y}_i$ deviate from the straight-line relationship. Consequently, the F test of this remainder mean square is used as a test of the linearity of regression; see Section 10.

Rule 3. Two comparisons, $L = \sum c_i \bar{y}_i$ and $L' = \sum c_i' \bar{y}_i$, are called *orthogonal* if $\sum c_i c_i' = 0$.

If this relation holds, then $nL^2/\sum c_i^2$ and $nL'^2/\sum c_i'^2$ are *independent* parts of the treatments sum of squares, each with 1 DF. The remainder of the treatments sum of squares, with $k - 3$ DF, is independent of these two components.

It follows that if we construct $k - 1$ mutually orthogonal comparisons, L, L', L'', ... (that is, with every pair orthogonal), their combined sum of squares,

$$\frac{nL^2}{\sum c_i^2} + \frac{nL'^2}{\sum c_i'^2} + \frac{nL''^2}{\sum c_i''^2} + \cdots$$

is exactly equal to the treatments sum of squares.

Note: In Rules 2 and 3 we often calculate a comparison from the treatment *totals*, that is, $L = \sum c_i T_i$. In this event the sum of squares is $L^2/(n \sum c_i^2)$.

The Latin-square experiment in Table 4 furnishes an example of a complete subdivision of the treatments sum of squares. Since the treatments were two doses of a standard (S) and two doses of an unknown (U) preparation of insulin, an orthogonal set of comparisons that is meaningful is that given in Table 5.

TABLE 5   Orthogonal Subdivision of Treatments Sum of Squares Applied to Results in Table 4 (Initial Variates)

	A S_1	B S_2	C U_1	D U_2			
Treatment totals	224	160	212	140	L	$\sum c_i^2$	$L^2/(4 \sum c_i^2)$
$U - S, a$	-1	-1	$+1$	$+1$	-32	4	64
Average slope, b	-1	$+1$	-1	$+1$	-136	4	1,156
Difference in slopes, ab	$+1$	-1	-1	$+1$	-8	4	4
							1,224* = treatments SS

* Same as doses sum of squares in Table 4.

Since the error mean square s^2 is 35.7 with 6 DF (from Table 4), there is no indication of difference either in average response or in slope between the unknown and the standard. The significant F value in Table 4 can be attributed to the difference in response to the higher and lower doses.

This example illustrates a 2×2 *factorial* experiment, in which the factors are two preparations each at two dose levels. Further examples of the breakdown of the treatment sum of squares in factorial experiments are given in Section 12.

6. Failures in the assumptions

As already noted, most of the assumptions in the analysis of variance concern the residuals. These are assumed to have zero means and constant variance and to be normally and independently distributed.

In addition, the assumption of additivity of treatment and group effects is made in the two-way and Latin-square designs.

In preparation for this paper the writer tried to recall past experiences in which analyses of variance gave badly misleading results and to ask himself, "What was the reason?" In recollection the culprits, in the order of seriousness of mistakes or of confusion that they caused, were as follows (other statisticians might report different lists).

1. The arithmetic was wrong, or the formulas were misunderstood. The remedy is, of course, careful checking of both arithmetic and formulas. In the analysis of variance, when obtained by computer, an excellent check on the sums of squares is agreement between the error sum of squares, found by subtraction as indicated in the preceding sections, and that found as the sum of squares of the residual elements. Mistakes by a factor of $\sqrt{10}$ made in reading square roots also are common.

2. One or more gross errors were present. By "gross error" is meant a recorded value that is badly incorrect for any reason, perhaps because a measurement was calculated, recorded, or copied wrongly, or because something went wrong in applying the treatment on this occasion. A gross error seriously distorts the mean of the treatment that it affects. It can also greatly inflate the error mean square, so that the standard errors computed for unaffected treatment comparisons are too large. General alertness in looking over one's experimental results naturally helps. In the two-way and Latin-square designs it is hard to detect gross errors by eye inspection of the results, since an unusually low individual value might represent a combination of a poor treatment and a poor group. For this reason the residual elements are the place to inspect for gross errors. One method of detection will be presented in Section 7.

3. The error variance σ^2 was not constant throughout the experiment. The available research suggests that heterogeneity of error variance does not greatly disturb F tests of the treatments sums of squares in the standard designs except sometimes in a one-way classification with markedly unequal sample sizes for different treatments (Scheffé, 1959). However, t tests and confidence limits for individual comparisons among treatment means can be more seriously affected. For instance, if two of the treatments are more stable in their effects than the other treatments, so that the error variance is small for these two treatments, use of the pooled s from the analysis of variance will overestimate the standard error of the difference between these two treatments. Reasons for non-constancy of error variance and methods of handling it are discussed in Section 8.

4. The errors e_{ij} on different units were correlated. This can have serious effects. In a one-way classification, if the terms e_i for different

replicates of a treatment have correlation ρ, the variance of the treatment mean $\bar{y}_t$ is $\sigma^2[1 + (n - 1)\rho]/n$ instead of σ^2/n, while the within-treatment mean square $\sum (y - \bar{y}_t)^2/(n - 1)$ estimates $\sigma^2(1 - \rho)$ instead of σ^2. If ρ is positive, it follows that the pooled value s^2/n underestimates the true variance of a treatment mean.

Errors that are positively correlated within a treatment can arise in practice for several reasons. If randomization is not used, the different replicates of treatment 1 being applied and processed first for convenience, there may be positive correlations because the most responsive units (the animals) were picked out first or because some other aspect of the conditions of application of the treatment was unusually favorable to a high response on all replicates of that treatment. Examples occur in agricultural crop experiments in which the replicates of treatment 1 are weighed on a day when the crop is quite wet and later treatments are weighed on a dryer day, and in experiments in which the measurement involves human judgment, treatment 1 being scored by one judge and other treatments being scored by other judges with different levels or standards.

If such positive correlations are present in the data, we underestimate the standard errors of treatment means and obtain too many apparently significant results. Since positive correlations are not detected or revealed in the statistical analysis, the principal safeguard is the use of randomization at any stage in the processing at which systematic sources of error may enter. Further, if several measurers are involved, each should measure the same number of replicates of all treatments, and he should not know which treatment he is measuring.

5. In the two-way and more complex classifications the treatment and group effects may not be additive. Roughly speaking, what happens then is that the residual from the additive model in, say, a two-way classification becomes $e_{ij} + h(\alpha_i, \beta_j)$, where $h(\alpha_i, \beta_j)$ represents the nonadditive component needed to make the model correct. The pooled s^2 becomes an estimate of $\sigma^2 + \sigma_h^2$. The pooled s^2/n is still approximately unbiased as an estimate of the variance of a treatment mean under the fitted additive model, but s^2/n is inflated in the sense that, if one could transform the data to a scale on which effects were truly additive, the term analogous to σ_h^2 would disappear, and one would legitimately obtain a smaller error variance. To put it in practical terms, undetected nonadditivity has two consequences: one does not estimate the differences between treatments as precisely as if one fitted the correct model, and one fails to learn that the differences between treatments are not constant from one replicate to another.

In the potato experiment of Fisher and Mackenzie nonadditivity was obvious, because the additive analysis-of-variance model produced *negative* figures for the estimated yields on a number of plots. For less extreme situations a test for nonadditivity that also provides a clue to the kind of transformation needed to attain additivity is presented in Section 9.

6. The reader may be surprised that nothing has been said about non-normality of the residuals. Several reasons can be suggested. First, analysis-of-variance procedures stand up fairly well under moderate amounts of nonnormality. Second, the standard tests for nonnormality — tests of skewness and kurtosis — are not effective in small experiments; thus, we lack powerful weapons for detecting the presence of non-normality. Third, the more harmful types of nonnormality, the so-called long-tailed distributions of errors, tend to produce both extreme observations, which may be picked up in tests for gross errors, and heterogeneity of errors. The latter arises because, as is the case in many nonnormal distributions, the variance is a function of the mean. Thus, in handling gross errors and variance heterogeneity statisticians hope that they are coping also with the more serious effects of nonnormality. It must be admitted, however, that we are not sure that we have the best approach to this general problem.

7. A test for outliers

As indicated in Section 6, the first step is to look over the residuals *d* from the fitted model. If the greatest residual appears suspiciously large on eye inspection, a check should be made to see whether any obvious mistake occurred in the experiment in connection with this observation. Sometimes a mistake is discovered such that the correct value can be found and inserted. Sometimes a mistake is discovered but no clue to the correct value; in this event the observation usually is deleted and treated as a missing value, as described in the textbooks (e.g., Bliss, 1967, and Snedecor and Cochran, 1967). Sometimes no mistake is unearthed. Any of three causes may account for a large residual: there actually is a mistake, a gross error, or there is no gross error but the distribution of errors is nonnormal and long-tailed, producing some high residuals, or there is nothing wrong, it is just one of those rare events.

At this point the investigator is likely to ask two questions: "What do I do when no mistake is unearthed?" and, an earlier question, "How do I decide whether the greatest residual looks suspiciously large?" As a guide, several tests for outliers are available. Most of these tests regard an outlier as suspicious if the probability of getting an outlier as large as it under the additive normal model is low, say 5% or less (the tests take account of the fact that the *largest* residual has been picked out).

We shall present a different approach, one due to Anscombe (1960). He regards outlier tests as equivalent to buying insurance against gross errors, since it is assumed that, whenever an outlier is detected, this observation is rejected. Now, any outlier test occasionally leads to rejection of a good observation and, when this happens, the treatment means are not as precisely estimated as they would be if the suspect had been kept. The insurance premium that one pays with Anscombe's test is defined as the percentage increase in the variance of the treatment means through the occasional rejection of good values in the routine use of the test. A 3% premium means that one is willing to incur on the average a 3% increase in the variance between the treatment means through this occasional rejection of good values.

The mathematical solution to this problem is difficult, and the procedure to be given is an approximation due to Anscombe and Tukey (1963). For the three standard designs the residuals d have the following form (there are k treatments and n replicates in the one-way and two-way classifications, and k replicates in the Latin square):

One-way: $\quad |d| = |y - \bar{y}_t|, \quad f = k(n-1), \quad N = kn$

Two-way: $\quad |d| = |y - \bar{y}_t - \bar{y}_g + \bar{y}|,$
$\qquad\qquad f = (k-1)(n-1), \quad N = kn$

Latin square: $\quad |d| = |y - \bar{y}_t - \bar{y}_r - \bar{y}_c + 2\bar{y}|,$
$\qquad\qquad f = (k-1)(k-2), \quad N = k^2$

The steps are as follows:

1. Find the one-tailed normal deviate z corresponding to the probability $fP/100N$, where P is the premium *in percent*.
2. Calculate $K = 1.40 + 0.85z$.
3. Calculate $C = K[1 - (K^2 - 2)/4f](f/N)^{1/2}$.
4. Reject the largest residual d if $|d|$ is greater than Cs, where s is the standard error per observation.

As an example, let us consider the one-way design in Table 1. The largest deviation is found to come from the observation -0.038 for log dose 0.30. This gives

$$d = -0.038 - 0.119 = -0.157, \quad s = \sqrt{0.00341} = 0.0584,$$
$$|d| = 2.69s$$

Further,

$$f = 30 \text{ (error DF)}, \quad N = 35, \quad f/N = 6/7, \quad \sqrt{f/N} = 0.926$$

1. With a 3% premium we have $fP/100N = 0.0257$ and $z = 1.948$.
2. $K = 1.40 + (0.85)(1.948) = 3.06$.
3. $C = (3.06)(1 - 7.36/120)(0.926) = 2.66$.
4. Since $|d| = 2.69s$, we are just in the rejection region.

Two possibilities now present themselves. If our guess is that there was a gross error, we reject the observation and use the missing-value technique. If we think it more likely that this is an indication of a long-tailed distribution of errors, we may, alternatively, replace the -0.038 observation with a less extreme one. The latter technique is known as Winsorization in honor of C. P. Winsor, who first suggested its use (see pp. 261, 266 for additional discussion). Finally, it might be remarked that an outlier of which no explanation is found always presents a tricky situation and that research toward improved methods of handling such a situation is continuing.

8. Nonconstancy of error variance

Nonconstancy of error variance can occur for several reasons. First, some treatments are more erratic in their effects than others, the error variance changing from treatment to treatment. Second, it is not uncommon to find that the error variance increases as the mean increases; thus, if there are large differences among treatment means, high-yielding treatments may have higher variances then low-yielding ones. Third, nonnormality in the distribution of the errors e_{ij} can also produce a relation between the variance within a treatment and the treatment mean.

If the heterogeneity is caused by erratic behavior of certain treatments, the variance of the comparison $L = \sum c_i \bar{y}_i$ becomes $\sum c_i^2 \sigma_i^2 / n$, where σ_i^2 is the variance within the ith treatment. In the one-way classification an unbiased estimate of this variance is given by $\sum c_i^2 s_i^2 / n$; s_i^2 is the mean square within the ith treatment and can be calculated and recorded separately for each treatment. For t tests and confidence intervals an approximate number of degrees of freedom may be assigned to this estimate of variance by the following formula (Satterthwaite, 1946):

$$\mathrm{DF} = (\sum c_i s_i^2)^2 / \sum (c_i^2 s_i^4 / f_i)$$

where f_i is the number of degrees of freedom in s_i^2.

This approach is not feasible with two-way classifications or Latin squares. With the two-way there are two possibilities. If the treatments that enter into $L = \sum c_i \bar{y}_i$ do not seem to differ much among themselves in their variances, one may calculate a pooled error mean square that applies to them by an analysis of variance in which the other treatments are omitted. If k' treatments enter into L, this error mean square has $(n - 1)(k' - 1)$ DF. Alternatively, one may calculate $L_j = \sum c_i y_{ij}$ separately for each group. Then L is the mean of the L_j, and an unbiased estimate of the variance of L is $\sum (L_j - L)^2 / n(n - 1)$. Unfortunately, this has only $n - 1$ DF.

When the heterogeneity takes the form of a smooth relation between the standard deviation σ_i within the ith treatment and the population mean μ_i of the ith treatment, one should try to express this relation in the form $\sigma_i = \varphi(\mu_i)$, where $\varphi(\mu_i)$ is a simple mathematical function. As an example, let us suppose that the variables e_{ij} have constant variance σ^2 but that the sources of experimental error operate in a multiplicative rather than an additive way. The replicates of the ith treatment then have the values $\mu_i(1 + e_{i1}), \mu_i(1 + e_{i2}), \ldots$, instead of our usual $\mu_i + e_{i1}, \mu_i + e_{i2}, \ldots$. The deviations from the population mean μ_i of this treatment are $\mu_i e_{i1}, \mu_i e_{i2}, \ldots$, with variance $\sigma_i^2 = \mu_i^2 \sigma^2$. Thus the relation in this example is $\varphi(\mu_i) = \sigma \mu_i$.

Given $\varphi(\mu_i)$, a transformation that puts the data on a scale in which the variance becomes approximately constant is to replace each observation y by the indefinite integral of $dy/\varphi(y)$. Since the integral of $dy/\sigma y$ is $(\log y)/\sigma$, we transform the data to logs before analysis. This variance-

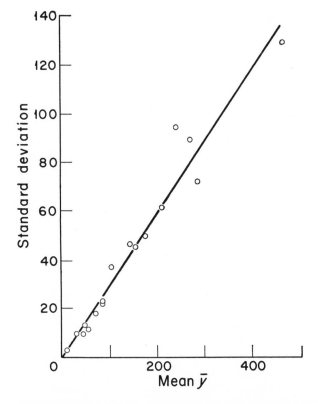

FIGURE 1   Standard deviation versus mean ratio of oviduct to body weight in groups of chicks given different doses of stilbestrol; fitted by a straight line with a zero intercept. From the groups in Table 3 (top) and three additional series.

stabilizing device is fairly crude, and sometimes the suggested transformation is revised if this seems to stabilize the variance more effectively. Thus, $\log (y + 1)$ is often used instead of $\log y$ for data that cover a wide range. If $\varphi(\mu_i) = a + b\mu_i$, a linear relation that does not go through the origin, the suggested transform is to $\log (y + a/b)$. Sections 13 and 15 illustrate the use of this type of transformation for two well-known nonnormal types of data, binomial percentages and counts (small whole numbers). Section 14 illustrates a different kind of transformation used with qualitative data.

The experiment of Table 3, on the oviduct response of four breeds of chicks, provides an illustration. For each breed and specified amount of stilbestrol a number of chicks, usually about twenty, were used. Consequently, we can calculate the standard deviation and the mean for each breed–amount combination. Figure 1 shows the plot of standard deviation versus $\bar{y}$ *before* the transformation to logs. Since the points lie close to a straight line through the origin, a log transformation is indicated.

9. A test for nonadditivity

The rationale of the following test for nonadditivity may be indicated by a consideration of the potato experiment of Fisher and Mackenzie. After criticizing the additive model they proceeded to fit a multiplicative model as more realistic. In our notation the product model is written

$$y_{ij} = \mu(1 + \alpha_i)(1 + \beta_j) + e_{ij}$$

where α_i might be called the deviation of row i from the mean of all rows and β_j a similar deviation. Expanding, we have

$$y_{ij} = (\mu + \mu\alpha_i + \mu\beta_j) + \mu\alpha_i\beta_j + e_{ij}$$

Note that the term within the parentheses is an *additive* model. Thus the nonadditive term that appears is $\mu\alpha_i\beta_j$. Apart from the multiplier μ, this is the product of the row deviation and the column deviation. In other words, nonadditivity of this kind is revealed by a linear regression of the residual elements d from the additive model on the product

$$(\bar{y}_t - \bar{y})(\bar{y}_g - \bar{y})$$

Tukey (1949), to whom this method is due, has shown more generally that with any kind of nonadditivity that is removable by a transformation to the scale y^p the residuals d from the additive model in an analysis of y have an approximately linear regression on $x = (\bar{y}_t - \bar{y}) \times (\bar{y}_g - \bar{y})$. The regression coefficient B_* is an estimate of $(1 - p)/\bar{y}$, so that the value of p needed to secure additivity is estimated by $1 - B_* \bar{y}$. In experiments of ordinary size this estimate is very rough; an average value over a series of experiments and the use of judgment are called for.

The technique may be illustrated from the data in Table 3, where the residual elements d and the variates $\bar{y}_t - \bar{y}$ and $\bar{y}_g - \bar{y}$ are shown. In this experiment the variate y is already in the log scale, this transformation being suggested (see Section 8) by the fact that in the original scale y' it was found that σ' was proportional to y' (Figure 1). Has additivity also been achieved?

In Figure 2 the residual elements d are plotted against x. The scatter about the line is so wide that a line with zero slope would fit almost as well. For a numerical test we compute the numerator and denominator of B_*. For the numerator we first compute the sum of products (SP) of the elements of each row in Table 3 with the variates $\bar{y}_t - \bar{y}$. In the first row we have

$$\sum y(\bar{y}_t - \bar{y}) = (0.74)(-0.370) + \cdots + (1.43)(0.360)$$
$$= 0.29755$$

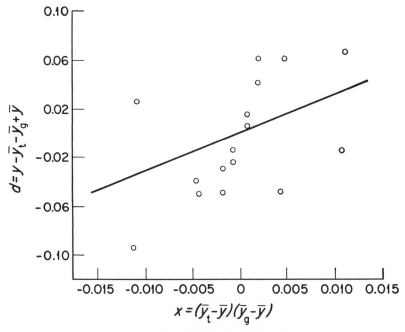

FIGURE 2   Tukey test for nonadditivity after transformation of the data in Table 3 to logarithms. The regression of the residuals in a cross-classification upon the product of the deviations of its treatment and its group mean from the general mean is shown.

The numerator of B_* is the sum of products of these quantities multiplied by the corresponding $\bar{y}_{\mathrm{g}} - \bar{y}$:

$\sum y(\bar{y}_{\mathrm{t}} - \bar{y})$	$\bar{y}_{\mathrm{g}} - \bar{y}$
0.29755	-0.030
0.26530	-0.005
0.34000	0.005
0.34335	0.030

Numerator $= \mathrm{SP} = 1.7475 \times 10^{-3}$

The denominator of B_* is the product of $\sum (\bar{y}_{\mathrm{t}} - \bar{y})^2 = 0.31155$ and $\sum (\bar{y}_{\mathrm{g}} - \bar{y})^2 = 0.00185$, which is 5.7637×10^{-4}. In the analysis of variance in Table 3 the contribution of nonadditivity, with 1 DF, to the error sum of squares is num.^{2}/den. $= 0.0053$. The remainder of the error sum of squares is $0.0340 - 0.0053$, with 8 DF, giving a mean square of 0.00359. The F ratio in the test for nonadditivity is $0.0053/0.00359 = 1.47$ with 1 and 8 DF, well below the significance level.

Bliss (1967) gives a time-saving way of making this test without finding either the row and column deviations or the residual elements. We let S_{t} and S_{g} denote the treatment and group (breed) sums of squares in the analysis of variance. For the denominator we take $S_{\mathrm{t}}S_{\mathrm{g}}$; this is N

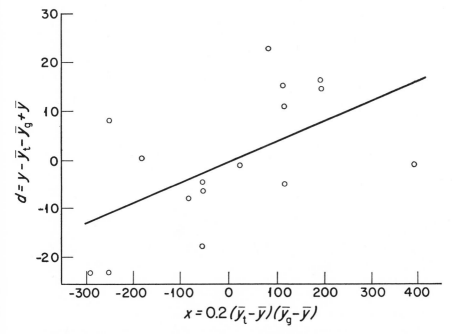

FIGURE 3 Tukey test for nonadditivity before transformation of the data in Table 3 to logarithms.

times the denominator given above. For the numerator we first multiply each row in Table 3 by the corresponding T_t, entering these products $\sum (T_t y)$ beside the column totals T_g. Now we form the sum of products of the entries in these two columns to get $\sum (T_g T_t y)$. For the numerator we calculate

$$S_* = \sum (T_g T_t y) - T(S_g + S_t + C_m)$$

where T is the grand total and C_m the correction for the mean. Since the quantity S_* is N times the previous numerator, B_* is $S_*/S_t S_g$, and the sum of squares for nonadditivity is $S_*^2/N S_g S_t$ (this calculation is illustrated numerically in Table 9).

The original data y' before transformation to logs gave an F of 3.86 with P about 0.08, as suggested by the plot of d versus x in Figure 3. The value of $1 - B_* \bar{y}'$ was about -0.2, suggesting that we replace y' with $(y')^{-0.2}$. A power of y' lying between -0.2 and $+0.2$ behaves rather similarly to $\log y'$, so that the log transformation that was made is not inconsistent with this suggestion. Sometimes nonadditivity is due to one or two outliers — a point worth keeping in mind.

10. Regressions in a one-way design

As described in Sections 2 to 4, an initial step in the analysis of variance partitions the total sum of squares of the deviations of the N responses from their overall mean $\bar{y}$ into categories that can be identified from the design of the experiment. In one-way classifications these are the sums of squares for treatments and for error. When the treatments mean square has more than one degree of freedom, comparisons between treatments may differ widely in significance. The F ratio for treatments tests the null hypothesis that the response under study is the same for all treatments. Even when this aggregate test is not significant statistically, one or more individual contrasts between treatments may be significant.

When treatments differ qualitatively, such as between different test species or between different lots of a hormone, significance testing will depend upon a posteriori comparisons of their respective means (comparisons such as these are considered in Chapter 3). In other experiments the comparisons of interest can be defined a priori and limited in number to the degrees of freedom between treatments. When these comparisons are mutually independent or orthogonal, the total of their separate sums of squares, each with 1 DF, is equal to the treatment sum of squares with $k - 1$ DF. In studies of the response to a hormone or drug the treatments may consist of the different dose levels. Although statistics has sometimes been misapplied to testing which responses from a succession of doses differ significantly, the real experimental objective is to determine an appropriate regression equation and its precision.

As a first step the data are plotted on cross-section paper and fitted with a smooth curve by inspection. From the shape of the curve and the scatter of the points about it scales that will reduce the regression to a straight line or to a simple curve may be selected for the abscissa and ordinate. Such a plot also serves as a check for outliers. Ideally, the response will be equally variable at all dose levels. Especially in border-line cases a plot of this type may suggest what transformation of the response will conform most readily to this ideal.

The treatments sum of squares is subdivided initially into a term, B^2, due to the slope of a straight line (1 DF) and a remainder term, $k - 2$ DF, that measures the scatter around the linear regression. The spacings between successive doses, the number of observations at each dose level, or both, may differ from dose to dose. In this most general case we may compute

$$[x^2] = \sum (n_t x^2) - (\sum n_t x)^2 / N \tag{9}$$

$$[xy] = \sum (x T_t) - \sum (n_t x) \sum T_t / N \tag{10}$$

$$B^2 = [xy]^2 / [x^2] \tag{11}$$

where n_t is the number of responses and T_t is the total of the responses y for each treatment or dose x. The square brackets denote a sum of squares or products about a mean. The slope is estimated as

$$b = [xy]/[x^2] \tag{12}$$

with an intercept estimated from the means $\bar{y}$ and $\bar{x}$ as

$$a' = \bar{y} - b\bar{x} \tag{13}$$

The calculation may be illustrated with data on the comb growth of capons in Table 2, where $y = \log$ (length + height) and $x = 1 + \log$ dose. The number of birds (n_t) varied from eight to ten between doses, four having been omitted because they were later shown to be regenerating testicular tissue. The analysis of variance in Table 2 has been extended in Table 6 by subdividing the sums of squares for doses into terms for slope and for scatter about the slope. The regression has been plotted in Figure 4. It is evident from the variance ratio for scatter ($F = 0.44$) that a straight line with the equation $Y = 0.2648 + 0.5245x$ adequately describes the effect of androsterone in this experiment.

When the k doses are spaced equally in the preferred units and the frequencies n_t of response are the same at each dose ($n_t = n$), the calculation of the regression can be shortened. It is also easy to test for

TABLE 6   Extension of Analysis of Variance of
Androsterone Experiment (Table 2)

Term	DF	SS	MS	F
Slope B^2	1	1.4102	1.4102	101.7
Scatter	3	0.0183	0.0061	0.44
Error	41	0.5684	0.01386	

Here $[x^2] = 5.1255$, Equation 9; $[xy] = 2.6885$, Equation 10: slope $b = 0.5245$, Equation 12; intercept $a' = 0.2648$, Equation 13.

curvature by isolating orthogonally the quadratic term in the parabola

$$Y = \bar{y} + B_1 x_1 + B_2 x_2 \qquad (14)$$

For the linear term, or slope B_1, successive values of x are coded to x_1. When k is an odd number, say 5, then x_1 is -2, -1, 0, 1, and 2. This is extended or shortened for other values of k with an interval between successive doses of $I_1 = 1$. For k even, say 4, x is coded to x_1 equal to

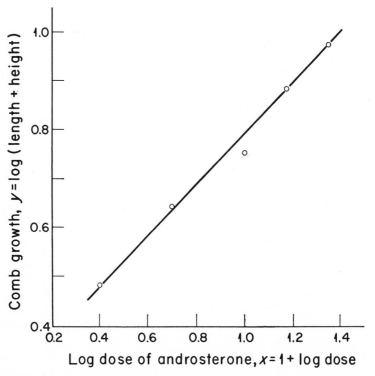

FIGURE 4   Regression of log growth of capon comb upon log dose of androsterone. From Table 6.

-3, -1, 1, and 3. This is extended similarly for other even values of k in steps of $I_1 = 2$ below and above the mean. In coded units of x_1 the slope is determined as

$$B_1 = \sum (x_1 T_t)/(n \sum x_1^2) \qquad (15)$$

Coded quadratic polynomials x_2, orthogonal with the linear x_1, are taken most readily from a table (Fisher and Yates, 1963; Bliss, 1967; Snedecor and Cochran, 1967). These and the intervals I_2 are given in Table 7 for

TABLE 7 Orthogonal Polynomials x_2 for Quadratic Curvature in Regressions with k Equally Spaced Doses

No. k of doses	Orthogonal polynomials for dose level								$\sum x_2^2$	I_2
	1	2	3	4	5	6	7	8		
3	1	-2	1						6	3
4	1	-1	-1	1					4	1
5	2	-1	-2	-1	2				14	1
6	5	-1	-4	-4	-1	5			84	$\frac{3}{2}$
7	5	0	-3	-4	-3	0	5		84	1
8	7	1	-3	-5	-5	-3	1	7	168	1

k of 3 to 8 dose levels. The regression coefficient for quadratic curvature in terms of x_2 is

$$B_2 = \sum (x_2 T_t)/(n \sum x_2^2) \qquad (16)$$

The sum of squares for slope and for curvature are computed as

$$B^2 = [\sum (x_1 T_t)]^2/(n \sum x_1^2) \qquad (17)$$

$$Q^2 = [\sum (x_2 T_t)]^2/(n \sum x_2^2) \qquad (18)$$

each with 1 DF. The remainder with $k - 3$ DF measures the scatter about the parabola, when Q^2 is large enough to rule out fitting a straight line.

When the regression is linear, the slope in coded units of x_1 may be converted to the original scale of x with

$$b = B_1/i_* \quad \text{if } k \text{ is odd}, \quad \text{or} \quad b = 2B_1/i_* \quad \text{if } k \text{ is even} \quad (19)$$

where i_* is the interval between successive values of x. If the quadratic term is required, the regression in x_1 and x_2 can also be transformed to units of x in a parabola. The dose giving a maximal (or minimal) response can be computed directly from the coded coefficients as

$$x_0 = \bar{x} - B_1 I_1 i_*/(2B_2 I_2) \qquad (20)$$

The subdivision of the sum of squares for treatments may be illustrated by the uterine weights of immature rats in Table 1 at five dose levels spaced equally on a log scale with seven responses y (coded) at each dose. As shown in Section 7, the first log uterine weight (-0.038) at $x = 0.30$ would be judged an outlier by two or more tests, so that the sample at this dose has been Winsorized (that is, the lowest value, -0.038, is replaced with the next to the lowest value, 0.100, and the highest value, 0.214, is replaced with the next to the highest value, 0.149, giving 0.903 as the total for the group).

With this adjustment the terms for linear slope and quadratic curvature have been computed (as if there had been no outlier) in Table 8 with the orthogonal coefficients x_i, leading to the first two variances, or mean squares, in the last column. The mean square for scatter with 2 DF and error variance s^2 with 28 DF are taken from the revised analysis

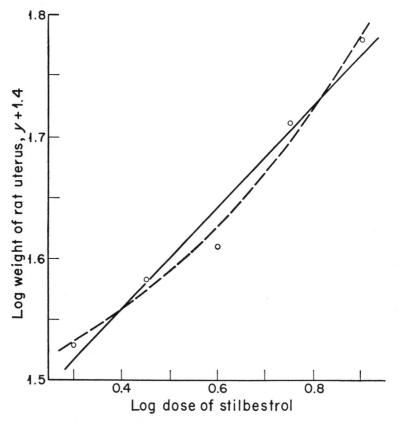

FIGURE 5   Log uterine weight of immature rats as a function of the log dose of stilbestrol, fitted with a linear regression (solid line) and with a parabola (broken line). From the data in Table 8.

of variance. Although $F = 2.19$ for quadratic curvature, this was not significant ($P = 0.16$), so the mean values, decoded by adding 1.4 to each mean, are plotted and fitted with a straight line in Figure 5. They have also been fitted with a parabola (broken line). Both equations are given in Table 8.

TABLE 8   Partitioning of Sum of Squares for Response to Stilbestrol (Table 1) after Winsorization of Responses for $x = 0.30$

Term	Coefficients x_i for x					$n \sum x_i^2$	$\sum x_i T_t$	$\dfrac{(\sum x_i T_t)^2}{n \sum x_i^2}$
	0.30	0.45	0.60	0.75	0.90			
Slope x_1	-2	-1	0	1	2	70	4.376	0.273563
Curvature x_2	2	-1	-2	-1	2	98	0.728	0.005408
T_t	0.903	1.271	1.463	2.167	2.643		scatter MS:	0.002100
$\bar{y}_t$ (decoded)	1.529	1.582	1.609	1.710	1.778		error s^2:	0.002467

Here $i_* = 0.15$, $B_1 = 4.376/70 = 0.062514$, $b = B_1/i_* = 0.41676$, $B_2 = 0.728/98 = 0.007429$, $\bar{y} = 8.447/35 + 1.4 = 0.24134 + 1.4 = 1.64134$. Straight line: $Y = 1.64134 + 0.41676(x - 0.60)$.   Parabola: $Y = 1.64134 + 0.062514x_1 + 0.007429x_2$.

11. Regressions in a cross-classification

When a particular treatment effect in a two-way design, such as a slope, accounts for a major part of the treatments sum of squares, it is prudent to test the consistency of this effect between replicate groups by isolating the interaction groups $\times$ slope. For a regression with k dose levels the numerator of the regression coefficient is computed separately for each group or replicate directly from the dosage units x or, if coded, from x_1 as

$$[xy] = \sum xy - \sum x \sum y/k \qquad \text{or} \qquad [x_1 y] = \sum x_1 y \qquad (21)$$

Their overall total from all replicates will be equal to the numerator of the overall or combined regression for the entire experiment. All will have the same denominator, either of the following:

$$[x^2] = \sum x^2 - (\sum x)^2/k \qquad \text{or} \qquad [x_1^2] = \sum x_1^2 \qquad (22)$$

The sum of squares for differences in slope (or the term for groups $\times$ slope) is then computed as either of the following:

$$[B_i^2] = \sum [xy]^2/[x^2] - B^2 \qquad \text{or} \qquad [B_i^2] = \sum [x_1 y]^2/[x_1^2] - B^2 \quad (23)$$

When subtracted from the error sum of squares, or sum of squares of groups $\times$ treatments, in the original two-way analysis of variance, the mean square for the remainder, or groups × scatter, is a new estimate of the residual, or error, variance s^2. If the mean square for groups × slope is significantly or substantially larger than the new error mean square, it is the error for the average B^2, unless the term for scatter is also significantly larger than the new s^2, in which case the error for the slope term depends upon the mean squares for both scatter and groups × slope. When the overall quadratic term Q^2 from the treatments sum of squares indicates a significant or nearly significant curvature in the regression, the interaction groups × quadratic curvature can be separated similarly from the interaction groups × treatment.

The calculation may be illustrated with the oviduct response of chicks to stilbestrol, Table 3. The mean response for the four breeds (groups) at each dose of stilbestrol (on a log scale) is plotted and fitted with a linear regression in Figure 6. The scatter of points about this line is so free from trend that separation of a quadratic term is unnecessary. Because of the even log spacing, $i_* = \log 2 = 0.3010$, the numerator of the slope has been computed for each breed with the linear polynomials x_1 equal to -3, -1, 1, and 3 to give the $\sum x_1 y$ in Table 9 and their sum over the four breeds.

The term for slope in the analysis of variance accounted for all but

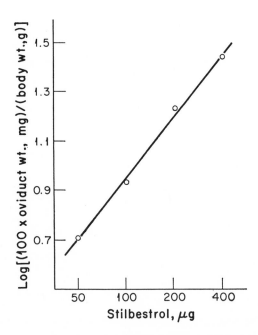

FIGURE 6   Mean log ratio of oviduct to body weight in four breeds of chicks as a linear function of the log dose of stilbestrol. From the data in Table 9.

TABLE 9 Regression Analysis of Log Oviduct Response of Chicks to Stilbestrol (Table 3)

Dose, µg	x_1	T_t	Breed	$\sum x_1 y$	T_g	$\sum (T_t y)$
50	−3	2.82	WL	2.38	4.18	19.1642
100	−1	3.72	WR	2.12	4.28	19.4652
200	1	4.92	RI	2.72	4.32	19.9360
400	3	5.74	Hy	2.74	4.42	20.3794
Total:	0	17.20		9.96	17.20	78.9448

Calculations:

$B^2 = 9.96^2/(4 \times 20) = 1.2400$,   breeds × slope $= 25.0648/20 - B^2 = 0.0132$,
$S_* = 339.617880 - 17.20(19.7436) = 0.027960$, $N S_g S_t = 0.147550$.

Analysis of variance:

Term		DF	SS		MS	F
Breeds		3	0.0074	$= S_g$	0.0025	0.66*
Dose, linear B^2		1	1.2400 ⎫			
Dose, scatter		2	0.0062 ⎬ $= S_t$		0.0031	0.82*
Breeds × slope		3	0.0132		0.0044	1.26†
Breeds × scatter		6	0.0208		0.0035	
	Total:	15	1.2876			
	C_m:	1	18.4900			
Nonadditivity		1	0.0053	$= B_*^2$	0.0053	1.47‡
Remainder		8	0.0287		0.0036	
Error		9	0.0340		0.00378	

* Denominator of F ratio is MS error.
† Denominator of F ratio is MS breeds × scatter.
‡ Denominator of F ratio is MS remainder.

0.5% of the sums of squares for treatments, the remainder being the scatter about the fitted line. By squaring the sums of products $\sum x_1 y$ for the four breeds and dividing their total by $\sum x_1^2 = 20$, the 9 DF for the interaction breeds × doses has been divided into a sum of squares for breeds × slope of $1.2532 - 1.2400 = 0.0132$ with 3 DF and a remainder for breeds × scatter of $0.0340 - 0.0132 = 0.0208$ with 6 DF. From their mean square it is clear that the log oviduct ratio increased similarly with the dose of stilbestrol in all four breeds of chicks.

12. Factorial experiments

An important design in which the treatment contrasts can be defined a priori is the factorial experiment (see Chapter 1, Section 2). In its simplest form this is a comparison of two preparations or treatments, each at two or more dose levels, in all possible combinations such as the 2×2, 2×3, and 2×4 designs. These are used quite typically in biological assays for measuring the potency of one preparation, the unknown, relative to a second preparation, the standard (see pp. 106–117). Dosages of both preparations are assigned the same spacing, usually on a log scale, and so far as advance information permits they are expected to produce similar responses at each level.

Each factorial effect is isolated from the sum of squares for treatments by means of orthogonal comparisons, which involve the linear and quadratic coefficients x_1 and x_2 in Section 10. The number of orthogonal comparisons is equal to the degree of freedom between treatments, and the sum of their respective variances is the same as the sum of squares for treatments.

The 2×2 factorial design is illustrated by the two-dose insulin assay of Table 4. Its three orthogonal comparisons in Table 5 represent the difference a, or $U - S$, in the mean response between the unknown, or test, preparation and the standard, the average, or combined, slope b for the two regressions, and the divergence ab in their slopes when fitted separately, or nonparallelism. Note that the variances in the last column sum to the total sum of squares between treatments in the original analysis of the Latin square. Each may be compared separately with the error variance $s^2 = 35.7$ given in Table 4. These contrasts and their F ratio lead to a test of assay validity and to quantitative estimates of relative potency and of the limits within which it has been determined (see pp. 108–111).

For a 2×3 factorial design for a parallel-line bioassay of corticotropin the five relevant contrasts are given in Table 10, a one-way

TABLE 10 Corticotropin Assay from Adrenal Ascorbic Acid in Hypophysectomized Rats with Dose Levels of 23.6, 59.0, and 147.5 µg Injected Subcutaneously*

Row	Factorial coefficients† x_i						$\sum x_i^2$	$T_i = \sum (x_i T_t)$	$\dfrac{T_i^2}{n \sum x_i^2}$
	S_1	S_2	S_3	U_1	U_2	U_3			
a	-1	-1	-1	1	1	1	6	-298	2,467
b	-1	0	1	-1	0	1	4	$-1,418$	83,780
ab	1	0	-1	-1	0	1	4	50	104
q	1	-2	1	1	-2	1	12	-240	800
aq	-1	2	-1	1	-2	1	12	-196	534
T_t:	2,536	2,180	1,802	2,379	2,146	1,695		Total:	87,685

* Data of Bliss (1956).

† Here $i = \log 2.5 = 0.3979$, $n = 6$, error $s^2 = 25,794/30 = 859.8$ (30 DF).

classification with $n = 6$ rats. The first three contrasts are analogous to those for the 2×2 factorial design. The remaining two contrasts correspond to quadratic curvature for testing divergence of the standard and unknown from a linear dose–response relation. For details see pp. 111–113.

A 2×4 factorial experiment compared the motility indices of fowl spermatozoa in two diluents, one with glucose constant at 2% and the other with sodium chloride constant at 0.13%, both at pH $= 7.1 \pm 0.1$. Four equally spaced levels of tonicity were tested with each type of solution upon five ejaculates in the two-way classification; see Table 11. The factorial coefficients for isolating the seven orthogonal contrasts between the eight treatments are given in Table 12.

TABLE 11 Motility Indices of Fowl Spermatozoa in Two Diluents at Four Tonicities at pH $= 7.1 \pm 0.1$*

Ejaculate no.	Glucose 2.0%				NaCl 0.13%				Total T_g
	50	100	150	200	50	100	150	200	
1	31	61	67	50	38	65	70	18	400
2	51	62	45	0	53	55	58	3	327
3	22	28	32	13	34	42	27	3	201
4	33	61	71	67	54	67	73	68	494
5	41	77	76	55	62	70	75	9	465
Total T_t:	178	289	291	185	241	299	303	101	1887

* Data of Wales and White (1958).

The contrast a between the two diluents corresponds to that between standard and unknown in the parallel-line bioassay, and contrasts b and q correspond to the combined linear coefficients and combined quadratic coefficients (Table 7) for $k = 4$ equally spaced dose levels. The coefficients in the first five rows of the analysis parallel those for the 3×2 factorial parallel-line bioassay of Table 10. The coefficients in the last two rows correspond to scatter about a parabola but have been replaced here with orthogonal coefficients for fitting the cubic term in a polynomial regression. The results of applying the orthogonal coefficients to the y's for each ejaculate and the totals for all ejaculates are given at the right in Table 12. The sum $\sum x_i^2$ in the divisor for each row, 8 or 40, is multiplied by $n = 5$ in computations of the overall, or combined, effect of a treatment and by $n = 1$ in tests of the agreement between ejaculates. For example, the contrast for the linear slope b was $393^2/(5 \times 40) = 772.245$ as the combined linear component (1 DF), and its sum of squares between ejaculates was $[(8^2 + 317^2 + 131^2 + 160^2 + 113^2)/40] - 772.245 = 3{,}129.830$.

These sums of squares have been entered in the analysis of variance in Table 13; the sum of squares for each treatment effect (1 DF) is in the third column, and that for its interaction with ejaculate (4 DF) is in the

TABLE 12   Factorial Analysis of Motility Indices of Fowl Spermatozoa (Table 11)

Factorial contrast	Coefficients x_i for four tonicities								$\sum x_i y$ for ejaculate no.					$\sum x_i T_t$	$\sum x_i^2$
	Glucose 2%				NaCl 0.13%										
	50	100	150	200	50	100	150	200	1	2	3	4	5		
a, diluent	1	1	1	1	−1	−1	−1	−1	18	−11	−11	−30	33	−1	8
b, linear slope	−3	−1	1	3	−3	−1	1	3	8	−317	−131	160	−113	−393	40
ab, diluent × linear	−3	−1	1	3	3	1	−1	−3	118	−23	85	64	195	439	40
q, quadratic term	1	−1	−1	1	1	−1	−1	1	−126	−113	−57	−50	−131	−477	8
aq, diluent × quadratic	1	−1	−1	1	−1	1	1	−1	32	1	7	−14	17	43	8
c, cubic term	−1	3	−3	1	−1	3	−3	1	−34	−59	−7	0	−51	−151	40
ac, diluent × cubic	−1	3	−3	1	1	−3	3	−1	36	59	−35	8	85	153	40
Total T_t:	178	289	291	185	241	299	303	101							
Linear for glucose	−3	−1	1	3	0	0	0	0	63	−170	−23	112	41	23	20
Linear for NaCl	0	0	0	0	−3	−1	1	3	−55	−147	−108	48	−154	−416	20

TABLE 13   Analysis of Variance of Motility Indices of Fowl Spermatozoa (Tables 11 and 12)

Term	DF	SS	MS	F	Interaction SS, 4 DF
Ejaculates	4	6,929.650	1,732.413	19.44	
a, diluent	1	0.025	0.025	0.00	319.350
b, combined linear	1	772.245	772.245	0.99*	3,129.830
q, combined quadratic	1	5,688.225	5,688.225	63.83	756.150
c, combined cubic	1	114.005	114.005	1.28	68.170
ab, diluent × linear	1	963.605	963.605	10.81	631.370
aq, diluent × quadratic	1	46.225	46.225	0.52	148.650
ac, diluent × cubic	1	117.045	117.045	1.31	215.230
Ejaculate × linear	4	3,129.830	782.458	8.78	
Other interactions	24	2,138.920	89.121		
Total:	39	19,899.775			5,268.750
Linear for glucose	1	5.29	5.29	0.01*	2,375.860
Linear for NaCl	1	1,730.56	1,730.56	5.00*	1,385.340

For 2% glucose $Y = 47.15 + 0.23x_1 - 11.925x_2$ and $x_0 = 125 + 0.96 = 125.96$; for 0.13% NaCl $Y = 47.20 - 4.16x_1 - 11.925x_2$ and $x_0 = 125 - 17.44 = 107.56$.

* For these F ratios the appropriate denominator is the corresponding interaction mean square, e.g., $0.99 = 772.245/(3,129.830/4)$.

last column. For a test of the homogeneity of the interactions in the last column the largest sum of squares was divided by the smallest, since all have 4 DF, giving $3,129.83/68.17 = 45.91$ as the maximum F ratio. The expected value of F at $P = 0.05$ for 7 and 4 DF is 33.6 (David, 1952). Accordingly, the five ejaculates differed more in the linear term than would be attributed to chance. This omitted, the next largest F ratio, $756.15/68.17 = 11.09$, fell well below its expected 5% level of 29.5 for 6 DF. These six interaction sums of squares, therefore, may be considered separate estimates of the same error variance, differing from one another only by chance. Since each is based upon only 4 DF, they have been summed to give a common strengthened error of $s^2 = 89.121$ with 24 DF for testing the significance of the corresponding six contrasts between treatments.

Only the quadratic term, q, and the interaction diluent × linear, ab, were significant. Because of its significant mean square, equal to 782.458 ($F = 8.78$, $P < 0.001$), the interaction ejaculate × linear was the appropriate error for testing the overall effect of slope ($F = 0.99$). Since this interaction was significant, it is of interest to test whether the slope varied more among ejaculates with the glucose than among those with the sodium chloride by subdividing the sum of squares in rows

$b + ab$ as shown in the lower parts of Tables 12 and 13. The variation among ejaculates in the linear term was significantly larger with both diluents than the mean square for other interactions ($F = 6.66$ for glucose and 3.89 for sodium chloride). However, it cancelled out any mean effect for glucose while leading, in the case of sodium chloride, to the second largest factorial sum of squares.

The quadratic term was highly significant and consistent both between diluents and between ejaculates, so that it provided a uniform denominator for computing the tonicity giving the highest motility. Since the linear term for the numerator of this estimate differed between diluents, the tonicity for maximal motility had to be estimated separately with the linear term for each diluent. Substituting in Equation 20 gives $B_1 = 23/100$ for glucose, $B_1 = -416/100$ for sodium chloride, and $B_2 = -477/40$ for their combined quadratic coefficient. The tonicity x_0 giving the maximal motility was determined as 125.96 for glucose and as 107.56 for sodium chloride. The two parabolas and their maxima are illustrated in Figure 7. The difference between these two tonicities, $125.96 - 107.56 = 18.40$, is an estimate of the significantly greater tonicity required with 2% glucose in the diluent than with 0.13% sodium chloride.

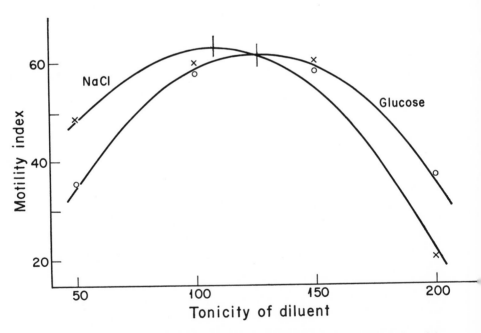

FIGURE 7   Mean motility indices of fowl spermatozoa as a parabolic function of the tonicity in two diluents. From the data in Table 12.

13. Analysis of binomial percentages

When the responses in an experiment are the percentages of animals that react, each is potentially a binomial proportion p with a sample variance pq/n that depends upon p. A direct analysis of variance of binomial percentages, especially if they were to cover a range wider than 30 to 70%, would not meet the assumption of homoscedasticity but would require weighting of each percentage by the reciprocal of its variance.

When treatments differ quantitatively in a sequence of increasing doses of a drug or hormone, successive percentages of response may represent proportionate areas from an underlying distribution of threshold susceptibilities. On this hypothesis each percentage response, when appropriately transformed, will plot as a straight line against a suitable function of the independent variate, usually its logarithm. If the underlying distribution is normal, the probit is the appropriate transformation. The information in each probit, however, also depends upon the parameter p, so that it, too, requires unequal weighting and does not fit the pattern of the analysis of variance.

A scale that is intermediate between no transformation and the probit is the inverse sine of the square root of the percentage. Its variance is constant in large samples when the size n_t of each test group is about the same. Within a range of 7 to 93% the angle is a nearly linear function of the probit. When predictions below 10% or above 90% are not a primary concern and n_t is constant ($n_t = n$), each observed proportion $\hat{p}$ is transformed to the angle

$$y = \sin^{-1} \sqrt{\hat{p}} \tag{24}$$

As $100p$ increases from 0 to 100%, the angle y for each percentage increases from $0°$ to $90°$ and may be read from a suitable table (Bliss, 1967; Snedecor and Cochran, 1967). The expected variance of y in large samples is

$$\sigma_y^2 = 820.7/n \tag{25}$$

when measured in degrees; it is $1/4n$ when measured in radians.

An approximate adjustment, which reduces the discontinuity near the ends of the scale, is to replace each observed percentage $100a/n = 100\hat{p}$ with an adjusted one,

$$\text{adjusted } \% = \frac{100(a + \frac{1}{4})}{n + \frac{1}{2}} = \frac{50(4a + 1)}{2n + 1} \tag{26}$$

before transformation to angles (Anscombe, 1954). When an analysis of variance has been computed in angles, its agreement with the expected binomial variance in Equation 25 can be tested with the sum of squares for error (with ν DF) by computing

$$\chi^2 = \nu s^2 / \sigma_y^2 \tag{27}$$

Even though χ^2 may be too large or too small for one to consider the test observations homogeneous binomial samples, the transformation is still valid for overdispersion or underdispersion.

The angular transformation may be illustrated with data on the dose–response curve for estrone in female rats that were born in January, spayed in May, and injected with two sequences of four doses of estrone between July and October, 1940. After each dose the response of a rat was called positive if in four vaginal smears on successive days epithelial or squamous cells predominated. Four cages, each of fifteen rats, were tested by means of two 4×4 Latin squares; the doses and number of positive responses in each test are shown in the upper part of Table 14. The responses with 1 to 4 or 11 to 15 positive were then converted to adjusted percentages, as defined in Equation 26, before being transformed

TABLE 14   All-or-None Dose–Response Curve for Doses A to D of Estrone in Repeated Tests with the Same Rats in Two 4×4 Latin Squares*

Dose and number a of rats positive in each cage of 15 rats in each test, after doses A = 2.208, B = 2.608, C = 3.008, D = 3.808 μg.

Cage no.	1, 7/1–5		2, 7/15–19		3, 7/29–8/1		4, 8/12–16		5, 8/26–31		6, 9/9–13		7, 9/23–27		8, 10/7–11		Tot.
						Injection no. and date										
457	A	1	B	6	C	10	D	14	A	5	B	5	C	10	D	14	65
458	B	3	A	4	D	13	C	7	B	7	A	3	D	13	C	9	59
459	C	7	D	11	A	5	B	8	C	12	D	12	A	6	B	7	68
460	D	11	C	10	B	9	A	6	D	14	C	7	B	11	A	5	73

Angular response in degrees from $\% = 100(a + \frac{1}{4})/(15 + \frac{1}{2})$. There may be occasional discrepancies in last digit owing to rounding error.

Cage no.	1	2	3	4	5	6	7	8	T_r	Dose x	T_t
				Injection no.							
457	16.5	39.2	54.8	73.5	35.2	35.2	54.8	73.5	382.7	A −0.222	259.4
458	27.3	31.6	67.6	43.1	43.1	27.3	67.6	50.8	358.4	B −0.077	344.0
459	43.1	58.4	35.2	46.9	62.7	62.7	39.2	43.1	391.3	C +0.047	407.2
460	58.4	54.8	50.8	39.2	73.5	43.1	58.4	35.2	413.4	D +0.252	535.2
T_c:	145.3	184.0	208.4	202.7	214.5	168.3	220.0	202.6	1545.8	Total:	1545.8

Calculations:
$x = 2(x' - \bar{x}')$, where $x' = \log$ dose; $\sum (xT_t) = 69.9340$, $8 \sum x^2 = 0.967408$, $\bar{x}' = 0.4548$, $\bar{y} = 48.306$, $b = 2 \times 69.9340/0.96741 = 144.580$.

* Data of Pugsley and Morrell (1943).

TABLE 15   Analysis of Variance of Estrone Experiment of Table 14

Term	DF	SS	MS	F	Cage no.	χ^2; $\nu = 14$
Cages	3	193.84	64.61	3.30		
Dates or tests	7	1,145.16	163.59	8.35	457	16.783
Dose, linear	1	5.055.53	5,055.53		458	16.471
Dose, scatter	2	7.07	3.54	0.18	459	40.588
Error	18	352.66	19.59		460	17.697
Total:	31	6,754.26	$\sigma_y^2 = 820.7/15$		Total:	91.539
C_m:	1	74,671.80	$= 54.71$			$P = 0.002$

Here $\chi^2 = \nu s^2/\sigma_y^2 = 6.446$; at $P = 0.99$, $\chi^2 = 7.015$ (18 DF).

to angles. The four dose levels in logarithms have been coded to deviations from their mean for computing the analysis of variance and the log dose–response curve in angles.

From F tests in the analysis in Table 15 the mean sensitivity of the rats, as measured from the just effective dose of estrone in each individual, differed between cages and more markedly between tests, when compared with the observed error variance with 18 DF. The dose–response curve was clearly linear in these units (Figure 8) with scatter around the line less than the error mean square. If the variation were binomial, the

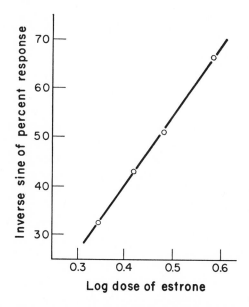

FIGURE 8   Regression of the mean inverse sine of the percentage of positive responses of castrated female rats upon four dose levels of estrone. From the data in Table 14.

observed $s^2 = 19.59$ would be of the same magnitude as its binomial expectation $\sigma_y^2 = 820.7/15 = 54.71$, but it was actually much less. To test the difference, the error sum of squares divided by σ_y^2 gave $\chi^2 = 6.446$, less than its expectation (7.015) for 18 DF at $P = 0.99$.

Underdispersion such as this may be attributed to balanced sampling. The same individual rats were tested on each occasion. If their inherent sensitivity p to estrone were to differ significantly, the variance in p, or $nV(p)$, could reduce the expected variance based upon the means $\overline{pq}$ for the individual rats to

$$E(\sigma^2) = n\overline{pq} - nV(p) \tag{28}$$

For a test of whether p did differ significantly between animals χ^2 was computed, in the right side of Table 15, from the number of positive reactions in the eight tests for each of the fifteen animals in each cage. From the total, $\sum \chi^2 = 91.54$ with 56 DF ($P = 0.002$), we would conclude that the level of susceptibility to estrone did differ, not only between cages but also between rats within cages, and that this reduced σ_y^2 below its binomial expectation in Equation 25.

14. Qualitative responses

Some endocrine responses cannot be measured on an objective scale, but they can be ranked or scored subjectively. To minimize observer's bias with either method, the responses to a series of treatments should be judged by the same observer and the treatments coded or otherwise concealed in a so-called "blind test."

Ranking has the advantage that it is independent of differences between observers in the numerical grade that each might assign to a particular response or to differences within groups in the degree of responsiveness. The responses in a given series might still be ranked in more or less the same sequence of intensities by different observers or by the same observer on different occasions, even though their scores were to differ appreciably. Ranking, however, takes no direct account of the size of the differences between responses, even though it may be easier to rank the extreme values in a series than those in the middle. This subjective experience is reflected in the transformation of ranks to rankits for analysis (Bliss, 1967; Fisher and Yates, 1963), a topic beyond the scope of this chapter.

An experiment that depended upon ranking is a comparison made by van Strik (1961) of the progestational activity of a series of synthetic steroids in immature female rabbits. An analysis in terms both of ranks and of rankits led to essentially the same conclusions.

In tests in which each animal can be used repeatedly scores of 1 or 0 have been proposed by Emmens (1957) and others as an alternative to the angular transformation for an all-or-none, or quantal, response. Each test animal would be scored either as 1 or 0, depending upon whether it reacted or not. In a comparison of intravaginal estrogen and proestrogen at four dose levels in spayed albino mice an analysis based upon 1,536 individual scores had a residual mean square for error one half of that observed between groups or between animals within groups. The F test for treatments (doses), however, was only slightly larger than in an analysis of the same experiment in angles based upon the group responses. In these units the error here was of the same magnitude as its binomial expectation, in contrast to the significantly smaller observed error in Table 15.

An extension of the scoring procedure, however, increased the sensitivity of this test. Vaginal smears were taken twice on the third day from the start of the test, there being very few positive smears at other times. Each mouse could be scored in each test as not reacting (0), reacting in only one smear (1), or reacting in both smears (2). The sum over twenty-four spayed mice in each of the eight groups in an 8 × 8 design has been analyzed both in angles and in units of this three-term scoring system, with the results shown in Table 16. The increased information from the

TABLE 16   Analyses of Variance Comparing Estrogen (S) and Proestrogen (U) in Mice in Two Units of Response*

Term	DF	Angles MS	F	Scores MS	F
Groups	7	74.250	2.22	22.980	1.63
Days	7	145.785	4.36	59.266	4.21
$U - S$	1	1,092.300	32.65	848.266	60.24
Slope	1	5,016.530	149.95	2,802.528	199.03
Parallels	1	14.365	0.43	55.278	3.93
Curvature	4	34.495	1.03	9.697	0.69
Error	42	33.454†		14.081	

*Data of Emmens (1957).
†Theoretical $\sigma^2 = 820.7/24 = 34.196$.

double scoring has increased the F ratios appreciably, most markedly in the test for lack of parallelism, although this was not significant in either unit.

15. Response in counts

The response in some endocrine research is recorded in counts, such as the number of mitoses per microscopic field in the vaginal epithelium of the mouse after intravaginal injections of estrogen (Martin and Claringbold, 1960). Of increasing importance are the instrumental counts of radioactivity in radioimmunoassays, numbered usually in the hundreds or thousands. Although commonly converted to percentages on some convenient scale, they potentially may be identified with a basic distributional pattern and analyzed more directly.

If the variation between replicate counts y' were completely random, the variance $V(y')$ between replicates should equal their mean $\bar{y}'$, which would identify the counts as samples from a Poisson distribution. In this case $s^2 = V(y')$ would increase with $\bar{y}'$ in a straight-line relation passing through the origin. The square root of each individual count, $y = \sqrt{y'}$, has a constant variance $V(y) = 1/4$ and is the appropriate unit for computing an analysis of variance or a relative potency. When the original counts y' are small, averaging $y' \leq 4$, a better approximation is $y = \sqrt{y' + 0.4}$, or, best of all, the maximum-likelihood solution given by Cochran (1940). A radioimmunoassay for human luteinizing hormone is analyzed in terms of $\sqrt{y'}$ in Chapter 24.

Alternatively, the standard deviation between replicate counts, $s = \sqrt{V(y')}$, may increase linearly with $\bar{y}'$, in which case each count y' is transformed to its logarithm. This relation holds equally in selecting a log transformation for a measurement, as in the oviduct response of chicks to stilbestrol (Figure 6). If the slope b of s upon $\bar{y}'$ has an intercept a' other than zero, the simplest distributional form is the negative binomial (Bliss and Fisher, 1953). The transformation that stabilizes the variance is then $y = \log(y' + a'/b)$ or $y = \log(y' + c)$. In a negative binomial distribution c is an estimate of $\frac{1}{2}k$, where k is its second parameter (Bliss and Owen, 1958). If the rate of decay in a radioimmunoassay were so rapid that its expectation changed appreciably between replicates, a logarithmic transformation of the counts might be preferred to their square roots.

DISCUSSION

FINNEY   As regards the rejection of observations, I distrust any slick, formal rule which calculates this and calculates that and then, if A is greater than B, throws the observation away. I doubt whether Professor Cochran meant anything quite so rigid, but I am afraid that he may have given that impression. I might, as a counter, state my own philosophy. I never like to reject an observation purely on my own responsibility. I want full discussion with the experimenter concerned, a policy that Professor Cochran implied, and I am reluctant to discard any observation *purely* on the basis of calculations. Consider an investigator who says, "Yes, this observation is obviously quite wrong, and I now see what happened. My assistant is notoriously untrustworthy and occasionally makes completely wild measurements." Cochran's rules may have helped to detect the flaw, but the investigator takes the decision to discard. (If an endocrinologist has an assistant who is liable to do such things rather often, possibly it is the assistant who should be rejected and not the observation.) On the other hand, the experimenter concerned may say, "Yes, this observation is obviously wrong. I now recognize that when we are measuring toward the lower end of the scale some important piece of instrumentation becomes unreliable, and we may record an excessively low value." That observation, -0.038 in Table 1, possibly has a much higher sampling variance than the rest, in which case a sensible decision may be to reject it and replace it with an expectation based on its being the smallest member of a sample of seven. (I think there are technical difficulties involved here if the experiment is more complicated in design.) Much more troublesome is the situation in which the experimenter says, "This figure looks completely absurd. I have no idea what is wrong with it, but I think it is wrong." One may imagine a table of weights of adult males containing one entry of 25 pounds; this may be a mistake for 250 or for 125 or for something quite different, but obviously it is not the weight of a normal human male. I would reject it, but should I reject 45 pounds, or 65 pounds, or 85 pounds? I don't know, and I don't think it is my job as a statistician to make the decision. If nothing is known about a reason for rejection, and the experimenter is not prepared to say, "This is so absurd that from my biological knowledge I insist on its being rejected," I would prefer to leave it in and not rely on an Anscombe, Tukey, or other rule.

I think something similar applies to transformation. The very interesting presentation of the analysis of variance lacked any mention of the fact that experiments seldom come singly or that, even if they come singly, there may be another one of the same series coming next month. One can have a rule for determining an appropriate transformation, and Professor Cochran stated that usually advocated. However, what is one to do when successive experiments of the same series indicate, as they are likely to do, different transformations? I am unwilling to analyze a relatively small experiment, look at the behavior of the variance, and say, "I think we should use the logarithmic transformation on this." Five weeks later another experiment in the same series may, by this same rule, suggest that the square-root transformation is the best, and a third experiment in the series may suggest another transformation. This probably means that no one experiment is sufficiently precise to indicate any transformation as quite clearly the best. I prefer to sacrifice a little on the quality of the transformation in the interest of having a consistent presentation of the series of experiments. One should also bear in mind that the investigator decides the scale of measurement in which he is interested. If he says that he is interested in the content of some constituent of a body fluid in micrograms per cubic centimeter or in the percentage of animals that show a particular reaction under experimental conditions, I am not doing a very satisfactory job for him if I present my results in terms of the inverse sine of the square root of his values. Yet too little is known, and even less is practised, of methods of inverting a transformation at the end of an analysis in order to return to the required scale.

COCHRAN   Nothing that Professor Finney has said about the rejection of observations is in contradiction to my views. He pointed out the importance of making an investigation before adopting any automatic rejection rule. The reason that there has been a demand for a routine rule is that in many cases such investigations are unhelpful. They fail to uncover information that enables us to substitute a more factually correct value. We then face the question of what to do. Some, like Professor Finney, lean toward a policy of reluctance to reject. Nevertheless, a gross error will make quite a difference in the conclusions. My judgment is that in such situations the routine use of the Anscombe-Tukey technique with a low premium will do more good than harm.

I should mention one other point. There is evidence that any rejection rule that rates a residual by its ratio to the standard error computed from the observations may not do well when there are two or three gross errors or outliers around. If there are two big errors, the standard error may be so inflated by the second gross error that one cannot even detect the first. In this situation, simple plotting of the kind that Dr. Bliss recommended or a test analogous to Daniel's half-normal plot method is likely to do the job better.

BLISS   Rejection of observations was introduced into the Pharmacopeia because on reviewing data derived from various sources we discovered that one statistician had rejected about a quarter of his data whereas another had rejected none. An objective criterion was needed.

SMITH   It was indicated that the rejection of an outlier very seldom leads one astray. In Figure 5 the rejection of the outlier may be misleading. As I understand this example, it represents a growth curve, that is, the effect of a drug, stilbestrol, on the weight of the rat uterus. This function will have an asymptote as the dose increases. It can't just go off helter-skelter. By rejecting that one point in the plot one gets a new value, which is higher than it was originally. Consequently, when one isolates a degree of freedom for a quadratic effect, one is using a curve that, in my view, is essentially incorrect in terms of the underlying model. Thus, there is good reason not to reject it. If it is not rejected, and a quadratic curve is fitted, the quadratic term will not be significant. This is not contrary to Dr. Bliss's position; I think he was merely illustrating the procedure for isolating a single degree of freedom. However, one should first state the mathematical model employed before discussing the rejection of outliers and segregating single degrees of freedom.

BLISS   I should expect this curve to have asymptotes at both the upper and lower extremities. If these doses were nearer the lower asymptote, I should expect curvature in just this direction. That is why I would interpret the rejection of the outlier as an adjustment in the right direction. On the insurance scheme, that first point would be still further off, since it would be replaced with the mean of the remaining observations.

SMITH   I would not do that; such an approach would never occur to me. I would either reject it or retain it. I agree with Professor Finney in that respect.

MCHUGH   I should like to ask Professor Finney two questions regarding transformations. I was interested in the Armitage-Remington example of the effect of a transformation of response in a 2 × 2 factorial experiment (p. 12). In the original scale there was no interaction; when square roots were taken, interaction appeared. Is this an example of what you find disturbing?

My second question concerns the choice of scale. I gather that you view this as not entirely a statistical issue. Do you tend toward the position that the experimenter's theoretical knowledge and experience are the essential criteria?

FINNEY   I would not imply that I never reject or never transform observations. I am pleading for a more critical approach to these problems. The Armitage-Remington illustration does not seem to me particularly relevant. Certainly, if a factorial experiment shows simple additivity on one scale, any nonlinear transformation will distort the addition to some extent. There was nothing atypical about the Armitage-Remington example; the same would almost certainly be true of any simple figures that might have been chosen to illustrate their argument. I would not go so far as to say that the experimenter should be solely responsible for the choice of scale. Perhaps this should be a joint responsibility. The statistician — here I run the risk of being provocative toward ninety per cent of the audience — has the advantage of objectivity. The experimenter has vested interests in the interpretation of his data. He may be tempted to find reasons for a transformation that supports his own hypotheses, and the restraining influence of the statistician may reduce the ill consequences of subjective judgments.

COCHRAN   I have two comments. First, with mild transformations, like the square root for counts and the inverse sine for percentages between 20 and 80, analyses in the original scale or in the transformed scale rarely produce material differences in the important conclusions. This is not so with a more severe transformation like the logarithmic one, which is, in effect, to say, "The world moves on a percentage scale and not on an absolute-difference scale."

Second, what does statistical theory say? It says that one must get one's model right. Transformations as such only enter the theory of estimation (the theory that promises to deliver good estimates) as an approximate means to an end. If one believes that the residuals in the original scale are normal, one does not transform to render a nonadditive model additive. One fits this difficult model with the original data by iteration on a computer. A transformation undertaken to make the model additive is theoretically justified as a good approximation only if it can be shown to retain residuals that are independent and approximately normally distributed. In Fisher's example, in which a multiplication model made more sense to him as a scientist, he did not transform. He analyzed the product model in the original scale.

BLISS   An an example of outliers, in an analysis in angles based upon groups of ten mice the protective action of pretreatment with conditioning injections of *Staphylococcus aureus* and of human or cow's milk was tested against later lethal levels of the same bacterium. From the number of survivors in each group the first working angles gave a chi square from the error term with 83 DF of 121.46 ($P = 0.0061$) or, in other words, one much bigger than its expectation. The residuals were then calculated, the two largest of the 83 DF were discarded, and the analysis was repeated with new working angles. The new chi square showed a probability of $P = 0.303$, in quite satisfactory agreement with the binomial expectation.

EMMENS   I should like to raise the question (which Haldane always used to answer negatively) of whether the majority of biological observations are normally distributed. The middle part may usually be, but many of us find so-called outliers among groups of data in which nothing is wrong, such as the heights and weights of humans. What does one do? Does one get the model right and have new distributions that allow for the nonnormality of many biological observations? Alternatively, does one adhere to the normal distribution and discard observations that don't appear to fit?

COCHRAN   Many of these methods have been developed partly because fitting the model with the correct nonnormal distribution of errors has so far proved too difficult. Computers will ease that process, but on a desk machine transformations, insofar as they increase proximity to normality, are useful.

EMMENS An outstanding feature of the nonnormality of many biological observations is not that they are skewed but that they have an unusual proportion of outliers. These may occur only occasionally, yet with sufficient frequency to cause worry about rejection. If the true distribution includes what would be called outliers in the normal distribution, what should one do?

COCHRAN With a long-tailed distribution of errors I do not recommend the Anscombe-Tukey rejection of outliers. One should either do the hard work of analyzing on a more realistic representation of the error distribution or transform to a scale in which one believes that one comes near enough to normality to permit the application of normal models. Another possibility is the device of Winsorization, though I have had insufficient experience with this technique.

RINARD It was stated earlier that additivity is an assumption necessary for the analysis of variance. From the experimenter's viewpoint non-additivity — that is, potentiation or inhibition — is often of great interest. Is the analysis of variance useful in detecting these types of interaction? Further, if it is useful and a transformation is undertaken to achieve homogeneity of variance, what happens to such interactions?

COCHRAN The kind of additivity that the analysis of variance requires is additivity of row and column effects, which will usually be treatment and replication, or group, effects. Effects on responses of drug potentiation or inhibition can be studied by response curves fitted to the treatment means or by an appropriate breakdown of the treatments sum of squares. Much of the data that I see are on the effects of inhibitors.

Concerning your second question we should have said more. I would transform to achieve additivity rather than to achieve equal variance. Additivity implies that life is being simply described. If the effect of one factor remains constant over all sorts of variations of the environment or of the levels of other factors, the work is quite easy. Even if that happens in a transformed scale, you have achieved a relatively simple description of a complex phenomenon.

RINARD It may be simple from the statistician's standpoint, but experimenters characteristically think in the original scale of measurement. I should hate to do an experiment, make a transformation to some unaccustomed scale, and thereby fail to detect some interesting hormonal interaction. I want to emphasize that there is danger that this will occur when an investigator looks at such transformed data. Experimenters who use the analysis of variance should be aware of what they are doing when they transform their data.

COCHRAN   That's a good point. However, if interactions are a mere artifact of the scale you are using, they are unlikely to be interesting from the point of view of pure science!

CHAPTER THREE

Multiple Comparisons

C. W. DUNNETT

1. Introduction

Many biological experiments are performed for the purpose of comparing the effects of two or more treatments. In the special case of only two treatment groups a commonly used significance-testing procedure for the comparison of means is Student's t test. This is a test of the null hypothesis that the difference between the treatments had no effect on the mean level of response in the two groups. The method can also be used to provide confidence limits on the true value of the effect of the change in treatment on the mean response level.

In the case of more than two treatment groups the t test for the null hypothesis of no treatment effect generalizes to the analysis-of-variance F test. However, the latter rarely provides an adequate basis for drawing inferences. If the F test is significant, further analysis of the data is necessary to determine which treatments differ; if it is not, it is still possible that certain treatment effects are present and can be detected. These are effects that failed to produce a significant value of the overall F ratio because they were, in a sense, averaged out in the treatments mean square by other treatment effects that were small or negligible. Whatever the outcome of the overall F test, it is usually necessary to make further comparisons between the treatment group means in order to detect those effects of concern to the experimenter.

The overall F test of the null hypothesis that none of the treatments under study affect the mean level of response entails a risk, α, of rejecting this hypothesis when it is true. This risk is usually chosen to be 0.05 or 0.01. However, with further comparisons between the treatment group means (such as testing the significance of the difference between selected pairs of treatment means and, more generally, of contrasts in the means) several significance tests will be performed. If each is carried out at the level α, the risk of obtaining one or more falsely significant values is higher than α. In fact, for m *independent* tests of significance at the level α the risk of finding at least one significant result when all the null hypotheses tested are true is $1 - (1 - \alpha)^m$; for example, for $m = 5$ and $\alpha = 0.05$ this risk is 0.23.

Statisticians are not in complete agreement whether this is cause for concern. Those who feel it is say that the value of α used for each test should depend on the number of significance tests made in the experiment, and in such a way that the overall significance level of the experiments is, in some sense, controlled. Methods of doing this are called *multiple comparisons procedures*. Those who adopt the opposite viewpoint argue that with separate experiments for testing each null hypothesis the value of α for each test would be constant; hence, why change α merely because all null hypotheses are tested in the same experiment? They would agree, however, that their view applies only to the so-called a priori comparisons or contrasts, namely those used to test null hypotheses formulated before an experiment was performed; a posteriori comparisons, which are those suggested by the way the treatment means turned out, can suitably be tested only by an appropriate multiple comparisons procedure. The reason for this stipulation is that comparisons selected after the data have been examined tend to be the more striking ones and, hence, the more likely to have been the result of chance fluctuations in the data. Thus their error rate will be higher than the error rate for contrasts selected independently of the data.

Fisher (1935) recognized the problem presented by multiple tests of significance within a single experiment. He recommended the use of ordinary Student t tests for determining the significance of contrasts after observing a significant F test. However, he advised changing the value of α for each test to α/m, where m is the number of tests to be done, after a significant overall F test. The practice of performing ordinary t tests after a significant F test is known as the least-significant-difference procedure. Ordinary t tests not preceded by an F test (the procedure recommended by the nonmultiple-comparisonists) are known as multiple t tests. Fisher's procedure for altering the level of significance according to the number of tests is an early example of a multiple comparisons procedure.

In this chapter some of the more widely used multiple comparisons procedures are described and are illustrated with a set of data kindly supplied by Dr. Sidney H. Ingbar. I wish to emphasize that the aim is to illustrate the procedures and their properties and not to advocate the use of a particular method in the analysis of these data. Only the experimenter can determine which method best suits his needs.

2. Tests of significance for contrasts, and error rates

Multiple comparisons procedures are applied to testing the significance of *contrasts* among treatment means. Denoting the set of treatment means by $\bar{y}_1, \bar{y}_2, \ldots, \bar{y}_k$, a contrast has been defined as a linear combination,

$$c_1\bar{y}_1 + c_2\bar{y}_2 + \cdots + c_k\bar{y}_k$$

in which $c_1 + c_2 + \cdots + c_k$ equal zero (see p. 42). A special case is the simple difference between two means, such as $\bar{y}_1 - \bar{y}_2$, which is obtained by taking c_1 equal to 1, c_2 equal to -1, and all remaining c's equal to zero.

A test of significance on a contrast determines whether the null hypothesis that its true value is zero can be rejected. For example, a test of significance on $\bar{y}_1 - \bar{y}_2$ tests the null hypothesis that the first two treatments have the same level of response, and a test of significance on the contrast $\bar{y}_1 - (\bar{y}_2 + \bar{y}_3)/2$ tests the null hypothesis that the mean level of response for treatments 2 and 3 is the same as that for treatment 1.

As a test of the significance of a contrast its value is compared with that of a certain "allowance": if the value of the contrast exceeds its allowance, it is significant at a chosen level of probability. The differences between the various multiple comparisons procedures lie in the way in which the appropriate allowances are determined.

Before we indicate how the allowances are calculated it is essential to understand the concept of "error rates." By "error" is meant the error of rejecting a null hypothesis when it is true (the so-called Type I error).

Tukey (1953) distinguished between three error rates; for our purposes, however, we need be concerned with only two of them, the comparison error rate and the family (or, more correctly, "familywise") error rate. A family is a set of comparisons, usually all the comparisons made in an experiment. It can also be a subset of these or, in principle, it may even be all the comparisons in a series of experiments. The determination of what constitutes a family is difficult and is a controversial issue among statisticians. This point is discussed in the last section of this chapter, and for further elaboration the reader is referred to Miller (1966, pp. 31–35).

The following definitions are based on a long series of such comparisons made over many experiments, when the null hypothesis for each comparison was in reality true:

Comparison error rate =
$$\frac{\text{number of comparisons leading to rejection of null hypothesis}}{\text{total number of comparisons}}$$

Family ("familywise") error rate =
$$\frac{\text{number of families in which one or more null hypotheses are rejected}}{\text{total number of families}}$$

Consider first a simple t test for comparing two treatment means. This consists of determining the difference between the two means and dividing by its standard error; if the result exceeds the appropriate critical value tabulated for the Student t distribution at the probability level α, the null hypothesis that the two groups have the same mean is rejected. Thus, the allowance for the difference between two means is the critical value of Student's t multiplied by the standard error of the difference between the two means. Such a test controls the comparison error rate at the level α.

Now consider the effect of performing multiple t tests in the same experiment, each one at the probability level α. Provided that the contrasts are selected in advance (that is, they are not determined on the basis of the results of the experiment), it will still be true that among many such tests in a large number of experiments a proportion α of those for which the null hypothesis is actually true will be falsely labeled significant. This outcome is not altered by the fact that the tests performed within the same experiment are correlated to some extent. Thus, for multiple t tests carried out at a fixed level of significance, α, the comparison error rate is controlled at the level α.

The family error rate takes into account the entire set of comparisons, the family being the unit. It measures the frequency with which families containing one or more comparisons falsely labeled significant occur among all families. This is appropriate in situations in which conclusions are based on the whole set of comparisons in the family. These are situations in which the existence of a single error within a family might jeopardize the conclusions. For example, suppose an experiment is performed to compare several treatments with a standard with the object of selecting one of them for future use. The family of comparisons of interest might consist of each treatment versus the standard. The experimenter would be led seriously astray if the comparison in error happened to be the one involving the selected treatment, since it could result in the standard's being replaced with a treatment that was not really superior to it. When the family error rate is controlled, the critical allowance depends upon the number of treatment groups but not upon the actual number of comparisons within the family. Thus, without affecting the nominal value of the error rate additional comparisons can be added after observation of how the data have turned out.

3. Calculation of allowances for multiple comparisons procedures

The method chosen for calculating the allowances depends upon which type of error rate is to be controlled and which type of contrast is of most concern. If only the comparison error rate is of interest, then the least-significant-difference procedure or the multiple t test is valid, no matter what type of contrast is to be tested. On the other hand, if the family error rate is to be controlled, the choice from among the several procedures available depends upon the type of contrast of greatest interest. The two most versatile are Scheffé's procedure (1953), based upon the F distribution, and Tukey's procedure (1953), based upon the Studentized-range statistic. In addition there are special-purpose procedures designed for particular types of contrast, such as that for a set of orthogonal contrasts, due to Tukey (1953), and that for multiple comparisons with a control or standard, due to Dunnett (1964). Procedures called *multiple range tests* are also popular when only comparisons between treatments taken in pairs are of interest. However, these do not control error rates in the same sense as the other methods. Of particular interest are the methods of Newman-Keuls (Keuls, 1952) and Duncan (1955).

We now proceed to show how the allowances are calculated in these various procedures. For further information it is suggested that the reader consult Miller (1966, Chapter 2) and Seeger (1966, Part III) or the original papers in which the methods were reported.

In what follows the $\bar{y}_1, \bar{y}_2, \ldots, \bar{y}_k$ refer to the observed treatment means and s^2 to an estimate of variance that is based on, say, f degrees of freedom. These quantities summarize the experimental results of interest for making the treatment comparisons, no matter what experimental design was used to generate the data. It will be assumed for simplicity of exposition that each treatment mean is based on the same number of observations and that the variances within the treatment groups are homogeneous. If that is not the case, the formulas will require modifications, which are described in the references given above.

The least-significant-difference and multiple t test procedures

The least-significant-difference procedure (LSD) and the multiple t test are simply the well-known Student t test already discussed. The allowance for a difference between two means, such as $\bar{y}_1 - \bar{y}_2$, is

$$\text{LSD} = t_\alpha s_\text{d} = t_\alpha \sqrt{2} s_{\bar{y}}$$

where t_α is the α point of Student's t distribution with f DF (degrees of freedom), s_d is the standard error of the difference, and $s_{\bar{y}}$ is the standard error of a treatment mean (equal to s divided by the square root of n, the number of observations per treatment). The allowance for any contrast $c_1\bar{y}_1 + \cdots + c_k\bar{y}_k$ is

$$\text{LSD} = t_\alpha s_\text{c} = t_\alpha \sqrt{c_1^2 + \cdots + c_k^2} s_{\bar{y}}$$

where s_c is the standard error of the contrast. Use of this procedure for a priori comparisons will lead to the occurrence of results falsely labeled significant in a proportion α of the comparisons; that is, the procedure controls the comparison error rate at the level α.

Scheffé's fully-significant-difference procedure

Scheffé's fully-significant-difference (FSD) method (1953) controls the family rate at any desired level α. This is achieved by replacing t_α in the formula for LSD with $\sqrt{(m-1)F_{\alpha,m-1}}$, where $F_{\alpha,m-1}$ is the upper α point of the F distribution with $m-1$ DF in the numerator and f DF in the denominator, m being the number of means involved in the family of comparisons ($m \leq k$). The allowance for any contrast is given by

$$\begin{aligned} \text{FSD} &= \sqrt{(m-1)F_{\alpha,m-1}}\,s_c \\ &= \sqrt{(m-1)F_{\alpha,m-1}(c_1^2 + \cdots + c_m^2)}\,s_{\bar{y}} \end{aligned}$$

Since it controls the family error rate at the level α for the totality of contrasts that can be formed from the treatment means, it is not necessary to specify in advance the particular contrasts; that is, contrasts suggested by the way the data have turned out (a posteriori contrasts) can be added and tested without their affecting the nominal value of the error rate.

Tukey's wholly-significant-difference procedure

Tukey's wholly-significant-difference (WSD) method (1953) also controls the family error rate. It is particularly suited when the chief interest is in testing all the differences between m treatment means, taken in pairs, because the allowances for these contrasts are considerably smaller than those of the FSD method. The allowance for a difference, such as $\bar{y}_1 - \bar{y}_2$, is given by

$$\text{WSD} = q_{\alpha,m}s_{\bar{y}}$$

where $q_{\alpha,m}$ is the upper α point of the distribution of the Studentized range for m means and f DF. Extensive tables have been provided by Harter *et al.* (1959). The method can be extended to test any contrast, the allowance for $c_1\bar{y}_1 + \cdots + c_m\bar{y}_m$ being

$$\text{WSD} = q_{\alpha,m}\frac{|c_1| + \cdots + |c_m|}{2}\,s_{\bar{y}}$$

where $|c|$ represents the absolute value of the constant c (the value of c with any negative sign changed to a positive sign).

Tukey's test for orthogonal contrasts

Another method, also due to Tukey (1953), controls the family error rate when the family consists of a set of orthogonal contrasts (as defined on p. 43, two contrasts, $c_1\bar{y}_1 + \cdots + c_k\bar{y}_k$ and $d_1\bar{y}_1 + \cdots + d_k\bar{y}_k$, where all the means are based on the same sample size, are orthogonal if $c_1d_1 + \cdots + c_kd_k$ equals 0). To give the required allowance, t_α in the formula for the LSD is replaced with $t'_{\alpha,m}$, the upper α point of the distribution of the Studentized maximum modulus (namely, the maximum of m independent normal variates with zero mean divided by an estimate of the standard error, where m is the number of contrasts in the orthogonal set). This distribution coincides with Student's t for a single comparison ($m = 1$), but its percentage points exceed those of Student's t for two or more orthogonal contrasts in the set. Tables for $\alpha = 0.05$ are provided by Pillai and Ramachandran (1954).

In this method the allowance for any contrast in a set of m mutually orthogonal contrasts is

$$A = t'_{\alpha,m}s_c = t'_{\alpha,m}\sqrt{c_1^2 + \cdots + c_k^2}\,s_{\bar{y}}$$

It can be extended to test other contrasts that can be expressed as linear combinations of the m contrasts in the orthogonal set without affecting the error rate. To see how this is done, denote by L_i the ith contrast in the set; let

$$L_i = c_{1i}\bar{y}_1 + c_{2i}\bar{y}_2 + \cdots + c_{ki}\bar{y}_k$$
$$d_i = \sqrt{c_{1i}^2 + \cdots + c_{ki}^2}$$

Then the allowance for any linear combination $p_1L_1 + \cdots + p_mL_m$ is

$$A = t'_{\alpha,m}(|p_1d_1| + \cdots + |p_md_m|)s_{\bar{y}}$$

Orthogonal contrasts arise in an analysis of variance when a treatments sum of squares is subdivided into orthogonal 1 DF components. An example, given on pp. 111–113, concerns a bioassay in which the treatments were a standard and a test compound, each at three dose levels. In the breakdown of the treatments sum of squares there were three orthogonal contrasts for testing assay validity: divergence, curvature for standard, and curvature for unknown. One way to obtain a single overall validity test is to add these three sums of squares and apply an F test with 3 DF in the numerator. Another way is to test the $m = 3$ contrasts separately by using this multiple comparisons procedure based on the Studentized maximum-modulus distribution; the latter will achieve the same probability of a Type I error as the F test but will have greater power to detect a failure in validity that has affected only one of the contrasts.

Comparisons with a control or standard

Often one of the groups corresponds to a control or standard treatment, and the comparisons of interest are those between each treatment mean and the control or standard mean. Let $\bar{y}_1$ denote the mean for the control or standard; the contrasts of primary concern are $\bar{y}_1 - \bar{y}_2$, $\bar{y}_1 - \bar{y}_3, \ldots, \bar{y}_1 - \bar{y}_m$. For control of the family error rate the upper α point of a multivariate Student t distribution is required in place of t_α in the LSD formula. Tables for α of 0.05 and 0.01 have been prepared by Dunnett (1964). When the required percentage point for m treatments, including the control, is denoted by $t''_{\alpha,m}$, the allowance is

$$A = t''_{\alpha,m} s_d = t''_{\alpha,m} \sqrt{2} s_{\bar{y}}$$

The same allowance can also be used to test the control against any weighted average of the treatment means.

Multiple range tests

The multiple range tests, known as the Newman-Keuls and Duncan procedures, may be considered modifications of Tukey's WSD procedure, although they were developed independently. They are used when the sole comparisons of interest are between the treatment means taken in pairs; more general contrasts cannot be tested.

In these procedures the k treatment means are ranked from the lowest to the highest:

$$\bar{y}_1 \leq \bar{y}_2 \leq \cdots \leq \bar{y}_k$$

To test the difference between any two means, say $\bar{y}_i - \bar{y}_j$, the WSD allowance is $q_{\alpha,k} s_{\bar{y}}$, no matter which pair is being compared. The Newman-Keuls procedure, however, uses $q_{\alpha,k'} s_{\bar{y}}$, where k' is the number of means lying between and including the two being tested (that is, $k' = i - j + 1$, where i and j represent the rank order of the two being compared). Thus, the Newman-Keuls allowance is smaller than that of the WSD method, except for comparison of the two extreme means, in which case they are equal. A proviso is that once a pair of means $(\bar{y}_j, \bar{y}_i)$ is tested and found to be nonsignificant, no other pair falling *between* $\bar{y}_j$ and $\bar{y}_i$ can be declared to be significant.

In Duncan's multiple range test the allowance is the quantity $q_{\alpha',k'} s_{\bar{y}}$, where k', as in the Newman-Keuls procedure, is the number of means between and including the two being tested, and α' is equal to $1 - (1 - \alpha)^{k'-1}$. This choice of the percentage point of the Studentized-range statistic is based upon the concept of "error rate per degree of freedom," introduced by Duncan (1955). This is a controversial concept among statisticians, but it has found considerable favor among statistical users, because it results in allowances that are smaller than those of the Tukey and Newman-Keuls procedures (considered by many people to be unduly conservative) but larger than those of the LSD method. Since the formula for α' results in values different from those normally provided in tables of the Studentized range, special tables have been constructed for use with this procedure (Harter et al., 1959).

4. An example

Description of experiment and preliminary analysis

The data used to illustrate the methods are given in Table 1. The purpose of the experiment was twofold: to determine the response of the thyroid iodide-transport mechanism (measured by the ratio of

TABLE 1   Analysis of Thyroid Serum Iodide Concentration Ratios

Data:

		Iodide level, μg		
	0	0.25	2.5	45
Without PTU	Group 1	Group 2	Group 3	Group 4
	184	87	92	146
	137	128	138	162
	207	172	117	119
	166	172	83	68
	276	81	152	141
	145	167	115	139
	197	130	99	164
With PTU	Group 5	Group 6	Group 7	Group 8
	215	204	245	260
	169	145	132	359
	274	317	291	196
	116	315	354	228
	209	282	629 (?)	222
	127	241	204	90
	214	141	249	475

Analysis of variance of log T/S values:

Source of variation	DF	SS	MS	F
Treatment groups	7	0.9644	0.1377	5.74 ($P < 0.001$)
PTU	1	0.6815	0.6815	28.4 ($P < 0.001$)
Iodide levels	3	0.0072	0.0024	0.10
PTU × I interaction	3	0.2757	0.0919	3.83 ($P < 0.05$)
Within groups	48	1.1521	0.0240	
Totals:	55	2.1165		

iodide concentrations in the thyroid and in the serum) to the acute administration of various doses of iodide in the rat, and to determine whether the effect of iodide, if any, can be prevented by propylthiouracil (PTU). Specifically, the experimenter asked the following questions:

A. Does any dose of iodide without PTU lower the T/S value significantly from the control values?

B. Do the different doses of iodide differ significantly in their ability to lower the T/S value?

C. Does PTU significantly affect the T/S values?

D. Does PTU prevent the effects, if any, of iodide on the T/S values?

The statistical analysis of the data begins with an analysis of variance. This provides an estimate of the error variance to be used in the multiple comparisons tests and yields an overall test of significance for the presence of treatment effects. However, it is necessary first to check that the assumptions of the analysis of variance are satisfied.

The most crucial assumption is the equality of the variances among the treatment groups. Bartlett's test for homogeneity of a set of sample variances (see Snedecor and Cochran, 1967, p. 296), applied to the eight treatment groups, turns out to be highly significant. Another test, due to Cochran (1941) and based on the ratio of the maximal variance to the sum of the variances, also gives a significant result. Regardless of the test used, there is a strong indication that the variances cannot be assumed to be homogeneous.

A plot (not shown here) of the standard deviation versus the mean for the eight treatment groups indicates that the standard deviation tends to be directly proportional to the mean, except for the last two groups, which had somewhat large standard deviations. This suggests that transformation to logarithms should help to stabilize the variance. After such transformation both Bartlett's and Cochran's tests were nonsignificant.

The experimenter has placed a question mark after one of the observations, indicating a possibly aberrant measurement. The application of a statistical outlier test (p. 47) to the transformed data failed to provide sufficient justification for discarding the observation; therefore, in the subsequent analyses *all* values shown in Table 1 are included.

The bottom part of Table 1 gives the analysis of variance of the log data. Its main purpose is to provide the variance value $s^2 = 0.0240$ used in determining the standard error of the treatment group means. The overall F test of the between-groups mean square is highly significant $(P < 0.001)$.

Since the eight treatments in the experiment form a 2×4 factorial arrangement (two levels of PTU by four levels of iodide), a natural subdivision of the treatments sum of squares is the orthogonal components corresponding to the levels of PTU, the levels of iodide, and their interaction, which are shown in the analysis-of-variance table. If desired, the latter two could be further subdivided into 1 DF sums of squares corresponding to particular orthogonal contrasts of interest. The testing of the various null hypotheses corresponding to these contrasts could be made by means of F tests, each with 1 DF in the numerator and each at some level of significance, α. These are equivalent to multiple t tests of the contrasts, and they control the comparison error rate at the level α. The probability that at least one of the null hypotheses will be wrongly declared significant may be considerably more than α; if this causes concern, Tukey's test for orthogonal contrasts may be used to provide control of the experiment error rate instead. Since in this example it is likely that other comparisons besides those corresponding to any orthogonal set will be of interest (see below), we shall not pursue this further here.

Contrasts of interest

For any set of k treatment means, where k is greater than 2 (in this example it is 8), the total number of contrasts that can be formed is infinite. In practice only a limited number will actually be of interest, but it can be considerable.

Table 2 presents a list of contrasts of possible interest. Although the list is lengthy, it is not intended to be exhaustive, and the reader might add others. Further, it is not implied that each contrast listed is necessarily of concern. Most are suggested by the specific questions posed by the experimenter; others, at least in part, by the way the means have turned out.

Consider question A, "Does any dose of iodide without PTU lower the T/S value significantly from the control values?" Let $\bar{y}_1$, $\bar{y}_2$, $\bar{y}_3$, and $\bar{y}_4$ be the means for the control group and three iodide levels without PTU, and let $\bar{y}_5$, $\bar{y}_6$, $\bar{y}_7$, and $\bar{y}_8$ be the means for corresponding groups with PTU; then this question suggests the three differences $\bar{y}_1 - \bar{y}_2$, $\bar{y}_1 - \bar{y}_3$, and $\bar{y}_1 - \bar{y}_4$. These are the contrasts defined as

$$\text{Contrast 1:} \quad c_1 = 1, \quad c_2 = -1, \quad \text{other } c\text{'s} = 0$$
$$\text{Contrast 2:} \quad c_1 = 1, \quad c_3 = -1, \quad \text{other } c\text{'s} = 0$$
$$\text{Contrast 3:} \quad c_1 = 1, \quad c_4 = -1, \quad \text{other } c\text{'s} = 0$$

and are the first three listed.

Next, consider question B, "Do the different doses of iodide differ significantly in their ability to lower the T/S value?" This suggests that each of the three iodide treatment groups (without PTU) should be

TABLE 2 Comparison of Multiple Comparisons Procedures for Testing Some Contrasts of Interest in the Data of Table 1

Col no.:	1	2	3	4	5	6	7	8	9	10	11	12	13	14	
		Contrast coefficients c_i ($i = 1,\ldots,8$)								**Value of contrast**	**Allowance for 5% error rates**				**Question**
		Iodide levels without PTU				Iodide levels with PTU					Comparison	Experiment			
Question	Contrast no.	0	0.25	2.5	45	0	0.25	2.5	45		LSD or multiple t	Scheffé's FSD	Tukey's WSD	Allowance	Method used
A	1	1	−1							0.153	0.166	0.326	0.262	0.201	Comparisons with a control, with $m = 4$
	2	1		−1						0.215	0.166*	0.326	0.262	0.201*	
	3	1			−1					0.149	0.166	0.326	0.262	0.201	
B	4		1	−1						0.062	0.166	0.326	0.262	0.200	Tukey's WSD with $m = 3$
	5		1		−1					−0.004	0.166	0.326	0.262	0.200	
	6			1	−1					−0.066	0.166	0.326	0.262	0.200	
	7		1/2	−1	1/2					0.064	0.144	0.282	0.262	0.200	
C	8	−1				1				−0.003	0.166	0.326	0.262	0.214	Orthogonal contrasts with $m = 4$
	9		−1				1			0.241	0.166†	0.326	0.262	0.214*	
	10			−1				1		0.385	0.166†	0.326†	0.262†	0.214†	
	11				−1				1	0.258	0.166†	0.326	0.262	0.214*	
	12	−1/4	−1/4	−1/4	−1/4	1/4	1/4	1/4	1/4	0.221	0.083†	0.163†	0.262	0.214*	
	13		−1/3	−1/3	−1/3		1/3	1/3	1/3	0.295	0.096†	0.188†	0.262*	0.214†	
D	14	−3	−1	1	3	3	1	−1	−3	−0.924	0.745*	1.456	2.099	0.916*	Orthogonal contrasts with $m = 3$
	15	1	−1	−1	1	−1	1	1	−1	0.370	0.333*	0.651	1.049	0.410	
	16	−1	3	−3	1	1	−3	3	−1	0.172	0.745	1.456	2.099	0.916	
D (alternate)	17	1	−1			−1	1			0.243	0.235*	0.461	0.525	0.284	Comparisons with a control, with $m = 4$
	18	1		−1		−1		1		0.387	0.235†	0.461	0.525	0.284†	
	19	1			−1	−1			1	0.260	0.235*	0.461	0.525	0.284	
Treatment means, $\bar{y}_i$:		2.262	2.109	2.047	2.113	2.260	2.350	2.432	2.371						

* Value of contrast exceeds the allowance for a 5% error rate.
† Value of contrast exceeds the allowance for a 1% error rate.

compared with each of the other two, to determine whether any are significantly different; this gives $\bar{y}_2 - \bar{y}_3$, $\bar{y}_2 - \bar{y}_4$, and $\bar{y}_3 - \bar{y}_4$, which are contrasts 4, 5, and 6. In addition, noting that the means for the lowest and highest iodide levels are almost identical, the experimenter might wish to compare the intermediate dose level with the average of the other two: that is, to test the significance of $(\bar{y}_2 + \bar{y}_4)/2 - \bar{y}_3$, which is contrast 7.

Question C, "Does PTU significantly affect the T/S values?" could be examined in several ways. One way is to compare corresponding levels of iodide in the presence and absence of PTU, which is to compare groups 5 and 1, groups 6 and 2, etc. These comparisons are indicated by contrasts 8, 9, 10, and 11. Alternatively, or in addition, the average of the four groups with PTU could be compared with that of the four groups without PTU (contrast 12), or the average of the three iodide groups with PTU could be compared with that of the three iodide groups without PTU (contrast 13).

The answer to question D, "Does PTU prevent the effects, if any, of iodide on the T/S values?" seems to require a posteriori comparisons, unless it is possible to formulate a priori (before observing the results of the experiment) what the effect of the iodide is likely to be. The data indicate that the most obvious effect of the iodide in the absence of PTU is an initial decrease in T/S at the low and intermediate dose levels, followed by an increase at the high dose level. If the mean responses are plotted against log dose, a marked curvature is readily apparent, particularly if the response for the zero dose is plotted as well, by placing it at some arbitrarily small dose level, say 0.025, in order to include it on the graph. From a table of orthogonal polynomials (p. 57) for four points one could obtain the contrast coefficients for the linear, quadratic, and cubic regression effects.[1] These same coefficients could also be used to determine the corresponding effects *with* PTU. In order to test whether these effects have been changed by the presence of PTU, one obtains contrasts 14, 15, and 16, contrast 14 representing the difference between the two linear effects (with and without PTU), contrast 15 the difference between the two quadratic effects, and contrast 16 the difference between the two cubic effects.

Alternatively, the experimenter might prefer not to consider any regression effect of the iodide dose level to answer the question, but, rather, to consider the effect of each dose separately. Now, the effects of

[1] Strictly speaking, the dose levels should be equally spaced on *some* scale, if we are to use these coefficients, but this is not actually necessary when we are not using them to calculate a dose-effect equation. In any case, a scale of measurement can always be *devised* on which the particular dose levels used in the experiment will appear as equally spaced.

the three dose levels of iodide in the absence of PTU are measured by contrasts 1, 2, and 3. Analogous contrasts involving $\bar{y}_5$, $\bar{y}_6$, $\bar{y}_7$, and $\bar{y}_8$ would measure the effects of the three dose levels of iodide in the presence of PTU. Contrasts made up of the differences between the corresponding effect contrasts in the presence and absence of PTU could then be used to test whether the presence of PTU has altered any of the individual dose effects; these are shown as contrasts 17, 18, and 19.

This makes a total of nineteen contrasts listed in Table 2. Of course, the choice is subjective, and one may wish to alter some or to condense them to a shorter list. The point to be made, however, is that in a set of treatment means a sizable number of contrasts of potential interest can be devised.

Column 10 of Table 2 lists the values of the contrasts. These are calculated by multiplying each set of contrast coefficients given in columns 2 to 9 (a blank being understood to represent $c_i = 0$) by the corresponding treatment mean and summing the products. For convenience in carrying out these operations the treatment means are listed in the last row of the table.

Allowances for controlling various error rates

In the previous section the LSD or the multiple t test was described as a procedure for controlling the comparison error rate, and Scheffé's and Tukey's tests, besides the two special-purpose tests, as procedures for controlling the family error rate. In the latter the family usually consists of the entire set of contrasts tested in the experiment, in which case the family error rate becomes an experiment error rate. In the present example, however, there is another possibility that may be considered. Since the contrasts to be tested fall naturally into distinct sets according to the particular questions which suggested them, each set may be considered a family, and the family error rate then becomes a question error rate. Both possibilities are illustrated below.

Whichever of the methods is used, the standard error $s_{\bar{y}}$ of a treatment mean is needed. This is calculated from s^2, the within-groups mean square in the analysis of variance in Table 1, by dividing by the number of observations in a treatment group and taking the square root:

$$s_{\bar{y}} = \sqrt{s^2/n} = \sqrt{0.0240/7} = 0.05856$$

The associated degrees of freedom are that for the within-groups mean square, 48.

Control of comparison error rate   To control the comparison error rate, the LSD method or the multiple t test is used. For example, if a comparison error rate of 5% is desired (leading to a rate of 5% for results falsely labeled significant), the value of t_α, obtained from tables of Student's t distribution for 48 DF and $\alpha = 0.05$, is 2.011. Multiplication by the standard error of each contrast gives the numerical values of the LSD allowances shown in column 11 of Table 2.

Control of experiment error rate   In order to control the experiment error rate at any specified level, for example 5% (in which case the number of experiments containing at least one comparison falsely labeled significant will be limited to 5% of the total), it is clear that larger allowances will be required than those provided by the LSD procedure.

In the previous section the two special-purpose procedures and Scheffé's and Tukey's methods were described as capable of controlling the experiment error rate. However, only Scheffé's FSD and Tukey's WSD procedures are applicable to the entire set of contrasts given in Table 2, the other two being appropriate only if all the contrasts in the set are of a certain type.

A calculation of the FSD allowance requires the value of $\sqrt{(m-1)F_{\alpha,m-1}}$, where m is 8, the number of treatment means. For a 5% experiment error rate the value of $F_{\alpha,m-1}$ for $m-1 = 7$ DF in the numerator and $f = 48$ DF in the denominator is 2.21, obtained from tables of the F distribution for $\alpha = 0.05$. Thus $\sqrt{(m-1)F_{\alpha,m-1}}$ is 3.93; multiplication by the standard error of each contrast gives the values of the FSD allowances shown in column 12 of Table 2.

The ratio of $\sqrt{(m-1)F_{\alpha,m-1}}$ to t_α represents the factor by which the LSD allowances must be inflated in order to give the FSD allowances. In the present example this inflation factor is $3.93/2.011 = 1.96$; thus, the size of the allowances is almost doubled, an indication of the price to be paid for controlling the experiment error rate by the FSD procedure, instead of controlling the comparison error rate.

If Tukey's WSD method is used, the value of $q_{\alpha,m}$ for $m = 8$ is required. From tables of the Studentized range for $m = 8, f = 48$ DF, and $\alpha = 0.05$ the value $q_{\alpha,m} = 4.48$ is obtained by interpolation. Multiplication by the standard error of a treatment mean gives the allowance for a simple difference between two means. For any other contrast this is multiplied by one-half the sum of the absolute values of the contrast coefficients. The results are given in column 13 of Table 2.

In the WSD procedure the inflation factor over the LSD allowance is $q_{\alpha,m}/\sqrt{2}t_\alpha$ for the contrasts, which are simple differences between two means. In this example the inflation factor is $4.48/(1.414 \times 2.011) = 1.58$, appreciably smaller than that in the FSD procedure. However, for other types of contrast it will be larger; for some it will even exceed that of the FSD procedure. Thus the choice between the FSD and WSD procedures for controlling the experiment error rate depends upon which contrasts are of most interest.

Control of question error rate   In controlling the question error rate it will be found that the allowances required are usually not as large as those needed in controlling the experiment error rate. One reason for this is that it is often possible to use one of the special-purpose procedures when the contrasts corresponding to a particular question are of a certain type. Another reason is that the number of treatment means involved in a particular set of contrasts may be less than the total number in the experiment.

For question A of the previous section contrasts 1 to 3 in Table 2 were suggested. This set involves multiple comparisons with a control, for which the method of comparisons with a control or standard is appropriate. Since four treatment means are involved, m is 4, and interpolation in the tables gives $t''_{\alpha,m} = 2.426$ for $\alpha = 0.05$ and $f = 48$ DF. Multiplication by $\sqrt{2}s_{\bar{y}}$ gives 0.201 as the allowance for each contrast in this set.

For question B the contrasts 4 to 6 in Table 2 represent all possible differences among the three means $\bar{y}_2$, $\bar{y}_3$, and $\bar{y}_4$, while contrast 7 is a more general contrast in the same three means. Thus Tukey's WSD method can be used, with $m = 3$ instead of the $m = 8$ required to control the experiment error rate, since only three means are now involved. For $m = 3$, $\alpha = 0.05$, and $f = 48$ DF the Studentized-range tables give the value $q_{\alpha,m} = 3.421$; multiplication by $s_{\bar{y}}$ gives the required allowance of 0.200, as shown in column 14 of Table 2. The same allowance applies also to contrast 7.

For question C it can be easily seen that contrasts 8 to 11 form an orthogonal set, for which Tukey's method for orthogonal contrasts is appropriate. Furthermore, contrasts 12 and 13 are linear combinations of the four contrasts in the orthogonal set, contrast 12 being an average of the four and contrast 13 being an average of three of them. As has been explained, the method for orthogonal contrasts is easily extended to cover these.

For this set of contrasts, 8 to 13, we refer to tables of the Studentized maximum modulus with $m = 4$, the value of $t'_{\alpha,m}$ for $\alpha = 0.05$ and for $f = 48$ DF being 2.58. Multiplication by $\sqrt{2}s_{\bar{y}}$ gives an allowance of 0.214. This allowance applies to contrasts 12 and 13 as well.

The set of contrasts 14 to 16 suggested by question D also forms an orthogonal set, so that Tukey's test for orthogonal contrasts is again appropriate. This time m is 3, since there are only three contrasts in the orthogonal set. Interpolation in tables of the Studentized maximum modulus gives $t'_{\alpha,m} = 2.475$ for $m = 3$, $\alpha = 0.05$, and $f = 48$ DF. This is multiplied by the standard error of each contrast, equal to $\sqrt{\sum c_i^2 s_{\bar{y}}}$, to give the allowances shown in Table 2.

The alternative set of contrasts proposed for answering question D, contrasts 17 to 19 in Table 2, requires a different procedure. Note that these three contrasts may be considered as three comparisons between treatment and control, $\bar{y}_1 - \bar{y}_5$ being the "control" and $\bar{y}_2 - \bar{y}_6$, $\bar{y}_3 - \bar{y}_7$, and $\bar{y}_4 - \bar{y}_8$ the three "treatments." Thus the method for obtaining the allowances from comparisons with a control or standard is appropriate, with $m = 4$, since the total number of "treatments," including the control, is four. As for the set of contrasts for answering question A, the value of $t''_{\alpha,m}$ is 2.426, but the standard error of each contrast is now $\sqrt{\sum c_i^2 s_{\bar{y}}} = 0.1171$, so that the allowance is 2.426 × 0.1171 = 0.284, as shown in Table 2.

Allowances with the multiple range procedures

The multiple range tests are used when each treatment mean in the set is to be compared with each of the others and these are the only comparisons of interest, when, in other words, there is no interest in more general contrasts involving three or more means. For the purpose of illustrating these methods we shall now assume this to be the case.

The eight treatment groups, denoted by the letters A through H, in order from lowest to highest are

C:	2.047
B:	2.109
D:	2.113
E:	2.260
A:	2.262
F:	2.350
H:	2.371
G:	2.432

Table 3 shows the allowances for comparing any two of the means in this set at the $\alpha = 0.05$ level. These were calculated for the multiple

TABLE 3 Comparison of Multiple Range Tests: Allowances for 5% Error Rate

Method	No. of means between and including two to be compared						
	2	3	4	5	6	7	8
Tukey's WSD	0.262	0.262	0.262	0.262	0.262	0.262	0.262
Newman-Keuls	0.166	0.200	0.220	0.235	0.246	0.255	0.262
Duncan	0.166	0.175	0.181	0.185	0.188	0.190	0.193

range tests as described in the previous section. For the Tukey procedure the allowance is constant, irrespective of which particular pair of means in the ordered set is being compared, since it is based on the Studentized-range statistic for $k = 8$ means. On the other hand, for the Newman-Keuls procedure the Studentized-range statistic is used for the number of means in the ordered set between and including the two being compared. For comparing the extreme means (in this case groups C and G) the allowance coincides with that of the Tukey procedure, but for comparing any other pair it is smaller, and for comparing two adjacent means it is equal to the LSD allowance.

The Duncan multiple range procedure has still smaller allowances. For comparing the extreme means, since $\alpha' = 1 - 0.95^7 = 0.302$, the upper 0.302 point of the Studentized range for eight means is used instead of the 0.05 point used in the Newman-Keuls procedure. For other comparisons both α' and k' decrease, depending upon the number of means between and including the two being compared. Ultimately, for comparing two adjacent means the allowance is equal to the LSD allowance.

A convenient format to use with either the Newman-Keuls or the Duncan procedure was suggested by Bliss (1967, p. 255). It is a two-way table that shows the differences between each pair of means in the upper right corner and the allowances corresponding to each difference in the lower left corner. Table 4 shows the Newman-Keuls allowances; Table 5 shows the Duncan allowances. Significant differences, marked with a dagger or asterisk, are obtained by comparing the observed differences in the upper right corner with the corresponding allowance in the lower left corner, beginning at the right edge and moving to the left or at the top edge and moving down. The proviso that two means contained within a nonsignificant pair of means cannot be judged significant implies that no observed difference below or to the left of a difference not marked with a dagger or asterisk can be called significant, even if it should happen to exceed its allowance. This applies to both the Newman-Keuls and the Duncan procedures. In Tables 4 and 5 a dagger has been used to denote a significant difference based on the $\alpha = 0.05$ allowances shown in the tables; an asterisk indicates that the corresponding $\alpha = 0.01$ allowance, not shown in the tables, is also exceeded.

Confidence intervals for contrasts

It has been assumed throughout that interest is in significance-testing. The experimenter's questions A to D are of the type that traditionally have been answered by significance-testing procedures. If they were rephrased to ask "How much?" instead of "Does it?" (for example, "How much does each dose of iodide lower the T/S value?"),

TABLE 4   Application of the Newman-Keuls Multiple Range Test to the Data in Table 1

Treatment group	Treatment group							
	C	B	D	E	A	F	H	G
C		0.062	0.066	0.213	0.215	0.303*	0.324*	0.385*
B	0.166		0.004	0.151	0.153	0.241†	0.262†	0.323*
D	0.200	0.166		0.147	0.149	0.237†	0.258†	0.319*
E	0.220	0.200	0.166		0.002	0.090	0.111	0.172
A	0.235	0.220	0.200	0.166		0.088	0.109	0.170
F	0.246	0.235	0.220	0.200	0.166		0.021	0.082
H	0.255	0.246	0.235	0.220	0.200	0.166		0.061
G	0.262	0.255	0.246	0.235	0.220	0.200	0.166	

* Exceeds allowance for $\alpha = 0.01$ (not shown in table).
† Exceeds allowance for $\alpha = 0.05$.

TABLE 5   Application of Duncan's Multiple Range Test to the Data in Table 1

Treatment group	Treatment group							
	C	B	D	E	A	F	H	G
C		0.062	0.066	0.213†	0.215†	0.303*	0.324*	0.385*
B	0.166		0.004	0.151	0.153	0.241†	0.262*	0.323*
D	0.175	0.166		0.147	0.149	0.237†	0.258*	0.319*
E	0.181	0.175	0.166		0.002	0.090	0.111	0.172
A	0.185	0.181	0.175	0.166		0.088	0.109	0.170
F	0.188	0.185	0.181	0.175	0.166		0.021	0.082
H	0.190	0.188	0.185	0.181	0.175	0.166		0.061
G	0.193	0.190	0.188	0.185	0.181	0.175	0.166	

* Exceeds allowance for $\alpha = 0.01$ (not shown in table).
† Exceeds allowance for $\alpha = 0.05$.

estimates instead of significance tests would be required. However, this introduces no new problem. The estimate of the value of each contrast is simply the observed value of the contrast, as given in column 10 of Table 2, and confidence limits are easily obtained by adding and subtracting the value of the allowance. There is the same choice between methods of determining the allowance in confidence-interval estimation as in significance-testing; the "confidence coefficient" $1 - \alpha$ may apply to each confidence interval separately or jointly to all the confidence intervals in a family. Thus, corresponding to the comparison, question, and experiment error rates of significance-testing procedures, we have comparison, question, and experiment confidence coefficients for interval estimation.

There is no confidence-interval procedure corresponding to either the Newman-Keuls or the Duncan multiple range test. Although limits could be calculated in the same way as in the other procedures, they would not constitute confidence intervals. Hence, these procedures are restricted to significance-testing situations.

Summary of results

Looking at the numerical results in Table 2, one can determine to what extent the experimenter's questions are answered.

For the first question it may be noted that one of the three comparisons of iodide level versus control (contrasts 1 to 3) is significant by the multiple *t* test. If these were the only significance tests, the result might be questioned on the grounds that iodide has been given three opportunities to exhibit an effect. In this case the two nonsignificant iodide levels are close to significance (by the multiple *t* test) and hence tend to support the evidence of a true effect of iodide. However, the multiple comparisons test for questions, designed to take account of the multiple significance testing, still shows significance for this dose level. On the other hand, neither of the multiple comparisons tests for experiments does.

In answer to the second of the experimenter's questions, none of the three dose levels of iodide even come close to being significantly different from each other by the multiple *t* test and, of course, neither do they by any of the multiple comparisons tests. Thus, although the data may suggest that the iodide effect is at a maximum in the neighborhood of the middle dose level, more precise experimental information is needed to establish whether this is so and, if it is so, the location of the maximum effect.

In answer to the experimenter's third question, there appears to be little doubt that the presence of PTU has affected some of the treatment responses. In the absence of iodide (contrast 8) there is no evidence that PTU had any effect. However, in the presence of iodide (contrasts 9, 10, and 11) its effect has been significant at all three dose levels, judged by either the multiple *t* test or the multiple comparisons test for questions. On the other hand, judged by either of the multiple comparisons tests for experiments the PTU effect is significant at one dose level and approaches significance at the other two.

The remaining two sets of contrasts, 14 to 16 and 17 to 19, compare the effects of the iodide in the presence and absence of PTU. In the first set the iodide effect is measured by its linear, quadratic, and cubic regression components, while in the second the iodide effects are measured by differences of each dose level from its control. Significant differences have been found in both sets by means of the multiple *t* test. In each case one of them remains significant when account is taken of the multiple tests performed in the particular set of contrasts (by the multiple comparisons procedure for questions), but none are sufficiently large to reach significance by either of the multiple comparisons procedures for experiments.

The multiple range tests (Tables 4 and 5) reveal significant differences between each of the groups B, C, and D on the one hand and groups F, G, and H on the other with the Newman-Keuls procedure and, in addition, between groups C and E and between groups C and A with the Duncan procedure.

5. Further discussion and comments

The purpose of this chapter has been to illustrate some of the more useful multiple comparisons procedures by using a set of data from an endocrinological experiment. As to which method is most appropriate for any particular set of data, there is room for discussion and even for debate.

In the analysis of an experiment involving multiple comparisons the most difficult problem is to decide what constitutes a *family* of comparisons. Viewpoints differ among statisticians. At one extreme is the nonmultiple-comparisonist, who would consider each separate comparison a family; in his opinion only the comparison error rate is ever of concern. At the other extreme is the strict multiple-comparisonist, who would insist that all comparisons made in the experiment constitute a single family and that a multiple comparisons procedure be used to control the experiment error rate.

In the example discussed in this chapter it seemed natural to take an intermediate position and to consider as a family the set of comparisons (or contrasts) corresponding to each question asked by the experimenter. In many situations this would lead to the use of the same procedure as that recommended by the nonmultiple-comparisonist. One such example arises in drug screening, in which several unknown compounds are compared with a control, to determine which ones appear to have sufficient biological activity to justify further investigation. It is clear that the error rate per compound is of prime concern, since it determines the proportion of inactives that will be passed by the screen. In fact, in each experiment there are as many questions of the nature "Does *this* compound have sufficient activity to justify further investigation?" as there are compounds to be compared with the control. Here the procedures involving question and comparison error rates coincide.

When error rates were defined in the second section of this chapter it was mentioned that they referred to errors under the null hypothesis, or

Type I errors. It should be stressed that another error that needs to be considered is that of *not* finding significance when the null hypothesis is false (the so-called Type II error). In other words, if there is a real treatment effect corresponding to a particular contrast, one should like that contrast to exceed its allowance. The probability of the latter's happening is referred to as the *power* of the test procedure.

It is unfortunate that, as the allowance is increased in order to control the family error rate instead of the comparison error rate, the power of the test decreases. Power should be considered at the time the experiment is being planned, and the size of the experiment (namely, the number of animals per treatment group) should be so chosen that treatment effects large enough to be of interest will have a high probability of detection. Once the experiment is completed, power can be increased only by increasing the value of α, the error rate (for a comparison or for a family, whichever is appropriate in the particular situation) under the null hypothesis of no treatment effect. One difficulty that arises in relaxing the value for α for the two special-purpose multiple comparisons procedures (Tukey's test for orthogonal contrasts and comparisons with a control) is the lack of extensive tables, since tables for the first of these have been constructed only for $\alpha = 0.05$ and tables for the second only for $\alpha = 0.05$ and $\alpha = 0.01$. Tables computed by Dunn and Massey (1965), however, are of some help, because they cover a wide range of values of α for a limited number of degrees of freedom (4, 10, 30, and ∞ DF) and for a limited number of tests to be done (2, 6, 10, and 20). For orthogonal contrasts one should use the value $\rho = 0$ in the tables of Dunn and Massey, and for comparisons with a control one should use the value $\rho = 0.5$.

DISCUSSION

INGBAR   I should like to express my gratitude to Dr. Dunnett for the extensive consideration he has given to my data. The physiology underlying the experiment is that when one administers different doses of iodide to animals, the thyroid gland forms differing amounts of hormone. With doses of 0.25, 2.5, and 40 µg the response is sharply biphasic, hormone formation first increasing and then decreasing. The question that we were asking (testing a hypothesis that others had made) was "To what extent does the dose of iodide determine the reduction in iodide transport?" We might well have expected the curve for iodide transport to constitute a mirror image of hormone formation.

With regard to that peculiar value of 629, we have never seen a value so high in experiments like this, in which literally thousands of rats were used. Therefore, I know that this value must have resulted from an error in technique, such as radioactive contamination. I would discard the observation regardless of what the statistics showed.

DUNNETT This constitutes additional information. The statistical outlier tests contain only the data from the current experiment. Therefore, I agree that if you feel that it should be thrown out, it should be thrown out.

BLISS From the means at the foot of Table 2 it appears that without PTU the T/S ratio falls below the control whereas with PTU it exceeds it. Consequently, when one adds the levels with and without PTU these opposing trends are averaged out. Although in the analysis of variance in Table 1 the interaction is quite significant, it has not been subdivided to show these opposed tendencies explicitly.

DUNNETT That is quite definitely true. I did not show a plot of these data against doses of iodide.

BLISS Wouldn't such a plot be more instructive and informative than a comparison of mean values?

BARTOSIK Further, it appears that the multiple comparisons tests ignore the obvious mirror-image effect of the dose–response curves.

DUNNETT In any dose–response experiment a plot of the mean values would certainly be informative. Following that, a comparison of mean values or certain linear combinations of them might be called for, to test for significant differences.

BLISS It seems to me that this could be looked at essentially as an a priori rather than an a posteriori set of comparisons.

DUNNETT I agree. Most of the comparisons listed in Table 2 are a priori comparisons. However, the point that I was illustrating is that there are more comparisons than there are degrees of freedom for treatments.

SMITH I wish to return to the problem of comparing several means. A type of problem that better illustrates multiple comparisons procedures is the following. One has seven completely different compounds and would like to examine the response to each with a view to making some judgment about which are better, which two go together, etc. The compounds are not associated by a scale such as log dose or anything else. For this problem the speaker has presented several different techniques of separating mean values. Remember that each technique is based upon a different set of assumptions. It is an understanding of these fundamental differences that will enable the experimenter to decide which procedure he should use.

GUILLEMIN   We have been employing the Dunnett multiple comparisons test to determine whether the response of any one experimental group differs from the control group. It was my understanding that with k groups one cannot use the classical Student t test. What is the proper method of making this comparison?

DUNNETT   If there is no relationship between the treatments, if they are included together in the experiment merely for reasons of economy, then the LSD method is appropriate. One is comparing each treatment with the control, and it is the comparison error rate that is of interest. The experiment error rate has no meaning whatsoever.

GUILLEMIN   And if they are related?

DUNNETT   If they are related it is different. Then I would, at least, consider a multiple comparisons procedure. However, in that case I would want to know the nature of the relationship between the treatments and the sort of conclusions that are to be drawn from the results of significance tests. If more attention is to be paid to the group differing most from the control, I would use the multiple comparisons test instead of the LSD, to assure myself that it differed significantly from the control. In Dr. Ingbar's experiment there are three dose levels, and we ask whether any one dose differs from the control. We give the iodide three opportunities by testing it three times against the control. In this case my method (multiple comparisons against a control) is appropriate.

HIRSCH   If one were not interested in *any* mean but only in whether *low* dose mean is different from the control, then one would be asking about a single comparison. In that case would the ordinary LSD be appropriate?

DUNNETT   Yes.

FORTIER   I am concerned with the assessment of the statistical significance of the pattern of a physiological response (for example, the plasma concentration of some hormone) over time, following some experimental stimulus. Mean hormonal concentrations and their standard errors would be obtained at various time intervals after application of the stimulus. It may be that none of the means compared singly against the baseline is significantly different, although their sequential pattern over time suggests a rise or fall from the baseline. In this case neither a t-test comparison of individual means nor a multiple comparisons test seems appropriate, since both fail to take account of this trend. What would be an appropriate significance test for the pattern, especially when it corresponds to a nonlinear curve?

DUNNETT   Perhaps a moving average of the observed means would be a more sensitive indicator of this type of change from control. It is necessary to fit a curve of some kind to the points. If there is no underlying model to suggest the form of the curve, I would suggest fitting a polynomial-regression curve. The coefficients in the resulting regression equation can be tested for whether or not they are significantly different from zero.

FORTIER   Would it not be difficult to find the appropriate tests of significance for such polynomial-regression curves?

DUNNETT   No. There are standard tests of significance that accompany the fitting of a polynomial-regression curve.

CHAPTER FOUR

Continuous-Response Assays

C. PHILIP COX

1. Introduction and definitions

The term *bioassay* will be used to characterize an experiment in which the observations are the responses of biological material, and which is aimed at estimating the potency of an unknown preparation (called U) relative to that of a maintained standard preparation (called S).

By a *continuous-response bioassay* we mean one in which the response may assume any value in its naturally occurring range, as distinct from a quantal-response assay, in which the response may assume one of a set of discrete values. In practice the results of conceptually continuous-response assays are, of necessity, recorded discretely, because the smallest measurement unit is finite. We shall assume, however, that the measurement interval is so small relative to the innate biological variability that our analyses are unaffected by such grouping into a discretely measured variate.

The next definition we shall need is that for *relative potency*. We can arrive at this by supposing that the same response y can be achieved by either a dose D_S of the standard preparation or by a dose D_U of the unknown preparation. Pairs of doses that give the same response are termed *equipotent*, and it is convenient to designate the equipotency by a superscript e. The Greek letter ρ is used for the population, or "true" value, of the relative potency. Thus,

$$\rho = D_S^e/D_U^e \tag{1}$$

The preceding definition leads to an important distinction between types of assay situation. It will be immediately clear that, if relative potency is constant, Equation 1 must hold for pairs of doses over a useful range of doses or, equivalently, of responses. We then have what is known as a *dilution assay*. This is one in which the unknown preparation may be regarded as a dilution of the standard preparation in an inert diluent. We next distinguish between an *analytical* dilution assay and an *equivalent* or *quasi* dilution assay.

An *analytical dilution assay* is one in which the response-producing constituents in the standard and the unknown preparations are the same.

In this case the relative potency is the reciprocal of the dilution factor. The concentration of the response-producing constituent in the unknown preparation is the product of the relative potency and the concentration in the standard preparation.

An *equivalent, comparative,* or *quasi dilution assay* is one in which the response-producing constituents in the two preparations are only qualitatively similar. An apparently constant relative potency can be estimated over some more or less local range of responses and experimental circumstances, although the response-producing constituents in the two preparations are not the same. Unlike estimations from analytical dilution assays, those from equivalent dilution assays will usually depend upon the particular experimental situation, materials, or techniques. Gaddum (1950) indicated that the result of an analytical dilution assay should agree (apart, of course, from sample variability) with that obtainable from chemical or physical determinations of relative potency. That this property does not necessarily, or even usually, obtain for equivalent dilution assays gives rise to important practical questions concerning, for example, the extrapolation of assay results, determined from small laboratory animals, to human therapeutics.

The common *indirect assay*[1] is one in which the ratio of equipotent doses is estimated from curves relating responses and doses for the two preparations. The two common kinds of indirect assays are the following.

Parallel-line assays: those in which the response is linearly related to the log dose.

Slope ratio assays: those in which the response is linearly related to the dose itself.

The different statistical treatments required for each of these assay types are the main concerns of the remainder of this chapter; for more detailed exposition the reader is referred to Bliss (1952), Emmens (1948), and Finney (1964).

2. Parallel-line assays

With parallel-line assays and a linear relation between response and log dose it can be shown that the assumption of similarity (see pp. 145–147 for derivation) leads to the log relative potency, given by

$$\log \rho = (\alpha_U - \alpha_S)/\beta \tag{2}$$

---

[1] It is useful to distinguish *direct* and *indirect assays.* A *direct assay* is one in which one can actually determine equipotent doses. We might envisage the infusion of adrenalin into experimental animals until the heart rate reaches some specified end point. Such assays do not appear to be commonly used in endocrine research. The analysis of direct assays is described by Finney (1964).

where α_U and α_S are the respective intercepts of the unknown and standard log-dose–response lines and β is the common slope. In practice an experiment is conducted in which responses y to a convenient selection of log dose values x for standard and unknown are observed and parallel lines are fitted to the dose–response curves. From the fitted lines one obtains estimates b for β, $\bar{y}_U - b\bar{x}_U$ for α_U, and $\bar{y}_S - b\bar{x}_S$ for α_S. These in turn yield an estimate of log relative potency:

$$\log R = M = (\bar{x}_S - \bar{x}_U) - (\bar{y}_S - \bar{y}_U)/b \qquad (3)$$

Subject to the usual assumptions that responses are normally distributed about their population means with a variance that is the same whatever the log dose, an interval estimate for $\log \rho$ (and hence for the relative potency itself) can be obtained by using Fieller's theorem for interval estimation of a ratio (Fieller, 1940; Finney, 1964, pp. 27–29).

Experimental designs for parallel-line bioassays are chosen for the following purposes:

1. To facilitate calculation of the estimates $\bar{y}_S - \bar{y}_U$ and b and the estimate of variance s^2.

2. To permit examination of the validity of the procedure by testing the relevance of the basic model to the specific biological situation. In particular, it is desirable to ascertain whether the experimental data are consistent with the assumption that the population log-dose–response lines are parallel and straight.

Two experimental plans commonly used for achieving these ends are the *four-point* and *six-point assays*. The choice between these two will depend on particular circumstances. Thus, for the same total number of observations the four-point assay gives the better precision for relative potency. This plan allows us to make a test of whether or not the lines are parallel, but it does not permit a test for curvature (that is, consistency with the assumption of *straight* lines). Both aspects can be tested if the six-point plan is used. Accordingly, we may regard the four-point plan as suited to a well-established assay, whereas in an early research situation, in which there may be less assurance about the dose–response curve, the six-point assay is the more informative.

The four-point parallel-line assay

Let us first look at the four-point parallel-line assay in a simple randomization design (see pp. 61–62 and p. 7). For this we observe an equal number of responses n at each of the four preparation × dose combinations comprising a low and a high dose for both the standard and unknown preparations. If subscripts 1 and 2 indicate low and high doses, respectively, we may designate the doses D_{S1}, D_{S2}, D_{U1}, and D_{U2}, using corresponding x's to denote log doses.

In the interests of precision and convenience we should use any available a priori information to choose doses such that:

1. The dose range is as wide as possible while remaining within the range for which the response is linearly related to log dose.
2. The difference between the mean responses $\bar{y}_S$ and $\bar{y}_U$ is small.

Additionally, in the interests of precision it is desirable that:

3. The log-dose–response line be as steep as possible.
4. The standard deviation s be as small as possible.

The last two desiderata may be combined in the statement that, insofar as experimental techniques and circumstances permit, we aim for a small value of the ratio $\lambda = s/b$, the ratio commonly used as an index of precision in reports of endocrinological assays. The index is useful in the comparison of alternative assay techniques. However, its basis as a measure of precision assumes that good assay conditions obtain and, in particular, that the difference between the mean responses is small; see pp. 148–150 and Finney (1964, p. 185) for further discussion on this point.

In planning it is also convenient to use the same ratio of upper to lower dose for the two preparations: that is, to take doses such that

$$D_{S2}/D_{S1} = D_{U2}/D_{U1}$$

Although large departures from this condition are not recommended, its fulfillment is not absolutely essential provided that the preceding desiderata are under good control. Attempts to achieve exactly the same ratio can lead to experimental inconvenience and may give rise to difficulties with variance heterogeneity. The relatively slight modifications for the analyses of the four-point and six-point assays with unequal dose ratios are described by Cox (1967). Here we shall proceed with the simpler case of equal ratios and equal numbers of observations.

The relative-potency estimate can be calculated from the mean responses to the preparation × dose combinations, but a convenient alternative is to use three orthogonal contrasts that can be calculated from the totals of the n responses in each group. These totals being designated S_1 and S_2 for the lower and higher doses of the standard and U_1 and U_2 for the lower and higher doses of the unknown, two of the three contrasts are

Preparations: $L_p = -S_1 - S_2 + U_1 + U_2$

Common regression (slope): $L_r = -S_1 + S_2 - U_1 + U_2$

These contrasts may be interpreted by noting that

$$L_p/2n = \bar{y}_U - \bar{y}_S \tag{4}$$

which is the difference between the mean responses to the two preparations, while, if the log dose interval is

$$d = \log (D_{S2}/D_{S1}) = x_{S2} - x_{S1} \tag{5}$$

then the common slope is

$$\frac{L_r}{2nd} = \frac{1}{2}\left(\frac{S_2 - S_1}{nd} + \frac{U_2 - U_1}{nd}\right) = b \tag{6}$$

which is, therefore, the average of the slopes of the two log-dose–response lines. Substituting in Equation 3 and taking antilogs then gives

$$R = (D_{S1}/D_{U1}) \text{ antilog } (dL_p/L_r) \tag{7}$$

The steps so far may be illustrated by using data, reproduced by kind permission of Dr. R. P. Rathmacher, for a four-point assay of luteinizing hormone in swine pituitary tissue by the method of ovarian ascorbic acid depletion, described by A. F. Parlow (1961). The doses used were the following:

Standard preparation, μg		Unknown preparation, mg/ml	
Lower	Upper	Lower	Upper
0.4	1.6	0.1	0.4

Five immature female rats were used in each group, and the total responses were

S_1	S_2	U_1	U_2
362	247	325	224

These give

$$L_p = -362 - 247 + 325 + 224 = -60$$
$$L_r = -362 + 247 - 325 + 224 = -216$$

The dose ratio is $1.6/0.4 = 0.4/0.1 = 4$, so that $d = \log 4 = 0.6021$ and, with $D_{S1} = 0.4$ μg and $D_{U1} = 0.1$ mg/ml, the estimated relative potency, from Equation 7, is

$$R = \frac{0.4}{0.1} \text{ antilog } \frac{(0.6021)(-60)}{-216}$$

$$= 4 \text{ antilog } 0.1673$$

$$= 5.88 \text{ μg/(mg}_{\text{tissue}}/\text{ml)}$$

We should remember, however, that this estimate entails the assumption that the two log-dose–response lines are parallel and straight. The assumption of parallelism can readily be examined in the analysis of variance, which in addition provides the estimate of variability required to calculate an interval estimate for the relative potency.

The usual analysis of a completely randomized experiment (one-way classification) giving sums-of-square components among and within groups is appropriate (see pp. 34–37). Since we have four groups, each with n observations, there are 3 DF (degrees of freedom) among the groups and $4(n-1)$ DF within the groups. The sum of squares among the groups is divided into three additive components. These represent the contributions of the contrasts L_p and L_r previously defined and of the third contrast L_d, defined as:

$$L_d = S_1 - S_2 - U_1 + U_2$$

This contrast, which is the interaction dose × preparations, provides the test for divergence; for, by writing

$$L_d = (U_2 - U_1) - (S_2 - S_1)$$

we can see that it is a quantity proportional to the difference between the slope of the line for the unknown and that for the standard preparation. (It may be noted that some writers refer to the divergence term defined above as *parallelism*; the term *divergence* has an advantage in that, as the quantity calculated increases, the departure from parallelism increases.) For Rathmacher's data we have

$$L_d = 362 - 247 - 325 + 224 = 14$$

The analysis of variance is calculated in Table 1; for significance tests the tabulated F value at the 5% level for 1 and 16 DF is 4.49. The significance of the between-preparations term indicates that in this experiment, owing to a lack of preliminary information about the unknown

TABLE 1   Analysis of Variance of a Four-Point Parallel-Line Assay in a Completely Randomized Design; Data from an Ovarian Ascorbic Acid Depletion Assay of Luteinizing Hormone in Swine Pituitary Tissue*

Term	DF	SS	MS	F
Between preparations	1	$L_p^2/4n = 60^2/20$	180	7.63
Common regression	1	$L_r^2/4n = 216^2/20$	2,333	98.86
Divergence	1	$L_d^2/4n = 14^2/20$	10	<1
Within groups	$4(n-1) = 16$	By subtraction = 378	$23.6 = s^2$	
Total:	$4n - 1 = 19$	$\sum y^2 - C_m\dagger = 2,900$		

* Data from Rathmacher.
† C_m, correction for the mean.

preparation, a larger difference occurred between the mean responses than was desirable for precision. Favorable to precision, however, is the highly significant value for the slope of the common regression, as instanced by the F ratio of 98.9, and, favorable to the assumption of parallelism, the divergence term was not significant, the corresponding F ratio being less than 1. Encouraged, therefore, to accept the relative-potency calculation above, we proceed to find an interval estimate. The interval estimate also is an indication of assay precision, a narrow interval indicating high precision, and conversely.

The interval-estimation formula, obtained by applying Fieller's theorem to the balanced situation we are discussing, gives R_L and R_H, the lower and higher limits of the interval, as

$$R_L, R_H = \frac{D_{S1}}{D_{U1}} \text{ antilog } \frac{d[L_p L_r \mp \sqrt{NF_c s^2(L_p^2 + L_r^2 - NF_c s^2)}]}{L_r^2 - NF_c s^2}$$

(8)

where, in addition to quantities previously defined, $N = 4n$ is the total number of observed responses, F_c is the appropriate critical value obtained from the F distribution table for 1 and $4(n - 1)$ DF, and s^2 is the mean square within groups from the analysis of variance. An alternative form of this equation (Cox and Ruhl, 1966) is based on F ratios from the last column of the analysis-of-variance table and is somewhat easier to compute:

$$R_L, R_H = \frac{D_{S1}}{D_{U1}} \text{ antilog } \frac{1}{F_r - F_c}$$
$$\times \left[\left(d\frac{L_p}{L_r} \right) F_r \mp d\sqrt{F_c(F_p + F_r - F_c)} \right]$$

(9)

where dL_p/L_r has previously been calculated and, from the analysis of variance, F_p is the F ratio for the between-preparations mean square and F_r is the F ratio for the common-regression mean square.

Returning to the example, for which we have

$$F_p = 7.63, \qquad F_r = 98.86, \qquad F_c = 4.49 \text{ (95\% interval)}$$

we find that

$$R_L, R_H = 4 \text{ antilog } \frac{1}{98.86 - 4.49} [(0.1673)(98.86)$$
$$\mp 0.6021\sqrt{4.49(7.63 + 94.37)}]$$
$$= 4.37, 8.20 \text{ μg}/(\text{mg}_{\text{tissue}}/\text{ml})$$

The six-point parallel-line assay

Although some differences in detail will be noted, the six-point parallel-line assay in a completely randomized design can be analyzed on essentially the same principles. The experimental plan is that a total of $6n$ experimental units are divided into equal groups to give n responses to each of the doses D_{S1}, D_{S2}, and D_{S3} for the standard preparation and D_{U1}, D_{U2}, and D_{U3} for the unknown preparation. As in the four-point assay, a constant dose ratio is used to give equal intervals between the log doses. There being six treatment groups, five intergroup contrasts can be calculated. The group totals being denoted by S_1, S_2, and S_3 for the standard and by U_1, U_2, and U_3 for the unknown, the contrasts can be obtained from the array of coefficients in Table 2.

TABLE 2   Orthogonal Contrasts and Analysis of Variance of a Six-Point Parallel-Line Assay in a Simple Randomization Design

Coefficients of contrasts:

| | | Response total | | | | | | SS of |
Term	Contrast	S_1	S_2	S_3	U_1	U_2	U_3	coefficients
Between preparations	L_p	−1	−1	−1	+1	+1	+1	6
Common regression	L_r	−1	0	+1	−1	0	+1	4
Divergence	L_d	+1	0	−1	−1	0	+1	4
Curvature, standard	Q_S	+1	−2	+1	0	0	0	6
Curvature, unknown	Q_U	0	0	0	+1	−2	+1	6

Analysis of variance:

Term	DF	SS	MS
Between preparations	1	$L_p^2/6n$	$L_p^2/6n$
Common regression	1	$L_r^2/4n$	$L_r^2/4n$
Divergence	1	$L_d^2/4n$	$L_d^2/4n$
Curvature, standard	1	$Q_S^2/6n$	$Q_S^2/6n$
Curvature, unknown	1	$Q_U^2/6n$	$Q_U^2/6n$
Within groups	$6(n-1)$	By subtraction	s^2
Total:	$6n-1$	$\sum y^2 - C_m$	

Instead of the curvature contrasts Q_S and Q_U as defined in Table 2 the contrasts for common curvature and for opposed curvature may be used:

Common curvature: $Q_S + Q_U$

Opposed curvature: $Q_S - Q_U$

The writer prefers to use separate curvature contrasts for the two preparations, not because they are a little quicker to calculate, but because the linear range for the standard, unlike that for the unknown, may be fairly well established.

The analysis of variance is shown in the bottom half of Table 2. The tests for the validity of the mathematical model are then made by comparing the analysis-of-variance F ratios with the tabulated critical value F_c, from the table of the F distribution with 1 and $6(n - 1)$ DF. Thus:

If $Q_U^2/(6ns^2) < F_c$,   we infer that no curvature in the log-dose–response line for the unknown preparation is manifest.

If $Q_S^2/(6ns^2) < F_c$,   we infer that no curvature in the response line for the standard preparation is manifest.

If $L_d^2/(4ns^2) < F_c$,   we infer that no departure from parallelism is manifest.

Provided there are satisfactory results from these tests, we can proceed to estimate the relative potency from the formula

$$R = (D_{S1}/D_{U1}) \text{ antilog } M \tag{10}$$

where

$$M = 4dL_p/(3L_r) \tag{11}$$

Finally, R_L and R_H, the lower and higher limits for the interval estimate, can be conveniently calculated (Cox and Ruhl, 1966) as

$$R_L = (D_{S1}/D_{U1}) \text{ antilog } M_L$$
$$R_H = (D_{S1}/D_{U1}) \text{ antilog } M_H \tag{12}$$

where

$$M_L, M_H = \frac{M}{1 - F_c/F_r} \left[1 \mp \sqrt{\frac{F_c}{F_p}\left(1 - \frac{F_c}{F_r}\right) + \frac{F_c}{F_r}} \right] \tag{13}$$

with, from the analysis of variance, $F_p = L_p^2/(6ns^2)$ and $F_r = L_r^2/(4ns^2)$.

Further design possibilities for parallel-line assays

From the foregoing it will be appreciated that the basis of the estimation procedure is the comparison of the mean responses to the preparation × dose level for treatment groups. The experiments may correspondingly be regarded as factorial arrangements. Thus, the four-point assay, as already noted (p. 61), is a 2 × 2 factorial arrangement in which the first factor is the preparation, being either standard or unknown, and the second factor is the dose level, being lower or higher. Similarly, the six-point assay may be regarded as a 2 × 3 factorial arrangement. The required comparisons may be investigated in any convenient experimental design to take advantage of particular possibilities for increasing precision (especially via the reduction of the variability affecting the treatment comparisons). In using such designs it should, however, be noted that the precision of the assay is importantly governed, not by the value of the estimated variance s^2 alone, but by the quantity $s^2 F_c$. If effective, restricted randomization designs reduce the value of s^2, but if, in consequence, the associated number of degrees of freedom is small, F_c may be so large that precision is not necessarily gained.

The randomized block naturally comes to mind as a design possibility. For example, if the experimental units are small laboratory animals, the use of littermates to comprise the blocks is often advantageous. Since with equal numbers of responses per group the required intergroup contrasts are free from block effects, the formulæ given above for calculating the relative-potency estimates are still applicable. Some differences arise, however, in the analysis of variance. The first of these is that an among-blocks term now appears in addition to other quantities calculated as previously described. Thus, for a four-point assay in which one response is obtained to each of the four preparation × dose combinations from each of a number, say k, of blocks, the analysis of variance will be structured as follows.

	DF
Among blocks:	$k - 1$
Between preparations:	1
Common regression:	1
Divergence:	1
Residual variance:	$3(k - 1)$
Total:	$4k - 1$

Another difference appears when it comes to the interval-estimate calculations. It is known that in the application of randomized block designs to comparative experiments the residual-variance sum of squares may be regarded as composed of the interactions blocks × treatments. Thus in the structure given above we would identify the $3(k - 1)$ DF for residual variance as composed of $k - 1$ DF for each of the interactions blocks × preparations, blocks × regression, and blocks × divergence. In the context of assays it has been shown (Finney, 1964, pp. 375–382) that the first two of these components may be substantially larger than the last because of differences between the assay slopes from one block to another. In such case the term blocks × divergence is the valid term for the s^2 required in the interval-estimation calculations (see p. 65). The point previously made about the number of degrees of freedom is, therefore, especially pertinent.

By way of illustration, data published by McKerns and Nordstrand (1955) from a four-point assay of corticotropin are used. These investigators actually observed duplicate responses per preparation × dose combination in each block. The mean square calculated from differences between corresponding duplicate responses provides the most satisfactory value of s^2 and one with a more reasonably large number of degrees of freedom. The writer would, in fact, recommend that, when randomized block designs are being considered for bioassay experiments, replicate responses within blocks be obtained if at all practicable; there are good grounds for making the same recommendation for comparative experiments themselves, so that model relevance may be examined.

For present purposes, however, we take the totals of corresponding duplicates to represent a single observation in order to illustrate the common case in which one response is observed per preparation × dose combination in each block.

The lower and upper doses were taken as 0.015 and 0.045 IU per 100 mg of adrenal tissue; the results from four randomized blocks and the analysis of variance are shown in Table 3.

TABLE 3   A Four-Point Parallel-Line Assay of Corticotropin in a Randomized-Blocks Design*

Data:

Block	Dose 0.015	Dose 0.045	Dose 0.015	Dose 0.045	Total
1	45.07	60.20	49.75	66.35	221.37
2	44.12	62.93	35.83	48.58	191.46
3	39.64	48.44	44.94	54.26	187.28
4	31.48	48.95	34.76	56.39	171.58
Total:	160.31	220.52	165.28	225.58	771.69
	S_1	S_2	U_1	U_2	

Analysis of variance:

Term	DF	SS	MS
Blocks	3	324.6848	
Preparations	1	6.2876	
Regression	1	907.6663	
Divergence	1	0.0005	
Blocks × preparations	3 ⎫	268.1467	44.69
Blocks × regression	3 ⎭		
Blocks × divergence	3	14.1146	4.70
Total:	15	1,520.9005	

* From McKerns and Nordstrand (1955).

The new feature is the calculation of the sum of squares, with 3 DF, for the term blocks × divergence. For this we first calculate divergence terms for each block separately. For block 1 we calculate

$$L_{d1} = 45.07 - 60.20 - 49.75 + 66.35 = 1.47$$

and, similarly, for the remaining three blocks:

$$L_{d2} = -6.06, \qquad L_{d3} = 0.52, \qquad L_{d4} = 4.16$$

The sum of squares for blocks × divergence is then obtained as

$$\tfrac{1}{4}(1.47^2 + 6.06^2 + 0.52^2 + 4.16^2) - 0.0005 = 14.1146$$

The divisor is 4 (the number of responses contributing to each of the squared quantities, such as 1.47^2), and the subtracted term is the sum of squares for the mean divergence previously calculated as $L_d^2/16 = 0.0005$. Finally, the sum of squares for blocks × preparations + blocks × regression is obtained by subtraction, so that the sum of all the component sums of squares is equal to the total sum of squares.

For the assay analysis itself it is strictly necessary only to calculate the sums of squares for preparations, regression, divergence, and blocks × divergence; the complete analysis has been presented here to indicate the effects of separating out the interaction blocks × divergence. In this example, although the term has an undesirably small number of degrees of freedom (3 only), the mean square is much lower than that obtained by including all the interactions; that is,

$$\frac{268.1467 + 14.1146}{9} = 31.36$$

For comparison it is interesting to note that the mean square for the intrablock replicate variability was calculated from the complete data as 13.13 with 16 DF.

The remainder of the assay analysis (for the case of no intrablock replication) would then proceed according to the previously described formulæ for the four-point assay, with $s^2 = 4.70$, 3 DF, and $F_c = F(1, 3, 0.05) = 10.13$, giving the results

$$R = 1.096, \qquad R_L = 0.853, \qquad R_H = 1.422$$

Since, as has been remarked, the assay analysis is based on the calculation of intertreatment comparisons and of an appropriate estimate of residual variability, most of the experimental design possibilities (see, for example, Cochran and Cox, 1957) can readily be used for bioassay experiments. Of these we may conveniently mention the crossover design discussed on pp. 206–209. This possesses the feature of differential precision in that the essential assay contrasts, L_p and L_r, are estimated with greater precision than is the divergence contrast, L_d. This design is therefore useful when, as a result of knowledge gained from previous assays, it is sufficient to "monitor" the divergence contrast, enabling most of the experimental effort to be devoted to the assay estimation proper. A further refinement in this context (Good and Stenhouse, 1966) makes allowance for the effect on the response in one period of the dose given in the preceding period.

Lastly, we should note the possibilities of incomplete-block designs for bioassay. Such designs are adapted to deal with situations in which the number of preparation × dose combinations to be investigated exceeds the number of experimental units in the available blocks. Finney (1964) may be consulted for an exposition of various incomplete-block designs in bioassay situations. One of these, which gives full accuracy to the estimation of the preparation and regression contrasts, has been described in detail by Das and Kulkarni (1966).

3. Slope ratio assays

When the response, instead of being linearly related to the logarithm of the dose, is linearly related to the dose itself, relative-potency estimations can be made from slope ratio assays. Perhaps the best known slope ratio assay in endocrinological research is that of Steelman and Pohley (1953) for follicle-stimulating hormone.

When linear dose–response relationships obtain for the standard and unknown preparations, the principles previously set forth for the parallel-line assay now show that the relative-potency estimate becomes

$$R = b_U/b_S \tag{14}$$

where b_S and b_U are the estimated slopes of the dose–response lines for the standard and the unknown, respectively. Experimental designs are therefore aimed at providing efficient estimation of these slopes and information that will permit testing for the relevance of the basic assay model. Then, if x denotes dose and y denotes response, the population lines for standard and unknown, respectively, may be written

$$y_S = \alpha + \beta_S x_S \quad \text{and} \quad y_U = \alpha + \beta_U x_U \tag{15}$$

As the equations show, we now assume that the biological situation can be described in terms of two lines that intersect the y axis at the same point, the point $(0, \alpha)$. This point is the mean response to zero dose and should, therefore, lie on both lines, although in an actual experiment, of course, we do not expect exact agreement. The relevance tests are designed to show whether or not the observations obtained are statistically compatible with the model (that is, do not depart from it by greater deviations than can reasonably be attributed to sampling variability).

These points are illustrated by the procedures required in the analysis of a five-point symmetrical slope ratio assay. It involves obtaining an equal number n of responses to each of the five preparation × dose combinations consisting of a zero dose and two equally spaced doses for the standard and unknown preparations. If x_S and x_U are the higher doses for the standard and unknown, respectively, the doses investigated are, therefore,

Zero	Standard preparation	Unknown preparation
0	$x_S/2,$ x_S	$x_U/2,$ x_U

For convenience the two lower doses for each preparation are each coded 1/2 and the two upper doses are each coded 1, and the entire analysis is carried out by using these coded values. At the conclusion of the analysis the relative potency and the limits of the interval estimate obtained are converted back to the original units by multiplying by the factor x_S/x_U.

Let us suppose that the totals of the n responses observed in the five groups are as follows.

	Zero or control	Standard	Unknown
Dose:	0	1/2 1	1/2 1
Total response:	C	S_1 S_2	U_1 U_2

The first step is to carry out the analysis of variance in order to make the validity tests, after which, if these are satisfactory, one proceeds to the estimation itself. There being five treatment groups, the analysis of variance is structured as follows.

	DF
Among groups:	4
Within groups:	$5(n-1)$
Total:	$5n-1$

The within-groups mean square in the analysis of variance provides the estimate of residual variability for use in making the relevance tests and in obtaining the interval estimate of relative potency. To obtain the relevance tests the among-groups mean square is now calculated in its partitioned form.

	DF
Standard and unknown preparation regressions:	2
Blanks:	1
Intersection:	1
Among groups:	4

The first item, with 2 DF, is the sum of squares due to the two regressions of response on dose, one for the standard preparation and one for the unknown preparation. The two components do not appear as individual degrees of freedom in the analysis, because their sums of squares are not simply additive. Instead of two separate regression lines, the assumed model represents two lines having one point in common, the zero dose point. The sum of squares on 2 DF, therefore, represents the sum of squares for the joint regressions, allowing for this common-point restriction. As an alternative procedure, these two degrees of freedom can be split into two additive components, one for the common regression and one for the difference between the standard and the test preparation regressions (Claringbold, 1959).

The sum of squares for intersection (or the mean square, since it has 1 DF) is a component that provides one of the two relevance tests allowed for by the five-point plan. In effect, separate lines are fitted through the responses to the nonzero doses for each individual preparation. The difference between the intercepts that these lines make on the y axis, squared and suitably scaled, constitutes the intersection mean square. If the situation is to be compatible with the basic model of two population lines intersecting on the y axis, this mean square should be small relative to the residual variability.

In addition, the point of intersection should be, not just anywhere on the y axis, but at the point that represents the response to zero dose. The difference between C/n, the estimated mean response to zero dose, and the estimated point of intersection should then also be small relative to the residual variability. The square of this difference gives rise to the sum of squares for blanks, the remaining component in the analysis of variance.

The actual calculations required for the analysis of variance and for the estimate of relative potency can be made in terms of the contrasts defined in Table 4. One carries out the relevance tests by comparing the F ratios $L_B^2/14ns^2$ and $L_I^2/10ns^2$ with the tabulated F value for 1 and $5(n-1)$ DF and, if the results are satisfactory, one proceeds to estimate the relative potency.

The contrasts L_S and L_U are directly proportional to the regression coefficients, and the estimate of the relative potency is, simply,

$$R' = L_U/L_S$$

in the coded units so that, in terms of the original units,

$$R = (x_S/x_U)(L_U/L_S)$$

The formula for interval estimation is somewhat more complicated than that for parallel-line assay because, as previously noted, the numerator

TABLE 4   Contrasts and Analysis of Variance for a Five-Point Slope Ratio Assay

Coefficients of contrasts:

Term	Contrast	C	S_1	S_2	U_1	U_2	SS of coefficients
Regression (S)	L_S	-15	1	17	-6	3	560
Regression (U)	L_U	-15	-6	3	1	17	560
Blanks	L_B	2	-2	1	-2	1	14
Intersection	L_I	0	2	-1	-2	1	10

Analysis of variance:

Term	DF	SS	MS
Regressions	2	$(1/6,125n) \times$ $[16(L_S + L_U)^2 - 50L_SL_U]$	
Blanks	1	$L_B^2/14n$	$L_B^2/14n$
Intersection	1	$L_I^2/10n$	$L_I^2/10n$
Within groups	$5(n-1)$	By subtraction	s^2
Total:	$5n-1$	$\sum y^2 - C_m$	

and denominator of the ratio estimate L_U/L_S are not statistically independent. General formulæ for the calculation are given by, for example, Finney (1964). A reasonably convenient form for calculation (Cox and Ruhl, 1966) is

$$R'_L, R'_H = \frac{16F_S R' - 9F_c \mp \sqrt{175F_c(2F_r - F_c)}}{16(F_S - F_c)}$$

where the subsidiary quantities required can be obtained as

$F_S = L_S^2/560ns^2$

$F_c = $ the tabulated F value for 1 and $5(n-1)$ DF

$2F_r = $ (sum of squares for regressions)$/s^2$ from the analysis of variance

Finally, the interval estimate in the original unit is obtained simply as

$$R_L = (x_S/x_U)R'_L \quad \text{and} \quad R_H = (x_S/x_U)R'_H$$

Data from Steelman and Pohley (1953) can be used to exemplify these procedures. In their example the doses investigated were 0.1 and 0.2 mg of the standard and unknown preparations of follicle-stimulating hormone in conjunction with 20 IU of human chorionic gonadotropin which, alone, constituted the zero dose. Ovarian weights for eight rats were observed in each group and, in the present notation, the total responses were as follows.

	Zero	Standard		Unknown	
Dose:	0	1/2	1	1/2	1
Total response:	346.5	540.1	895.4	452.9	567.4

Calculated in accordance with the contrast scheme in Table 4, the required contrasts are

$$L_S = 9{,}549.2, \quad L_U = 4{,}346.8, \quad L_B = 169.8, \quad L_I = -153.6$$

The analysis of variance entries are the following.

Regressions: $(1/49{,}000)[16(13{,}896)^2 - 50(9{,}549.2)(4{,}346.8)] = 20{,}697.10$
Blanks: $169.8^2/112 = 257.43$
Intersection: $153.6^2/80 = 294.91$

By taking $s^2 = 516.63$, as given by Steelman and Pohley (1953), the analysis of variance can then be constructed as:

	DF	SS	MS
Regressions:	2	20,697.10	
Blanks:	1	257.43	
Intersection:	1	294.91	
Residual variability:	35	35(516.63)	516.63

Since the F ratios for both blanks and intersection are less than unity, the relevance tests are satisfactory, and we can proceed to estimate the relative potency. Because $x_S = x_U$ in this case, we have

$$R = \frac{4{,}346.8}{9{,}549.2} = 0.46$$

For the interval estimate we have

$$F_S = (9{,}549.2)^2/(4{,}480)(516.63) = 39.40$$
$$F_c = F(1, 35; 0.05) = 4.12$$
$$2F_r = \frac{20{,}697.10}{516.63} = 40.06$$

Hence,

$$R_L, R_H = \frac{16(39.40)(0.46) - 9(4.12) \mp \sqrt{1{,}754.12(35.94)}}{16(35.28)}$$

$$= 0.16, 0.73$$

It may be noted that Steelman and Pohley do not give the interval estimate in this form. Instead, they use an approximate formula to find the standard deviation of R. With t for 35 DF as 2.03, the corresponding interval estimate would be

$$R_{\mathrm{L}}, R_{\mathrm{H}} = 0.46 \mp (2.03)(0.1328) = 0.19, 0.73$$

so that the approximation gives a slightly narrower interval than the accurate limits that we obtained. Another difference from the analysis given by Steelman and Pohley is that, whereas they present an analysis for unequal numbers of responses in the treatment groups, we have here taken advantage of the equal numbers to obtain a more streamlined analysis.

Finally, it may be noted that, if a number of such analyses are required, and ready access to an electronic computer is not available, nomographic methods (Clarke and Hosking, 1953; Clarke, 1955) provide simple, quick, and usually sufficiently accurate procedures for both the point and interval estimations in slope ratio assays.

Acknowledgment

I am grateful to Miss Jan Bates for her skilled technical assistance in the preparation of the foregoing.

DISCUSSION

RODBARD   My question concerns the criteria for making a choice between the use of the four-point log dose parallel-line assay and the five-point slope ratio assay, when both may be applicable. We have been analyzing data from the Steelman-Pohley assay as if it were a parallel-line assay, disregarding the control values. Does the omission of the control observations result in a loss of precision?

COX   Strictly, if the lines are straight when the log dose is used, they are not straight when the dose is used, and conversely. Examination of data may guide us on this, and I personally think that there are grounds for regarding the Steelman-Pohley assay as a log dose parallel-line assay. Further, some data I have seen suggest there may even be a case for transforming the response because of greater variability at the higher doses. As for precision, when one discards the control values, one loses, not only the precision, but the effort invested in the animals. If the slopes are steep, however, the precision loss may not be serious.

BORTH   With respect to the choice between the slope-ratio and the parallel-line models, my impression is that quite often the data do not permit a decision as to whether regression on dose or on log dose better approximates a straight line. In such case it does not matter much for the estimate of relative potency. There might be a difference in precision, and I would make this the criterion for choice. If the evidence of a straight-line relationship between dose and response is quite clear, then one can make a case for using the computation system for parallel-line assays by converting both the response and the dose to logarithmic scales. If you have a straight line $y = a + bx$, then you also have a straight line $\log (y - a) = \log b + \log x$, and I think this has some practical advantages.

COX To complement the remarks of the last speaker, I should say that one ought to obtain a great deal of data as a basis for arbitration. I do think one ought to avoid looking at separate sets of data and using a slope ratio model one time and a parallel-line model another time. These days computational simplicity need not be the criterion for the decision; rather, we should get as close as possible to the biological situation. By taking log response and log dose it is possible to convert a slope ratio model into a parallel-line model. However, unless the lines go through the origin, the intercept, which is another parameter, may need attention.

ALBERT I should like to underscore everything that Dr. Cox has just said: the answer to Dr. Rodbard's question is to obtain sufficient data to establish the nature of the dose–response curve. We have obtained twenty-eight dose–response curves by using the Second International Reference Preparation for Human Menopausal Gonadotrophin. These describe a beautifully symmetrical sigmoid curve, for which the parallel-line model is most suitable. In addition, we have similar data for such gonadotropic preparations as NIH-HPG-UE, NIH-HPG-UPM-1, NIH-FSH-S2, and NIH-FSH-S1. If you do this for the substance with which you are concerned, the choice of computation method becomes clear.

ROSEMBERG The first example (p. 109) raises a point that has bothered me for some time. I do not see the ovarian ascorbic acid values for the control animals; the only responses shown are for two dose levels of the standard and two of the unknown. How do we decide whether the response corresponding to the low dose of the standard, in this case 0.4 μg, differs significantly from that of the control animals? Can the statisticians give us a formula that is applicable to any assay?

COX It depends, of course, on how we define "formula." I, myself, would not like at present to reply "yes."

ROSEMBERG   Arbitrarily, we consider only a response mean that exceeds that of the control animals by two standard errors as significantly different. Is that wrong?

COX   Actually, there are two different but related problems: the detection of minimal doses, with the underlying concept of sensitivity, and the determination of the potency of the unknown relative to the standard after a fairly extensive examination of the dose–response relationship.

ROSEMBERG   Yes, I understand that. I still don't know how to solve the problem, because the responses depend upon the sensitivity of the animals in different laboratories. However, in these data the responses to the low dose of the standard are nearly those found in control animals. I think that we must resolve these questions; otherwise, estimates of potency will differ from one laboratory to another.

GUILLEMIN   In my opinion no assay is valid at all unless the mean response to the low dose of the standard or unknown differs significantly from that of the saline control. What we do, upon completion of the analysis of variance of all of the data, is to apply the multiple-comparison test of Dunnett. Each treatment mean is compared with that for the saline control. The experiment is regarded as a possible bioassay only if the low doses of the standard and the unknown differ significantly. If they are different, we recalculate the analysis of variance, omitting the saline control.

FINNEY   I think that Dr. Guillemin has uncovered a confusion between experimentation made for studying the dose–response curve and the use of that curve in an assay. In an assay it does not matter what your controls would do, or even whether you have any. More worrisome is the use of a four-point assay in a situation that evidently contains grave danger of curvature. What has been said, in effect, is that the response curve for the standard is virtually horizontal at low doses (approximately less than 0.4 μg) but that at higher doses it turns downward, giving a section that is almost linear on a log scale. The response curve for the unknown must therefore be a similar curve displaced by a constant difference of corresponding log doses. For assay purposes the nearly horizontal region is of little interest. It may be perfectly correct, but it has very low discriminatory power. The nature of an assay is the use of differences in response to indicate differences between doses. If changes in response over a range of doses are small, therefore, they are of little use as indicators of dose differences. If one likes to expend a few animals in merely locating the horizontal region, one may do so, but that will not help the precision of the assay. More important is the question of whether there is reasonable linearity and slope from doses of 0.4 μg upwards.

Unless there can be great confidence in this at the time an assay is planned, at least three doses of each preparation should be located on the presumed linear section, one of which can be omitted from analysis if it chances to be too low.

COX I entirely agree. I was assured that there had been extensive preliminary investigations of dose–response curves. It may be that the assay is unstable and that there is curvature. However, Rathmacher did consider these points before deciding on four-point assays as his routine.

EMMENS A further difficulty is that unless the responses to the low doses of standard and unknown are significantly different from those in the unstimulated animal, one may get a spuriously low slope or a departure from parallelism. If neither differs from the control, the slope will be spuriously low. If one of them differs and the other does not, non-parallelism will result. One must know enough about the dose–response relation to be sure that one is avoiding these difficulties.

HIRSCH In our assays we, like Dr. Rosemberg, reject subthreshold responses, that is, means not significantly different from that for controls. However, supramaximal responses may present an additional problem. How should we deal with a response mean not significantly different from that for maximal response?

ALBERT Our procedure is as follows. When for the standard or the unknown a mean response falls on either the upper or lower asymptote, we simply discard it and use the remaining points as a parallel-line assay, that is, as a 1 + 2 assay instead of the original 2 + 2 or as a 2 + 3 instead of the original 3 + 3, and so forth.

BIRMINGHAM May I ask a question regarding the pooling of insignificant interactions with error? I work with a four-point assay in which I have only duplicate determinations, yielding four degrees of freedom for the error variance. However, if (in accordance with the recommendation in some texts) I were to pool the sum of squares for parallelism with that for error, I would gain an additional degree of freedom. This would improve the estimate of precision and narrow the confidence interval.

COX Not all statistics texts make such recommendations. There are various schools of thought, which divide practitioners of the art into the sometimes-pooling, the always-pooling, and the never-pooling. There is, I think, room for informed subjective judgment here. For example, if I know that a situation is one of analytical dilution assay, then I am inclined to pool. If I suspect that the constituents of the unknown preparation are not the same as those of the standard, then I am inclined not to pool. In the latter situation one will generally find that the divergence interaction is at least slightly larger than the residual error. The decision to pool or not to pool should not be taken merely to scrape the barrel for an extra degree of freedom when, in reality, a larger experiment may be required.

MUSSETT   The slopes in the second example, if calculated from the total responses, are almost identical for the two preparations, and the resulting variance for parallelism is significantly less than the residual error. Is this not odd, since the individual slopes vary enormously from one block to another?

COX   It is true that in this case the average divergence was surprisingly small. I do not, myself, know the McKerns and Nordstrand assay. However, these investigators did helpfully publish their original data, which well illustrate this point. If the regressions vary gently from block to block, a significantly subnormal divergence term is quite possible. So there is nothing really incompatible about that. Moreover, it was just one assay that they reported. It may be that in other circumstances they obtained greater divergence. I would regard this, charitably, as a random occurrence on this particular occasion. If it happened frequently, then perhaps we should be a little more suspicious.

ARMITAGE   I should like to raise a computational point. I am intrigued by Equations 8, 9, and 13. I haven't seen this formula before. Could I introduce a caveat here, that with this formula one ought to calculate the F ratios pretty accurately? If they are calculated only to one decimal point, will there not be too much inaccuracy in the fiducial limits? I wonder whether Professor Cox hasn't fallen into such a trap in Table 1, where his residual mean square is given to three digits, as 23.6. However, one of the F ratios is calculated to four and almost five digits. Is there spurious accuracy in these fiducial limits?

COX   Very likely there is. If one is going to use this formula, it is wise to calculate the F ratios a little further than is customarily done in significance testing. The data shown were rounded for presentation purposes; I like to carry what I consider a generous number of decimals and then round the figures off at the end, to be consistent with the accuracy of the original data. On your first point, however, I think two decimal places suffice. In fact, I've examined several cases, and it appears that one will not often be seriously misled with just one decimal place.

EMMENS   If there is a large variation in slope from block to block, isn't there danger that the small selection of blocks has, in fact, given an abnormal estimate of slope? Should not the slope variation somehow come into the determination of the fiducial limits?

cox I would refer you to Finney (1964), whom I find quite convincing on that point. If in an assay the relative potency is constant, then, although the blocks × regression variability enters into both the L_p and L_r contrasts, the term disappears in the construction of the interval estimate when Fieller's theorem is used. This may be shown by finding the expected mean squares. Dr. Bliss has noted that there might be some grounds for using the larger error, because one might not have a completely valid assay, and the larger mean square would give an appropriately wider interval. However, if one is prepared to say that the assay is valid, then, in the absence of intrablock replication, blocks × divergence is the appropriate error mean square. The point perhaps deserves consideration in other contexts, particularly in reference to quasi dilution assays.

CHAPTER FIVE

Quantal-Response Assays

BYRON W. BROWN, JR.

1. Introduction

Nature of the quantal assay

In the quantal assay the subject is given a predetermined dose of the preparation under test and is observed to see whether or not a specified response occurs. Thus, the observation is dichotomous rather than quantitative.

It is assumed that each subject has its own individual tolerance to the preparation. If a dose below the subject's tolerance is administered, there will be no response; if above, a response will occur. The tolerance itself is not observable.

It is seldom possible to test the subject at more than one dose. However, the underlying assumption of a tolerance for each subject and a distribution of such tolerances over the population of subjects is borne out by the observation of a sigmoid dose–response curve. This curve rises from zero percent response in a group of subjects tested at an extremely low dose to one-hundred percent response in a group of subjects tested at an extremely high dose.

The strength of a preparation is often characterized by the median tolerance, or the dose that induces 50% responses. This is called the LD_{50} (lethal dose) or, in cases in which the response is not death, the ED_{50} (effective dose). In the analytical dilution assay there are two dose–response curves, one for the standard and one for the test preparation. When plotted on the log dose scale these curves are identical in form but are horizontally transposed. In that case the log relative potency of test to standard is given by the distance between log LD_{50}'s.

Examples

One of the oldest and most familiar examples is the mouse convulsion assay for insulin. It was the consideration of this test that led to some of the basic research on quantal-assay methodology. In order to make the definition of the convulsion response objective, the mice are placed on a slanted screen and the response is defined by loss of footing.

Another quantal assay that has been in use for many years is the Allen-Doisy test for estrogens. The experimental animal is usually the mouse. The response is the appearance of cornified epithelial cells in vaginal smears taken at a specified time after estrogen administration.

The assay of gonadotropins is customarily quantitative, being based on the uterine weight of weanling mice. However, the assay is sometimes rendered quantal, the dichotomous response being defined by weight or by such characteristics of the hypertrophic uterus as edema and hyperemia.

2. Assay procedures

Purposes

The objective of the quantal assay may be to estimate the LD_{50} of a preparation. The usual design comprises a series of dose levels with subjects completely randomized among the dose levels. More complicated experiments will involve the comparison of one or more preparations with a standard, or a series of determinations with the use of the same substance in relation to time or to some other quantitative variable, such as a dose of an inhibiting or blocking agent.

A distinction should be made between the research and the pilot assay. In the research assay publication is intended, and the assay must stand by itself, furnishing sufficient internal evidence of validity to afford credence without appeal to supplementary data. Pilot assays are done for the information of the investigator, for exploratory purposes, or for routine checks on laboratory procedure. Here the investigator uses the data to make some judgment. He is free to depend on previous information in interpreting the results. These need not stand alone but can be assessed in conjunction with previous data and even with non-quantifiable impressions.

Dose range and dilution factors

The dose levels chosen for a preparation should range between a lowest dose, to which virtually no subjects will respond (say less than 10%) and a highest dose, to which virtually all subjects will respond (say at least 90%). Since the LD_{50} and the slope of the dose–response curve will be unknown, the dose levels must extend over a range sufficiently wide to cover various contingencies.

The dilution factor must be sufficiently small to place several doses in the range of intermediate response.

Fixed and sequential designs

In most quantal assays the various doses are administered and responses observed almost simultaneously. The doses are determined before the experiment begins, and subjects are assigned to these doses in a completely randomized way. However, it can be advantageous to treat the subjects sequentially, basing the dose for the next subject partly on the results up to that point. The rest of this chapter will be restricted to the nonsequential choice of dose levels. Some aspects of sequential designs are discussed in Chapter 11.

Size of experiment

The total number of observations per preparation in a quantal assay will depend on the precision desired, the parameter to be estimated (such as LD_{50}, potency, and regression of potency on some other variables) and the type of assay (such as pilot or research). Sample sizes will range from a dozen or so (5 animals at each of 3 doses, or 2 animals at each of 5 doses) to hundreds (50 animals at each of 6 to 8 doses). A simple method of determining sample size to assure desired precision is discussed in Section 5.

3. Analysis of assay data

Graphical procedures

With any extensive set of data, say fifty observations at each of six or eight doses, spanning the range from low to high percent response, it is easy to plot the percent responses against dose or log dose, smooth the data with a curve drawn by eye, and read off the LD_{50}. Generally the tails of the dose–response curve will be symmetrical when plotted against log dose. Further, when the percent response is plotted on normal or logistic probability paper against log dose, the curve will often appear linear over a wide range. The results of an assay of estrone (Biggers, 1950) are given in Table 1. The plot (Figure 1) of these data,

TABLE 1   An Assay of Estrone*

Dose, 10^{-3} µg	Number of mice	Mice responding, %
0.2	27	14.8
0.4	30	43.3
0.8	30	60.0
1.6	30	73.3

* Assay of Biggers (1950).

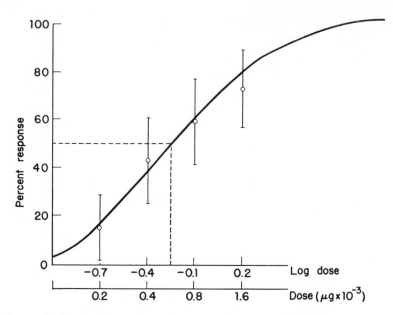

FIGURE 1   Dose–response curve for an assay of estrone. Observed proportion responding ± 2 standard errors. Curve fitted by eye. The dashed line indicates the log dose corresponding to 50% response. Data from Biggers (1950).

with 95% confidence limits for each group, gives an estimate of -0.25 for the log LD_{50}. The confidence limits for each dose group convey some impression of the statistical reliability of this estimate.

The disadvantages of the graphical estimate are its subjectivity and its lack of a measure of reliability. The problem of subjectivity is frequently solved by using any one of the several LD_{50} estimates requiring only simple arithmetic. The *Reed-Muench estimator* is popular. In addition, various simple interpolation or *moving-average procedures* are available. If some measure of reliability can be obtained by appropriate replications within the design, any of these estimators can be useful.

Spearman-Kärber estimator

If a standard error for an LD_{50} estimate must be computed internally from a single series of data, the simplest approach is the Spearman-Kärber procedure. If the log doses are denoted by $x_1, x_2, \ldots, x_k$ and are equally spaced d units apart (dilution factor 10^d), and if the observed proportion of responses at x_i is denoted by p_i, then the Spearman-Kärber estimate of the log LD_{50} is

$$\bar{x} = x_k + d/2 - d \sum_{1}^{k} p_i \tag{1}$$

The LD_{50} itself is estimated from the antilog of $\bar{x}$.

If the sample sizes are denoted by n_i, the standard error of $\bar{x}$ is

$$SE(\bar{x}) = d \sqrt{\sum_1^k \frac{p_i(1 - p_i)}{n_i}} \qquad (2)$$

and 95% confidence limits on the log LD_{50} are

$$\log LD_{50} = \bar{x} \pm 2 \, SE(\bar{x}) \qquad (3)$$

For the data in Table 1 the Spearman-Kärber estimator is calculated as shown in Table 2.

TABLE 2   Calculation of the Spearman-Kärber Estimate of the LD_{50} and Its 95% Confidence Interval from the Data in Table 1

$x = \log_{10}$ dose	p	$p(1 - p)/n$
−0.7	0.15	0.0047
−0.4	0.43	0.0081
−0.1	0.60	0.0080
+0.2	0.73	0.0066
	1.91	0.0274

$$\bar{x} = 0.2 + 0.15 - 0.3(1.91)$$
$$= -0.22, \quad \text{from Equation 1}$$
$$SE(\bar{x}) = 0.3 \sqrt{0.0274}$$
$$= 0.05, \quad \text{from Equation 2}$$
$$\bar{x} \pm 2 \, SE(\bar{x}) = -0.32, -0.12$$
$$LD_{50} = \text{antilog } \bar{x} = 0.60 \times 10^{-3} \, \mu g$$
$$95\% \text{ limits} = \text{antilog } [\bar{x} \pm 2 \, SE(\bar{x})]$$
$$= 0.48, 0.75, \times 10^{-3} \, \mu g$$

If the potency of one preparation relative to a standard is desired, the log potency is the difference in Spearman-Kärber estimates, and the standard error is the root sum of the squared standard errors for the two log LD_{50}'s.

Note that the Spearman-Kärber procedure requires no prescription of the mathematical form for the dose–response curve and, hence, is non-parametric. Nevertheless, it yields estimates that are almost as reliable as those obtained with parametric methods by using, for example, probits or logits (see Maximum-Likelihood Procedures, below).

The reasoning behind the Spearman-Kärber procedure is not clear from Equation 1. An equivalent formula, less convenient for computation, shows the nature of the estimator more clearly. If the observed p_i

are plotted as a cumulative frequency or ogive, starting from approximately 0 and rising to 1, it can be seen that the corresponding histogram could be computed by subtracting a p_i from the succeeding p_{i+1} to obtain the estimated proportion of tolerances in the interval (x_i, x_{i+1}).

The mean of the histogram could then be computed by assigning the estimated proportion of tolerances in the interval to the midpoint:

$$\bar{x} = \sum (x_i + d/2)(p_{i+1} - p_i) \tag{4}$$

If the estimated proportion of tolerances below the first level, p_1, is assigned to $x_1 - d/2$, and the proportion above the last level, $1 - p_k$, is assigned to $x_k + d/2$, then Equation 4 is equivalent to Equation 1. The Spearman-Kärber estimator is thus the quantal analogue of an arithmetic mean.

Least-squares procedures

Inspection of the curve relating percent response p_i to log dose x_i suggests that the LD_{50} be estimated by fitting a regression line. Several regression procedures have been advocated. These range from a simple, unweighted, least-squares computation (fitting a straight line for p_i's in the 10 to 90% range versus x_i) to some rather elaborate, nonlinear, weighted least-squares methods, with complex justification. The unweighted least-squares estimate is clearly disadvantageous because of its failure to take into account the heteroscedasticity among binomial percentages, as has been previously discussed (p. 67).

The most appealing least-squares procedure is the following. For a model that assumes that the subject-to-subject tolerances follow the logistic distribution the logit of p_i, that is,

$$y_i = \log_e [p_i/(1 - p_i)] \tag{5}$$

is approximately linearly related to log dose:

$$y_i \approx a + bx_i \tag{6}$$

The weights (approximating the inverses of the logit variances) are

$$w_i = n_i p_i (1 - p_i) \tag{7}$$

Thus, the straight-line estimates of intercept a and slope b are

$$\bar{y} = \sum w_i y_i / \sum w_i, \qquad \bar{x} = \sum w_i x_i / \sum w_i \tag{8}$$

$$b = \frac{\sum w_i(x_i - \bar{x})(y_i - \bar{y})}{\sum w_i(x_i - \bar{x})^2}$$

$$= \frac{(\sum w_i)(\sum w_i x_i y_i) - (\sum w_i x_i)(\sum w_i y_i)}{(\sum w_i)(\sum w_i x_i^2) - (\sum w_i x_i)^2} \tag{9}$$

$$a = \bar{y} - b\bar{x} \tag{10}$$

The estimate of log LD_{50} is that value of the log dose x at which the logit is zero, that is, $-a/b$. The standard error of the estimate is

$$SE(-a/b) = \frac{1}{b} \sqrt{\frac{1}{\sum w_i} + (\bar{y}^2/b^2)\left[\frac{1}{\sum w_i(x_i - \bar{x})^2}\right]} \qquad (11)$$

When the dose–response function is logistic in form, this least-squares estimator will be fully efficient for large samples. Relative to its competitors, the estimator also functions well for small samples. Empirical sampling experiments (Monte Carlo procedures), with average squared error as the criterion, indicate that a and b are at least as good estimates as those obtained by the maximum-likelihood method. However, $-a/b$ seems to be slightly inferior.

Returning to the data in Table 1, the least-squares computations based on the logit are outlined in Table 3.

TABLE 3   Calculation of the Weighted Least-Squares Estimate of the LD_{50} and Its 95% Confidence Interval by Assuming a Logistic Response Model and Using the Data in Table 1

x	n	p	$y = \log_e [p/(1 - p)]$	$w = np(1 - p)$
-0.7	27	0.15	-1.73	3.44
-0.4	30	0.43	-0.28	7.35
-0.1	30	0.60	0.41	7.20
$+0.2$	30	0.73	0.99	5.91

$$\sum w = 23.91 \qquad \bar{x} = -0.20, \text{ from Equation 8}$$
$$\sum wx = -4.89 \qquad \bar{y} = 0.03, \text{ from Equation 8}$$
$$\sum wy = 0.79 \qquad b = 2.78, \text{ from Equation 9}$$
$$\sum wx^2 = 3.17 \qquad a = 0.60, \text{ from Equation 10}$$
$$\sum wxy = 5.87$$

$$\log LD_{50} = -0.22 \qquad\qquad LD_{50} = 0.61$$
$$SE(-a/b) = 0.07, \text{ from Equation 11} \qquad 95\% \text{ limits} = 0.43, 0.85$$

Maximum-likelihood procedures

Most statisticians agree that the basis for statistical analysis must be the likelihood function, that is, the probability of the observations for various possible values of the parameters. In the case of quantal assay the fundamental question is, "Which value of the LD_{50} makes the observed data most likely?"

The maximum-likelihood estimate of the LD_{50} under the normal model or some similar model (the normal model assumes an underlying normal distribution for the subject-to-subject tolerances) is less easy to compute than the Spearman-Kärber or the least-squares estimate. Under the normal model the maximum-likelihood procedure is called probit analysis. The computation entails repeated, or iterative, weighted least-squares analysis.

The Spearman-Kärber and the noniterative least-squares procedures seem to yield virtually the same estimates as the more basic maximum-likelihood method, with essentially the same estimate of reliability. Therefore, it seems reasonable to use these simpler procedures. However, if the investigator has access to a computer, the maximum-likelihood calculations should be used.

4. Validity tests

Dependence and binomiality

There is an extensive literature on the choice of dose–response function and on nonparallelism and its implications. However, there is little discussion of the most basic and most frequently violated assumptions in quantal-assay inference, namely that the observed proportions are binomial variates, are mutually independent, and show expectations lying on a smooth dose–response curve.

Among the uninitiated there is a tendency to apply the quantal-assay model to situations in which the observations are not, in fact, quantal variables. For example, an investigator who observes the percent decrease from control level (in some serum component) may mistakenly regard the average percent decrease as a proportion based on quantal responses, when it is a mean of quantitative variates on a percent scale.

A more subtle and more frequent mistake is to regard the fraction of responses among animals in a dose group as binomially distributed when the group is composed of subgroups that are caged together and that are unlikely to be independent. It is important to remember that the model calls for a random allocation of animals to dose groups and randomization of any other important factors. Any clustering of factors, such as that likely to result from caging together all animals of a dose group, invalidates the correspondence of model to experiment. For example, caging together all animals in a dose group tends to make reliability poorer than that indicated by the binomial model analysis.

Judgment as to the conformance of model to experimental procedure is a matter of experience and statistical understanding. The chi-square test of homogeneity provides some statistical guidance, but it must be used with care. It can fail to detect differences that are critical, and in large experiments it can detect disturbances that should be ignored. A more reasonable approach is to estimate the amount of heterogeneity, or deviation from the model, by special study. One can then redesign either the assay, to circumvent any problems that come to light, or the analysis, to take the disturbances into account.

Parallelism

Significance tests and estimation procedures for detecting departures from parallelism exist but must be used with a great deal of judgment. The discussions in Chapters 4 and 6 of fundamental validity and of parallelism in quantitative assays apply generally to quantal assays.

Mathematical form for the dose–response function

For the Spearman-Kärber procedure it is not necessary to specify the mathematical form for the dose–response function. For the least-squares and likelihood procedures the mathematical form must be specified. However, most work seems to indicate that, unless the sample sizes are huge, with dose levels far out in the tails, the results depend only very weakly on the model used. In other words, among the usual models employed for quantal assay the wrong model can be used without much penalty.

5. Planning a quantal assay

Prior information

It is impossible to design a fixed-sample-size assay to achieve some specified precision unless certain information is available. This information must be in the form of bounds on the various parameters in the model. The slope of the dose–response curve and the LD_{50}'s must be roughly specified. This information may come from the literature, from reasoning by analogy to similar material, or from pilot studies with the same material.

The design for estimation of the LD_{50} of a single preparation will be discussed herein. Similar reasoning applies to the design of an assay for potency. For the former we assume that prior information indicates that the mean of the tolerance distribution (denoting the log LD_{50} by μ) lies somewhere in a range between two numbers μ_1 and μ_2; that is,

$$\mu_1 \leq \log LD_{50} \leq \mu_2$$

In addition, we assume from prior information that the standard deviation of the dose–response curve lies in a range between σ_1 and σ_2; that is,

$$\sigma_1 \leq \sigma \leq \sigma_2$$

This standard deviation may be interpreted as roughly one third to one sixth of the "range" of the dose–response function, or the distance between the log doses yielding virtually 0% response and those yielding virtually 100% response.

Determination of doses and sample size per dose

Suppose the LD_{50} is to be reliably estimated to within R-fold of its true value (that is, the estimate of $\log LD_{50}$ is to be within $\log R$ of the true value with high probability, say 95%). In order to design the assay the range of doses, their spacing, and the number of observations at each dose must be specified.

For any estimation procedure it is prudent to use a range of doses that ensures a low dose with a low probability of response and a high dose with a high probability of response. This will be secured, even under the worst contingencies, by choosing

$$x_1 = \mu_1 - 2\sigma_2 \quad \text{and} \quad x_k = \mu_2 + 2\sigma_2$$

To ensure negligible bias due to a coarse dilution factor, the doses should be spaced no more than 2σ apart. Thus d, the distance on the log scale, should be

$$d = 2\sigma_1$$

For convenience, a simple approximation to the standard deviation of the Spearman-Kärber estimator can be used in determining the number n of observations at each dose level:

$$SD(\log LD_{50}) = \sqrt{d\sigma/2n}$$

Setting two standard deviations equal to the desired error limit, $\log R$, yields

$$\log R = 2\sqrt{d\sigma/2n}$$

Solving for n, setting $d = 2\sigma_1$, and taking σ at the conservative level of σ_2 give

$$n = 4\sigma_1\sigma_2/\log^2 R$$

Note that x_1, x_k, and d can be rounded for convenience in making up the dilutions, and n will be rounded to the integer next above it.

For an example of the computations involved suppose it is desired that an assay of the ED_{50} of an estrogen preparation be precise within 1.6 times the true value ($\log 1.6 = 0.20$) with 95% probability. Suppose we know that the $\log ED_{50}$ is in the range

$$-1.00 \leq \mu \leq 0.0$$

and σ is in the range

$$0.40 \leq \sigma \leq 0.60$$

The low and high doses should be, approximately,

$$x_1 = -1.00 - 1.20 = -2.20$$
$$x_k = 0.0 + 1.20 = 1.20$$

The dilution factor should be

$$d = 2(0.40) = 0.80$$

Thus, the log doses should be

$$x_i = 1.20, 0.40, -0.40, -1.20, -2.00, -2.80$$

and the number of subjects at each dose level should be

$$n = 4(0.40)(0.60)/(0.20)^2 = 24$$

Bibliographical notes

The most comprehensive discussion and bibliography on the statistical aspects of biological assay are given by Finney (1964). Brief elementary introductions are given by Emmens (1950, 1962). For the endocrinologist the latter two books have the advantage of specific orientation toward hormone assays. Loraine and Bell (1966) also give a brief discussion of hormone-assay methodology.

There are a number of papers that provide some basis for choosing the Spearman-Kärber estimator in preference to the more complicated least-squares estimators. Armitage and Allen (1950) analyze a series of experimental data to demonstrate that the various procedures lead to essentially the same results. Bross (1950) performed Monte Carlo experiments to demonstrate that the Spearman-Kärber estimator has a distribution at least as favorable as its competitors for several dose-level designs and sample sizes. Finney (1950, 1953) and Brown (1961) carried out additional theoretical work that demonstrates the conditions under which the Spearman-Kärber estimator exhibits properties comparable to those of the maximum-likelihood estimator.

Finney (1964), Emmens (1950, 1962), and Brown (1966) provide guidance on planning quantal assays.

DISCUSSION

HERBST With regard to the use of the Spearman-Kärber estimator, the speaker indicated that the percent responding should vary from 10 to 90. Are there difficulties if the percentages vary, say, from 20 to 60? Under what circumstances is the Spearman-Kärber estimator not applicable?

BROWN   Actually, the data in the example I cited, with 73% response at the high dose, do not conform to the conditions that I set forth. Here I might doubt the propriety of using the Spearman-Kärber method. However, there is Monte Carlo work that indicates that the Spearman-Kärber method works well, even in these borderline situations. Indications are that it works better than some of its competitors, including the maximum-likelihood estimator, in terms of bias and variance. With the borderline data that I used the Spearman-Kärber estimate was -0.22; the least-squares method with the use of empirical observed logits also gave an estimate of -0.22. Moreover, the maximum-likelihood procedure yielded an estimate of -0.22. However, the agreement will not always be this satisfactory. There is cause for worry in a situation like this, but no procedure will perform better than the Spearman-Kärber estimator, unless the sample size is very large. When the sample size is in the hundreds or thousands, the method of maximum likelihood enables one to estimate the LD_{50} by extrapolation, even from doses in the tail of the tolerance distribution. However, such extrapolation is dangerous, because the choice of model is critical.

MILLER   Would you please elaborate on validity testing in quantal assays?

BROWN   Quantal-assay validity implies tolerance distributions on the log scale that have the same shape and equal standard deviations but are translated (that is, occupy different positions on the abscissa). The test for parallelism tests whether the standard deviations of the two tolerance distributions, that for the standard preparation and that for the unknown, are equal. Of course, the tolerance distributions themselves are not observable. What one sees are estimates of the corresponding dose–response curves. If one could measure the tolerances of the animals, then one would test for equality of the variances of the two distributions with a standard F test. It is well known that in this case large samples and knowledge of the underlying distribution (normal or nonnormal distribution) are required. With quantal responses even larger samples are required.

The information contained in a single quantal assay is rarely sufficient to permit assessment of its validity. Although validity tests can be performed, their power usually is too small to warrant the effort. A conviction of validity must be derived from analysis of a long series of assays.

BLISS I have two comments. First, the comparison of dosage-effect curves based upon a quantal response has not been considered directly. Their analysis poses many of the problems that arose with quantitative assays. The general practice has been to transform the data (by using logits, probits, or angles) to fit straight lines relating the transformed responses to· the log dose and to test agreement of the observed responses with the fitted lines. Frequently these lines fit well and are parallel. Many of the techniques described for quantitative assays (Chapter 4) are applicable. As regards choice of transformation, the angle usually gives satisfactory results when the percentages vary within the range of about 7 to 93. This leads directly to an analysis of variance, as in the example cited on p. 68. The logit and probit transformations are almost impossible to distinguish in the range of 2 to 98%. They require differential weighting and an iterative solution, which are computational disadvantages relative to the angle. The data in Table 1 cover so restricted a range, 15 to 73%, that there is little to gain from any transformation of the response. In this case working with the raw percentages would give nearly the same result.

My second comment is that interest does not always center on the ED_{50} or LD_{50}. Sometimes an extreme percentage is important. For example, in sterilization tests for fruit flies the quarantine officials desired 0% survival. It took some arguments to convince them that it is impossible to measure 0 or 100%. Another example that arises in therapeutics is determination of the "safety margin," that is, the difference between curative and lethal doses. Here interest might center on estimating the ED_{99} (the dose that cures 99%) and the LD_1 (the dose that kills 1%). Actually the ED_{95} and the LD_5 are preferable and more realistic points.

BROWN It's true that the Spearman-Kärber procedure does not yield a comparison of the slopes of the two dose–response functions. There is a Spearman-Kärber procedure for estimating the slope, but it hasn't been fully investigated. With the probit, logit, or some other transform the slopes can be separately estimated and compared. You are correct in that extreme differences will be detected. However, what I meant in my previous remark is that there can be important differences between the two slopes that cannot be detected with these estimates. There may be serious invalidity, but the data in most of the smaller assays are just insufficient to detect this.

I agree that there are situations in which interest is in the tails and not in the LD_{50} or in the potency. However, this is quite a different problem. It requires either very large sample sizes at the extreme doses or extrapolation that depends critically on the chosen mathematical form for the dose–response function. It is a very difficult situation — maybe hopeless!

EMMENS There is another important modern situation in which the tails of a distribution of this kind matter. Among women taking oral contraceptives there are only a few pregnancies per thousand women-years of exposure. It is of great interest to drug firms to know whether one formulation allows double the number of pregnancies that another one does. Another point is the increasingly common use of factorial designs. This is where analysis by probits or logits or any other "its" becomes extremely tedious, unless the investigator has access to a computer. To sit down at a desk calculator with something like a 2 × 2 × 3 × 4 factorial — well, if anybody's not tried it, just let him have a go at fitting probits and see how he gets on. The now almost classical example of probit planes (Finney, 1952) takes me six hours to do, and that's a fairly simple factorial. So what we have done is to devise short-cut methods. The shortest method is simply to use zeros and ones. We are fully aware of the accompanying snags, but the results are quite re-assuring. We have never obtained an answer substantially different from one derived by the use of probits or angles. If someone wishes to use probits or angles, he should do the zero-one estimation first (a matter of minutes rather than hours) and use the results as a first approximation for the probit or angular transformation. I have never yet needed to perform a further cycle of iteration.

TAYLOR For many years I have had the feeling that the full maximum-likelihood estimates, either logit or probit, were a waste of time. It can be shown that the estimates obtained by means of the minimum logit transform have the same asymptotic properties as maximum-likelihood estimates. If one is faced with data in which there are some embarrassing 0 or 100% responses, then one has to make some modifications. Some results of Berkson (1955) indicated that the very rough approximation of moving the 0 and 100% responses up or down half a unit and then continuing with a single iteration provides very good estimates.

BROWN Berkson's work is somewhat difficult to evaluate in that he never really investigated the LD_{50}. He estimated the intercept and the slope, a and b, but not the negative ratio of the two, $-a/b$, that is, the LD_{50} estimate. I believe he showed that the mean squared error (the difference between the estimate and the true value squared and averaged over repeated samplings) done by the simple method is good relative to the maximum-likelihood estimates. As a matter of fact, I believe he would claim that the minimum logit transform estimate is better than the maximum-likelihood estimate. Cramer (1964) did the same as Berkson but looked at the minimum-transform estimate of the LD_{50}

and compared it with the maximum-likelihood estimate. He concluded that it was slightly inferior. Neither has discussed the differences between estimates relative to their standard errors. Actually, these differences are quite small relative to the total standard error.

On the basis of published Monte Carlo sampling experiments and mathematical investigations I am quite willing to use the Spearman-Kärber estimator or the one-step least-squares estimator for most practical situations.

CHAPTER SIX

Invalidity in Bioassays

JEROME CORNFIELD*

1. Introduction

The mathematical treatment of experimental results in biological assay has both probabilistic and nonprobabilistic components. The probabilistic components have always been of special interest to statisticians. The appropriate formalization of the quantitative aspects of a bioassay, however, is nonprobabilistic in nature and will be considered first as a necessary background to a discussion of invalidity.

We start with the concept of a dose–response curve, which we consider simply a description of experimental results. There is a dosage scale D and a biological response y, and we assume that experimental results are described by a well-behaved dose–response curve of the form $y = f(D)$. In traditional bioassay this function, f, is entirely empirical. It has nothing like the law of mass action behind it. Although it may in fact be a consequence of just such a physical or chemical principle, the only characteristic necessary to a justification of its use is that it provides an economical description of experimental results.

We next take the assumption of *similarity*, which is basic to the theoretical formulation of the bioassay. We visualize two agents, the standard and some unknown, and introduce a constant, ρ, which we call the relative potency. The similarity assumption states that we can produce the same response y whether we give D units (cubic centimeters, milligrams, etc.) of the standard or ρD units of the unknown for all the values of D. This assumption would be correct if, for example, the standard and unknown consisted of the same "effective constituents" suspended in inert diluents but in different proportions. Thus, if we have $\rho = 2$, then 1 cm³ of the standard and 2 cm³ of the unknown give the same response; that is, the standard is twice as potent as the unknown, since it causes the same response in only half the amount. An assay for which this assumption holds is often referred to as an *analytical dilution assay*.

If the similarity assumption does hold, some fairly strong conclusions follow. Note first that ρ is a constant that characterizes the two

* The preparation of this paper was supported by Research Grant G.M.-15004 of the National Institutes of Health.

preparations and not the biological system used for assaying them. If the condition of similarity is satisfied, the relative potency should be the same no matter what the animal and no matter what the biological end point. If, in fact, one were concerned with some active substance suspended in a diluent that was inert for all possible biological systems exposed to it then this might be a reasonable assumption. One would expect to find the same results whether one assayed the substance in mice or rabbits or guinea pigs or, indeed, used a chemical assay.

Given the assumption of similarity and the dose–response curve for the standard, then, knowing ρ, one can reconstruct the curve for the unknown. One can map each point on the standard dose–response curve onto that for the unknown. For any point on the standard curve with coordinates (D, y) the corresponding point on the unknown has coordinates $(\rho D, y)$. It is easy to see by proceeding in this way that, if there is a lower or upper asymptote for the standard, the unknown must have the same asymptotes, although not necessarily at the same values of D. If one knows ρ and the dose–response curve for the standard, the condition of similarity enables one to deduce the dose–response curve for the unknown. In practice the inverse problem is the one of interest: given the dose–response curves for both standard and unknown and the similarity assumption, what is ρ?

Consider now the special case in which the standard dose–response curve is linear in log dose, that is, one in which

$$y = \alpha_S + \beta_S \log D_S \tag{1}$$

or, with $x_S = \log D_S$, in which

$$y = \alpha_S + \beta_S x_S \tag{2}$$

where logarithms are to base 10. Then, as is well known, the condition of similarity implies that the dose–response curve for the unknown is also linear in log dose and is parallel. The algebraic basis of this statement is simple and illuminating. We begin with the linear log-dose–response curve in Equation 1. The similarity assumption states that if one substitutes ρD_U for D_S one will obtain the same response y. The response associated with D_U units of the unknown must then be given by

$$y = \alpha_S + \beta_S \log \rho D_U \tag{3}$$

where y is the same as in Equation 1. Now,

$$\log \rho D_U = \log \rho + \log D_U \tag{4}$$

so that

$$y = \alpha_S + \beta_S \log \rho + \beta_S \log D_U \tag{5}$$

Thus, letting

$$\alpha_U = \alpha_S + \beta_S \log \rho \tag{6}$$

the equation for the dose–response curve for the unknown must be

$$y = \alpha_U + \beta_S \log D_U \tag{7}$$

which is a straight line with the same slope but with a different intercept. This is why the condition of similarity implies parallelism. What is more, it is easy to see from Equation 6 that, if α_S, α_U, and β_S, but not ρ, are known, then

$$\log \rho = (\alpha_U - \alpha_S)/\beta_S \tag{8}$$

This is the basis of the usual bioassay calculation.

Of course, one does not actually know the constants α_U, α_S, and β_S, but, given appropriate observations (and appropriate assumptions), one can estimate them and, hence, estimate the relative potency (see Chapter 4, Section 2). In such estimates three assumptions are customarily made: constant variances at the different dose levels, linear log-dose–response curves, and similarity. In my own experience I have found all three to be satisfied only once or twice and so have usually been compelled to determine what steps to take when they are not. The following sections consider cases in which one or more of these assumptions does not hold, cases of "invalidity."

2. Inequality of variance

Consider first the assumption of constant variance. To correct for inequality of variance one usually seeks some transformation that may restore constancy; that is, instead of working with y one works with some function of y, such as the log or the square root, and hopes that such a transformation will restore the equality. Unfortunately, variance-equalizing transformations may not preserve linearity. Nonlinearity introduces even more serious complications than unequal variances. My own view is that inequality of variance is the usual situation and that the most straightforward approach is simply to adopt the more complicated computational procedures required when variances are unequal.

What are these more complicated procedures? I believe that the last word on this subject has not been said. The general outlines of what to do, however, are fairly clear and, moreover, are accepted by all statisticians. It is agreed that the method of least squares should be used for fitting dose–response curves. It is also agreed that Gauss was right, well over a hundred years ago, when he said that, in general, with unequal variances one should fit curves by minimizing a *weighted* sum of squares, where the weight for the mean at a dose level is the reciprocal of its variance. There is some difficulty in applying this principle, however. It turns out that what is meant by variance is not the actual variance observed but the true variance that would be observed with an indefinitely large number of observations. This, of course, is not known to anyone. The practice of many bioassayists, when it is clear that the variances are varying by dose level, is to plot the variance against log dose or response and then determine the weights by using a free-hand or computed curve. Since the exact values of the weights employed in such calculation often have only small effects on the estimate of potency, the results are often quite satisfactory. Obviously, this is not an optimal procedure, but it does seem superior to assuming equality of variance when there is evidence to the contrary.

3. Inequality of variances and the index of precision

Inequality of the variances at the different dose levels also has a bearing on the distinction sometimes made between precision and sensitivity (see Chapters 18, 19, and 20). Sensitivity, defined somewhat loosely, is a measure of the smallest quantity of the unknown (or, alternatively, the smallest value of ρ) detectable by a given assay system. Once the inequality of variances is admitted, however, sensitivity so defined becomes indistinguishable from precision.

To show this we must first define the index of precision. One is given a known linear log-dose–response curve for the standard that is constant under repetitions of the experiment. One has a single observation of the response to one unit of the unknown and wishes to compute the amount of standard contained in that one unit. There is no problem in deciding how to do this. One uses the linear dose–response curve as a calibration curve and reads off the dose required to give the observed response y. The response y is, of course, subject to some variation, because the animals vary in their responses to one unit, or because the measurement process is variable, or for some other reason. One therefore ascribes to this quantity y a variation, say σ, where σ is the standard deviation of y. One now asks what the computed amount of standard would have been if $y + \sigma$ had been observed. The difference between the dose estimated for response y and for response $y + \sigma$ is, clearly, the error in estimated dose induced by variations in y. If one draws the graph and goes through the elementary geometry it becomes clear that this error is simply σ divided by β, the slope of the dose–response line; see Figure 1. This quantity, usually denoted by λ, is the index of inherent precision. Clearly, λ is the standard error of the logarithm of the amount of standard in one unit of the unknown, estimated from a single observation by

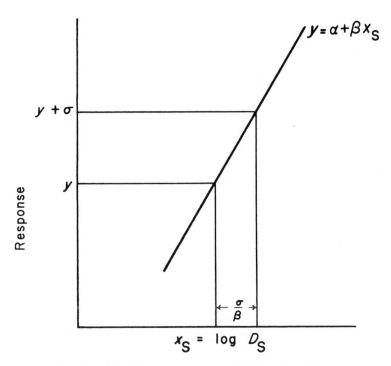

FIGURE 1 Graphical representation of index of precision.

means of a known dose–response curve. If an investigator says "My λ is 0.3; what's yours?" then what the 0.3 means, operationally, is that the log dose estimated from a single observation has a standard error of 0.3. Log dose is, of course, a calculating device, and interest really centers on the estimated dose and its error. For these one simply takes antilogs. Now, antilog 0.3 is 2, which means that with a single observation, in terms of standard-error units, one can come within two times the true value. That is to say, the true dose has a chance of approximately 0.68 of being from half to twice the estimated dose. The index λ is thus simply the standard error of the log dose, and its antilog has an appropriate interpretation in the original units.

If variances are not constant but are smaller at high dose levels than at low, then λ is not a constant but varies at different points along the dose–response curve. It was a characteristic of one of the first bioassays in which I was involved, the use of eosinophil counts in the assay of cortisone, that the larger the fall in eosinophil count, the smaller the variance. Large falls were, of course, associated with large doses of cortisone (Rosemberg et al., 1954). Consequently, large doses were estimated with more precision than were small doses. It just happened to be a biological fact and could not be rationalized away. Thus, the distinction between indexes of precision and sensitivity disappears, once allowance is made for the possibility that the index of precision is larger for the smaller doses. Another reason for the nonconstancy of λ is that the dose–response curve cannot really be linear over the entire range of doses, so at a sufficiently low dose there may be no slope at all (see next section). A suitable extension of the notion of λ, in which, not the slope, but the derivative at a dose level is used, shows that at sufficiently low doses λ explodes and becomes infinite. There is no precision at all at that point. This, however, is also a measure of the loss of sensitivity. As the λ becomes unbearably large, the ability to detect any unknown at all disappears.

4. Nonlinearity

We come now to the question of nonlinear dose–response curves. It seems to be a fact of most, if not all, biological assays that there is a lower limit to the response: that even if one gives no dose at all, there is a finite value of y. Similarly, there seems to be an upper limit: no matter how high the dose, the response cannot increase above a certain level. Thus, there are upper and lower limits. Some rough kind of sigmoid dose–response curve seems to be characteristic. The linear log-dose–response curve is an approximation for a restricted range of doses. This is well understood, and in using linear dose–response curves everyone knows that they must be used only in the applicable range. But, like many things in bioassay, it is easier said than done, and a certain amount of subjectivity in determining the applicable range necessarily arises. It would, therefore, be desirable if there were ways of avoiding this determination by routinely fitting nonlinear dose–response curves. Even ten years ago this was something from which most statisticians and all biologists shrank, since nonlinear dose–response curves present difficult computational problems. At least four parameters are needed to describe such a curve: one for the lower limit, one for the upper limit, one for the slope, and one for the average height. At least two of them enter nonlinearly. No theoretical problems are involved in fitting such a curve; it is merely a lot of work. The general availability of computers and of routine procedures for fitting nonlinear curves now makes this approach feasible. I have not spent any time with actual bioassay data in attempting to fit four-parameter sigmoid curves, but I should think that anyone concerned with this type of problem and having access to a computer and such curve-fitting procedures might well benefit from systematic exploration of the possibilities. Computer-based procedures tend to look better before they are tried than after some experience has been accumulated. Nevertheless, the possibilities are too real to be neglected.

5. Lack of similarity

I became involved with the problems posed by lack of similarity when an investigator with whom I had worked in the past, Dr. Grant Liddle, showed me some assay results that were giving him trouble. He had been studying four synthetic analogues of natural steroids. Up to that time it had been observed that any steroid that was potent in markedly lowering the eosinophil count also was potent in suppressing adrenocorticotropic hormone, as measured by a lowering of the urinary excretion of 17-hydroxycorticosteroids, and in its effect on blood glucose levels. The curious thing about three of the synthetic analogues was that, although they seemed to be very effective in suppressing the hormone, they appeared to have no effect whatsoever on eosinophils or blood glucose.

It may be noted immediately that if this was, in fact, the case, it was definitive evidence against the similarity assumption, since similarity implies a relative potency that is independent of the biological response used for estimation. In the assay for adrenocorticotropic hormone the log-dose–response lines were parallel, but this was not true of the eosino-phil or hyperglycemic responses. In fact, for these other two responses only one of the synthetic analogues produced a dose–response curve with a slope, while the other three yielded lines that were essentially flat. There were thus two independent indications that the similarity condition did not hold — which was not, of course, surprising, since the four analogues are chemically different.

The statistical problem presented was that of developing a quantitative expression of these findings without assuming parallelism or any other attribute implied by similarity. This seemed particularly important because of the critical reaction to a preliminary presentation of results by investigators familiar only with the traditional bioassay outlook, namely, that since the dose–response lines were not parallel, the assay was invalid, and it was improper to consider potency. This seemed to us a somewhat inflexible reaction to straightforward and reproducible bio-logical results. We therefore developed an analysis that took account of the fact that in the absence of similarity potency can vary, not only with the assay system, but also with the dose level (Cornfield, 1964).

The general tenor of the results (Kendall et al., 1963) may be conveyed by considering two of the analogues: ΔFF,[1] which was treated as the

[1] Abbreviation for 9α-fluoro-$11\beta,17\alpha,21$-trihydroxy-$\Delta^{1,4}$-pregnene-3,20-dione.

standard, and mesylate. In the response, the suppression of adreno-corticotropic hormone, for which the two dose–response lines were parallel, mesylate was estimated to be 1/55 as potent as ΔFF; that is, 55 times as much mesylate as ΔFF was required to get the same hormone suppression. This was true at all dose levels. However, in the hyper-glycemic response the potency of mesylate relative to ΔFF depended on whether 60, 160, or 640 mg were given. The potencies at each of these three dose levels were estimated as 1/75, 1/206, and 1/866. Although they vary tenfold, they are all below the potency of 1/55 obtained with the hormone response. No matter what the dose level, therefore, the potency of mesylate is higher as judged by the suppression of the hormone than it is as judged by hyperglycemia. Of course, it would have been preferable for the potencies to be constant at the different dose levels, so that we could have used a single number, but that was simply not the case. The appropriate way to describe the data seemed to be the way that we did it.

To define potency as a function of dose level or of response one applies the definition of relative potency as the ratio of doses that give equivalent responses. The algebra involved in implementing this idea is extremely simple. The two dose–response lines are

$$y = \alpha_S + \beta_S x_S \qquad \text{and} \qquad y = \alpha_U + \beta_U x_U \qquad (9)$$

for standard and unknown. If the two responses are equal, then the two y's must be equal. One thus finds pairs of values x_S and x_U that lead to the same value of y by equating $\alpha_S + \beta_S x_S$ with $\alpha_U + \beta_U x_U$. Remembering that log relative potency is defined as the difference between x_S and x_U that leads to the same y, one solves for $x_S - x_U$ to obtain

$$\log \rho = x_S - x_U = \frac{\alpha_U - \alpha_S}{\beta_S} + \left(\frac{\beta_U}{\beta_S} - 1\right)x_U \qquad (10)$$

If the lines are parallel ($\beta_U = \beta_S$), making the second expression on the right-hand side equal to zero, then the log relative potency is independent of x_U; that is, Equation 8 holds. If the lines are not parallel ($\beta_U \neq \beta_S$), then the relative potency depends on x_U. Log relative potency can also be written as a function of x_S or of y. The latter function is derived from the second equation, Equation 9, by solving for x_U as a function of y and substituting in Equation 10, giving

$$\log \rho = \left(\frac{\alpha_U}{\beta_U} - \frac{\alpha_S}{\beta_S}\right) + \left(\frac{1}{\beta_S} - \frac{1}{\beta_U}\right)y \qquad (11)$$

Having made this much progress in the problem presented by Dr. Liddle, I began to wonder how frequently the similarity condition had been found violated. A far from exhaustive search through the literature revealed the following examples (Cornfield, 1964).[2]

[2] In the quotation "ACTH" stands for "adrenocorticotropic hormone."

...(a) the potency of many of the early preparations of ACTH was markedly influenced by the route of administration, apparently because the ACTH preparations were inactivated locally by tissues when administered extravascularly, with the amount of tissue inactivation varying greatly from one ACTH preparation to another and one recipient to another (Forsham et al., 1951). (b) digitalis potency depends upon the assay species, apparently because digitalis is a complex mixture of many glycosides, each with special species effects and present in varying proportions in different samples (Perry, 1950). A difference of as much as a 10-fold between the results of an intravenous cat assay and oral assay in man has been reported (Gold et al., 1940). (c) potency of one purified tuberculin preparation relative to another can vary by 2-fold, depending upon whether tested on BCG vaccinated persons or upon guinea pigs or cows (Fisher, 1949). (d) some of the collaborative assays of International Standards have shown considerable variation in potency from laboratory to laboratory (Mussett and Perry, 1955, 1956), and numerous investigators performing repeated assays of the same substance have reported significant variations in potency, not attributable to variations in administered dosage (Sheps and Munson, 1957). (e) in the presence of varying amounts of an inhibitor log dose-response lines for test and standard need not be parallel even when the test substance is a dilution of the standard (Thompson, 1948).

Additional examples are given by Bliss and Cattell (1943).

In thinking about these examples it did not seem surprising to me that the condition of similarity was frequently violated, because bioassay procedures are often used when some agent is in process of purification. The very fact that it is in process of purification means that interfering substances may be present and that the assumption of an effective constituent suspended in an inert diluent may be grossly untrue. When the agent is so highly purified that the assumption becomes reasonable, one may have reached the point at which the chemist steps in and performs the assay. What has saved the situation is that nonparallelism is not a sensitive index of dissimilarity and that, in fact, few bioassays are sufficiently large to detect any but the most flagrant departures from parallelism. Failures to detect departures from parallelism are often simply a measure of the lack of power of the experiment, not of their actual absence.

The effect of dissimilarity depends upon the biological purpose that the assay is serving. If it is being used as a research tool for investigating the effect of variations in the experimental conditions on, say, blood levels of a hormone, then dissimilarity is only one of many unknown sources of error present, and it is a fact of biological experience that significant progress in understanding an agent can still be made. On the other hand, if one is concerned with biological standardization and must provide unitage as a guide to dosage, the departures from similarity may be more serious. If, for example, the departures are as large as those encountered in Dr. Liddle's work, one might seriously consider not putting unitage on the bottle at all. Physicians somehow decide on dosage despite wide departures from the conditions of similarity, as, for example, in the case of digitalis. It may be that even in biological standardization one can live with dissimilarity.

6. Conclusion

Some and perhaps many of the conditions regarded as necessary to provide "valid" bioassays may be violated in practice. This means, not necessarily that the underlying observations are incorrect or not reproducible or that no statistical analysis of results is possible, but often only that some suitable generalization of traditional statistical treatments must be sought.

DISCUSSION

MUSSETT   First, I can hardly wait to ask what useful purpose we expect to serve by issuing International Standards without a labeled potency. Second, the solutions given for dealing with invalidities seem to call for more and more sophisticated analyses. I have been thinking in the opposite direction. Third, does the analysis of variance serve any useful purpose in bioassay? It yields tests of validity and of the residual error for use in the calculation of the fiducial interval of potency. If the curvature term is significant, a transformation may be indicated but is unlikely to alter the results very much. This is certainly true with regard to potency estimation when the responses to the preparations are fairly well matched. Furthermore, the analysis of variance is not a particularly sensitive tool for detecting departures from parallelism. If an assay is relatively imprecise, even gross nonparallelism can be overlooked by examination of the parallelism term in individual analyses of variance for separate assays. For example, in the collaborative study of corticotropin (Bangham, Mussett, and Stack-Dunne, 1962) there were twenty-nine Sayers assays (injection by the subcutaneous route in gelatin), and only three displayed significant nonparallelism at the 1% level. However, repetition of the assay within each laboratory enabled us to examine the distributions of slopes for the two preparations. From this analysis a clear-cut difference in slope emerged, significant for every laboratory. This result could have been overlooked if we had considered only the individual assay analyses. Conversely, there are assays with responses that are very consistent, either because the system is highly reproducible or because the measurement of response is crude. For example, in the British Pharmacopœia assay of heparin (1963, p. 1137) the clotting times may be virtually identical within a treatment group. We have already encountered the assay with zero residual error! Here the analysis of variance breaks down completely.

Turning now to the analysis of variance as the source of a residual-error term to be employed in estimating potency limits, there are again deficiencies. Heterogeneity among potencies is commonplace in collaborative work or even within a laboratory, if conditions are changed between assays. Under these circumstances, the use of an intra-assay variance estimate is misleading. Because such an intra-assay error term takes no account of interassay variation, it leads to spuriously narrow limits of final potency. Hence, I wonder whether we should do an analysis of variance at all in bioassay.

My own current thoughts and practice are as follows. One of the basic concepts of the statistics of bioassay, that the preparations being compared should contain the same active principle and behave like dilutions of one another, is unsound or, at any rate, impractical. More often than not the preparations under comparison vary in composition. If one were dealing with pure chemicals, there would be no need for biological assay. One must therefore expect nonparallelism and variations in the unit of activity from one assay system to another, and the more refined the assay techniques become, the more rapidly we shall become aware of these discrepancies.

In the Division of Biological Standards we no longer discard individual assays on the grounds of nonparallelism, unless it seems likely that some error, say in dilution, has been made, but we assess slope differences by examining the distribution from a series of assays. All attempts to disguise nonparallelism by narrowing the dose range or using, for example, some highly selected strain of animal are resisted.

Relative potencies and their limits of error, derived in a single laboratory by the use of a standardized assay procedure, cannot be validly used for prediction except under those same conditions. It is only in a large-scale collaborative assay that an attempt can be made to assess possible variations in a universal potency, and in arranging such collaborative work we endeavor to include as many widely differing assay methods as possible.

CORNFIELD I tend to share your feelings concerning the analysis of variance. One can sometimes use it as an elegant means of analyzing data, but the situations in which it can be employed tend to be rather limited. In bioassay my major interests are the estimation of potency, the error with which that potency is estimated from internal variations within the experiment, and the validity of the assumptions required to obtain those two estimates. You have brought out the important point that there is no substitute for repeating one's work under different conditions. When this is done, one usually finds more variation than that predicted from the error estimated from a single assay. However, in order to determine whether the variations between repetitions are in excess of expectation, one must have obtained the error for each individual assay. To this extent internal error analysis serves a useful purpose. However, since the analysis of variance is merely *one* of the ways of performing this internal error analysis, and perhaps one lacking in sufficient generality, one should not insist that it is the key to bioassay.

As regards the trend toward increasing sophistication, this is characteristic of techniques in every field, not because sophistication is an end in itself, but because unduly simplified techniques can be misleading. I, myself, feel that this trend is at least partly praiseworthy and in any event inescapable.

Concerning the bottle without the label, I cannot answer your pointed question. However, let me ask one in return. When the potency of, say, digitalis varies tenfold, depending on the animal used, which number would one put on the label?

BANGHAM   I am quite unable to tell you which number to put on the label of that bottle of digitalis.

With regard to assay invalidity, I should like to examine some of the assumptions made in classical comparative bioassays. To estimate potency, one needs a biological standard that is sufficiently similar to the test material to permit an analytical dilution assay. As one whose responsibility it is to provide standards, I should like to draw attention to the problem of determining when two materials are so different that they cannot validly be compared. It is on this evidence that the decision is made about whether a new standard should be provided. This is a real problem, both to the investigator handling his own materials and to control authorities whose job it is to provide or approve official standards. Both groups are faced with a number of materials representing a spectrum of minor dissimilarities. Preparations of hormones may differ if they come from different species, tissues, or body fluids, and they exist in different degrees of purity. For example, there are synthetic polypeptide hormones of various chain lengths for which bioassays may be needed for control tests. By what criteria does one decide whether separate standards are needed for peptides in which the length of the chain containing the active site may differ by only one or two amino acids? This is not merely a hypothetical difficulty: there are about six synthetic peptides described, each with the same "corticotropic" active moiety and differing only in chain length. Since each may have some subtle and as yet unrecognized difference in biological effect, should separate standards be prepared for each? Is it safe to assume that quantitative or qualitative differences that may be negligible or undetectable in assay animals will not appear with quite unpredicted biological effects in man? There are also synthetic analogues of hormones in which substituted amino acids radically alter the biological activity, sometimes in a most bizarre way. What criteria of dissimilarity does one set for deciding when a new standard should be established?

Orthodox bioassayists would, no doubt, prefer to decide on the basis of invalidity detected in one or more bioassay systems. It is easy to test for and recognize nonparallelism in the assays (normally only one or two) carried out in a research laboratory. Sometimes, however, nonparallelism is detected only after the results of many assays have been combined. Invalidity expressed by heterogeneity of estimates within a laboratory may be spotted by the observant worker who assays the same material repeatedly. However, heterogeneity among laboratories or among methods is not so often seen or tested for, at least by those laboratories which do not perform a great number of assays. Invalidity becomes much more readily apparent when large-scale collaborative assays are carried out on materials in stable and homogeneous form. This is seen all too often in international collaborative assays performed to establish an international standard. The precision obtained by a combination of assay data almost always reveals unsuspected invalidities, suggesting dissimilarity between one international standard and its replacement. This is a salutary reminder that invalidity is usually buried by the level of precision that is considered to be acceptable in practice. Many research laboratories do not or cannot set up standards for their own materials which give invalid assays against an established standard. In seeking a means of expressing relative potency one tends to resort to a system of "conversion factors." From all that is known about the variability of biological substrates it follows that such a factor applies only to the preparations and specific assay conditions (method, procedure, animals, times, etc.) on which the observations have been made. It cannot be too often emphasized that it is not valid to transfer the factor to other laboratory preparations or assay methods without demonstration of statistical validity in each instance.

Indispensable as the use of the factor is for research within a laboratory, statements of potency have general validity only if they are expressed in terms of a similar stable and homogeneous preparation that other laboratories can use. It is a sobering thought that the labor of demonstrating that two preparations are slightly dissimilar biologically often exceeds the work of establishing yet another standard.

CORNFIELD The general question of standards is interesting and perplexing. In the early days of bioassay the proposal was to proceed without standards and to use animal units. Unitage was defined in terms of the amount of agent necessary to cause a given response in a given animal and exhibited marked variability. It was proposed that the way to eliminate the effect of variation in animal response was to develop a stable laboratory standard, against which unknowns could be compared. A reduction in variation has, in fact, been observed by bioassayists dealing with situations in which the conditions of similarity are satisfied. But when the conditions of similarity are *not* satisfied, I wonder whether any gain results from running concurrent standards. There is no theoretical reason why there should be. The question appears to be largely a factual one, whose answer may vary from one assay system to another. Having been raised on the concept that animal units were unreliable and that it was naive to use them and that the only proper way to do a bioassay was to use an appropriate standard, I was taken aback when I was working with an investigator who was assaying a certain digestive enzyme. His problem was how the secretion responded to such changes in experimental circumstances as diet. He said to me, "Sorry, no standard. I can't get any standard," and what we did was to return to animal units. What may be an inferior procedure in other circumstances may still permit progress to be made.

I thought I detected a suggestion that the concept of potency was applicable to a dilution assay and not to a comparative assay. I should like to know why the concept is applicable to one type of assay and not to the other. The computations can be performed in both. One may, of course, say that, given a dilution assay, the number is reproducible and, given a comparative assay, it is not. This may or may not be true. Again, it is a factual question to be settled by experimentation. There are many comparative assays in which two quite different chemical substances are being compared and the dilution assumption is not satisfied, but in which, nevertheless, potency calculations are reproducible. I would therefore argue that the conversion-factor approach, which is a useful way of quantifying certain kinds of results, is applicable to any numbers that can be put into that framework. Whether those numbers are biologically reproducible is an entirely different question, which is answerable only by experimentation.

Finally, there is one other point I should like to raise, because it often arises in routine assays of a single substance. Suppose one has a bioassay system in which there is evidence that the condition of similarity obtains and in which parallelism is to be expected. It is a common practice to perform tests of the parallelism assumption nevertheless, and to reject assays in which departures from parallelism at some significance level are found. The function served by these rejection procedures is not at all clear. In a bioassay system in which the condition of similarity is satisfied and the hypothesis of parallelism is tested at the 5% level, in the long run 5% of the assays will be rejected. I doubt whether anything is gained by rejecting assays that are fully as good as the 95% retained.

BORTH   We should not forget that the term bioassay has *assay* in it. *To assay* means to determine the amount of a substance in a mixture. To the question of how much, there exists only one correct answer. Moreover, since the advent of what Dr. Albert calls "high-precision rats" variation is no longer the main argument against animal units, or it may not be, under certain circumstances. The point remains, however, that hormones have a way of producing different effects, which are used as end points, and that animal units based on different end points are simply not comparable with one another. There is no way of relating, say, "rat units" to "frog units" or "adrenal ascorbic acid units" to "adrenal weight units" except by using a standard or reference preparation.

ALBERT   I should like to mention some data collected by Dr. Rosemberg and me concerning the ventral prostate weight bioassay for luteinizing hormone (LH). This assay, developed by Professor Greep, is more than twenty years old and has been used by many workers (Greep et al., 1941). Dr. McArthur employed it to demonstrate for the first time the ovulatory surge of LH during the menstrual cycle; it has been used as a guide in the purification and isolation of LH and in many studies of a physiological nature. It consistently behaves as a graded parallel-line assay of the comparative type, in which the untransformed response is a linear function of the log dose, and parallelism is not in question in ordinary computational procedures. When an endocrinologist encounters nonparallelism under such circumstances, he is annoyed for at least two reasons: first, he is usually unable to handle the data, and second, if he wishes to incorporate his data in a paper submitted to a journal, he knows that the reviewers will spot the nonparallelism immediately. They will reject the assay as invalid, and the report as incompetent. Sometimes I think that reviewers of papers on endocrinology have all taken the same course in biostatistics and remember by association the pair of words "bioassay, parallelism" and the automatic reply "nonparallelism, rejection."

Dr. Rosemberg and I (Albert et al., 1965) were interested in the biologic characteristics of certain assay systems for luteinizing hormone and human chorionic gonadotropin. In the course of this work we tannated ovine LH and tested the tannated product against the untannated material at the same dose levels, the assay now being somewhat between the dilution and the comparative type. We performed the standard parallel-line assay calculations and found the test for nonparallelism to be highly significant.

Figure 2 illustrates nonparallelism with the gonadotropin. The slope of the tannated gonadotropin is 2.6 times that of the free. We always include a blank, which is uninjected, hypophysectomized rats. Seven days after hypophysectomy the control ventral prostate weights are

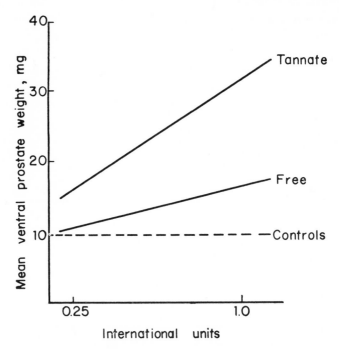

FIGURE 2   The effect of tannation on the bioassay of HCG.

between 7 and 10 mg. We always try to have at least one dose yield responses 100% greater than controls since, if we always work at this level, we can easily determine specific activities. Thanks to the availability of highly inbred, uniform rats of "reagent-grade purity," the response is a variable of known and well-behaved dimensions. Since the free and tannated gonadotropins give different slopes, one way to compare them is to determine the intercepts at some fixed level of response (twice the control level). This gives specific activities, and their ratio is used as a potency ratio.

This is experimentally induced nonparallelism in a previously parallel-line assay. It is not a random phenomenon, such as one might encounter upon repetition. It can be induced at will. Moreover, it has an important meaning for the index of discrimination and hence is of biologic usefulness. We would not discard this assay as invalid. Therefore, it would be helpful if statisticians could provide a new model. It should be one that would enable us to calculate the potency ratio and its error, serve as a tool for the study of bioassay systems, and provide a "number" for reasonable communication among investigators.

CORNFIELD   Methods now described in the literature present at least one way of systematically handling nonparallel-line assays. I published one possible procedure for the case in which there are multiple observations at different dose levels on the same experimental animal (Cornfield 1964). Cox and Leaverton (1966) have published a closely related procedure.

BLISS   I want to comment on the digitalis assays. As I understand the comments on tests for invalidity, we seem to be comparing different methods of assay and not a single type of preparation within a single method. I was involved in the development of a method of digitalis assay for the United States Pharmacopeia. Digitalis is a plant extract with more than one active ingredient; about 80% is digitoxin, but there are other ingredients that are also quite active. The first assays were performed on the frog and were statistically satisfactory. However, a complication arose in that a sample of digitalis taken from the shelf six months after the original assay exhibited a lower potency when tested by the frog method but not when employed clinically in man (Miller, 1944). Manufacturers consequently added an excess, so that a sample selected six months later and tested for labeled potency would not be rejected and the company penalized. This led to overpotent materials' being placed on the market. It was pointed out that if the cat were used as the assay animal, the response would be nearer to that of man. We therefore arranged a collaborative assay on cats (Bliss, 1944). The first proposal was to send a single sample of digitalis to everyone who would report its "just toxic" dose in cats. This was subsequently modified, and we sent both a standard and an unknown for a comparative test. The results demonstrated that the comparison was necessary because of the variation in animals and in technique from one laboratory to another. The present technique involves an intravenous infusion in the pigeon, which, like the cat, yields a response resembling that of man. In the biological assay of drugs it is essential that there be agreement between the response of the test animal and that of the species to which the drug is to be administered. Finally, bioassays should follow a single method before one speaks of invalidity. Invalidity should be restricted to the use of a common method and the same animal and not be extrapolated to differences in animals or in method. Many drugs and hormones contain so many impurities that one cannot literally adopt the assumptions underlying analytical dilution assays.

CORNFIELD   I was interested to hear the origin of that cat assay. My only comment is that, clearly, in the case of such a situation as that presented by digitalis, we are quite prepared to live with gross violations of the similarity assumption. My plea is that we adopt a similar point of view toward other manifestations of departures from similarity, such as nonparallelism.

FINNEY   I agree very strongly with almost all that the speaker has said. I want to mention a more general moral that seems to me important. I believe the analysis of variance to be a superb instrument for the examination of a single experiment, a single set of data in isolation. This is largely what it was produced for, and this is the purpose for which its use is usually described in textbooks on statistical method. Unfortunately, statisticians have written practically nothing on the general principles of putting together information from whole series of experiments. Especially is this true when the experiments are not a planned collaborative series but have developed casually as the biologist learns more about his material, and as the statistician learns more about how to handle that material. Many misunderstandings over questions of transformation, rejection of data, invalidity, dissimilarity, and the like stem from the fact that we are talking about different things. The formal presentations, with the solitary exception of the present one, have been concerned almost entirely with planning and analyzing a single experiment in isolation. A statistician may be able to advise on analyzing a particular series of experiments. Yet in our profession we have little idea of how to lay down formal principles for analyzing and interpreting somewhat unplanned series of experiments. Had Liddle's experiment, which was described to us, lacked a previous history, I think it would have been set aside as uninterpretable, although it would not have been thrown into the wastepaper basket as invalid. Only because the speaker was building on a long experience could he usefully put forward the kind of interpretation he did. Perhaps statisticians should more consciously try to refine, from the practice that has developed in particular case studies of combining information from groups of experiments, general principles that would help investigators.

CHAPTER SEVEN

Covariance Analysis in Bioassay and Related Problems

D. J. FINNEY

1. Introduction

The term *bioassay* is often used very broadly. I shall here restrict it to the employment of biological material (whether whole living organisms or pieces of tissue) for the estimation of the relative potency of two or more chemical compounds (therapeutic drugs, pesticides, etc.). I have discussed more fully elsewhere (Finney, 1964) the distinction between an experiment of which the purpose is to compare the effects on animals of alternative forms or doses of a drug and an experiment in which the responses of the animals are of no interest except in so far as they facilitate the estimation of equally potent doses of two forms of the drug. Only the latter is properly described as a bioassay. The two types of experiment may happen to be very similar in their execution; the logical difference can be vital in all discussion of optimal design and, of course, determines almost every aspect of statistical analysis and interpretation.

Nevertheless, the special statistical technique of *covariance analysis*, a procedure for using the internal evidence of the records of an experiment for improving the precision of numerical conclusions, is applicable to every kind of experiment in which analysis of variance is the central statistical method. My purpose is more to present the covariance technique than to discuss bioassay. I shall therefore begin with a detailed account of the use of covariance in the analysis of a very simple experiment that was not an assay. I want to show the technique in relation to other aspects of multivariate analysis, for which purpose I try to classify statistical variates (Section 2) and types of problem (Section 5). After establishing the form and purpose of the method I illustrate its use in bioassay computations.

2. Classes of variate

For convenience of discussion, I distinguish four different classes of variate. Any experiment that has involved exact numerical recording must have at least one variate of class 1 (and may have more); if it involves any comparison between alternative treatments, it must also have at least one variate of class 2; it need not have any of classes 3 and 4.

Class 1 variates (responses)

These I term *responses*, denoting them by y; they are the measurements that most directly interest the investigator (weight of an organ, contraction of a piece of tissue, survival time). If several distinct responses are measured for each subject in an experiment, they may be identified as y_1, y_2, y_3, etc., with $y \equiv (y_1, y_2, y_3, \ldots)$ still used to represent the set of variates.

Class 2 variates (treatments)

An experiment is usually planned to compare two or more treatments applied to subjects. Variates that measure or otherwise distinguish *treatments* are denoted by x_1, x_2, x_3, etc., or simply by x denoting either the whole set or the sole variate in this class. If the treatments are different doses (concentrations or weights) of a drug, x can represent the dose numerically. If the treatments are two qualitatively different materials (e.g., two drugs or diets) or procedures (e.g., two forms of surgery), x can be assigned values -1 and 1 for the two. If there are more than two qualitatively different treatments, several x-variates must be used (in fact, one fewer than the number of treatments); thus for four treatments A, B, C, and D one can use

	x_1	x_2	x_3
A	0	0	0
B	1	0	0
C	0	1	0
D	0	0	1

Alternatively one can use

	x_1	x_2	x_3
A	-1	0	-1
B	1	0	-1
C	0	-1	1
D	0	1	1

The essential requirement for the separate x-variates is that there shall not exist any linear function of them that is zero for all treatments. For example, in an experiment with equal numbers of subjects on each of four treatments,

	x_1	x_2	x_3
A	1	1	1
B	−2	0	2
C	1	−2	−5
D	0	1	2

is not permissible, because in each row

$$x_1 - 2x_2 + x_3 = 0.$$

Furthermore, this paper is not intended as a guide to the choice of the best treatment variates. The imposition of various constraints on the arbitrariness allowed by the rule just stated can simplify the interpretation, facilitate the computations, and reduce the risks from errors of numerical rounding in large analyses. For example, convenience and ease of interpretation are increased, if for each variate the numerical values are small, and if each variate totals to zero when summed over all subjects. The use of these x-variates and its relation to the more usual way of analyzing for treatments are illustrated in Section 7.

Class 3 variates (classifications)

In many experiments the subjects either deliberately or inevitably fall into groups that may differ consistently in respect of a response variate (even though no treatment effects are responsible), though these differences are of no intrinsic interest to the investigator. For example, animals of both sexes may be used, or animals from several different litters, in order to meet the requirements of total numbers, although no conclusions in respect of sex or litter differences are sought. Again, the exigencies of experiment may demand that responses be measured by several persons or on several occasions; personal differences or time trends that are irrelevant to the purpose of the experiment may occur and must not be ignored.

The subject of experimental design is largely concerned with these *classifications* and, especially, with so relating them to the structure of an experiment that they interfere as little as possible with the study of treatments. This is usually achieved by balancing treatments over classifications: one does not assign treatment A entirely to male mice and treatment B entirely to female mice but, instead, tries to have each sex represented in the same proportion for every treatment. The ideal is that of the complete balance of treatments over each classification known as *orthogonality*. However, if several classifications are simultaneously involved, or if the investigator has severe constraints on his materials, full orthogonality may be unachievable. Many types of experimental design have been devised to meet such situations. So far as analysis of results is concerned, the general situation can be met by invoking *classification variates*, here denoted by $u = (u_1, u_2, u_3, \ldots)$. These may be defined essentially as are the treatment variates, though in analysis they are used more like variates of class 4.

Class 4 variates (concomitants)

In many experiments additional measurements for each subject are available and are known to be independent of the treatments applied. The knowledge is usually based on the fact that the measurements antedate the randomization that determined the allocation of treatments. For example, weights or blood pressures of animals may have been measured before an experiment began. Variates in this class are *concomitants*; they will be denoted by $z = (z_1, z_2, z_3, \ldots)$.

Commonly a concomitant is logically paired with a response variate in the sense that these are measurements of the same property of a subject (for example, body weight) before and after treatment. This is by no means essential; it is obviously impossible for, say, weight of liver! However, when a choice is available to the experimenter, he will very reasonably choose to have concomitant variates either in this direct correspondence with response variates or alternatives that may be broadly indicative of initial values: body weight before experiment might be used as a concomitant for the final weight of an organ which cannot be measured twice.

3. Example

As an example, consider the results of a simple experiment, summarized in Table 1. Two drugs were to be compared in respect of their effectiveness in reducing blood pressure. A set of twenty animals was used; ten chosen at random received the first drug, and the remaining ten received the second. The blood pressure was measured before and after administration of the drug. Thus the variates are:

    y: final blood pressure of animal,
    x: drug administered ($x = -1$ or $x = 1$),
    z: initial blood pressure.

This experiment had no classification variate (other than that represented by the drug). Unfortunately, the publication from which the results are taken (Kodlin, 1951) does not record the species of animal, the units of measurement of blood pressure, or any further information about the drugs; nevertheless, the data illustrate statistical method so well that they are chosen for use here.

The choice of animals for each drug was random. The difference between drugs in respect of any effects they may have on blood pressure

TABLE 1 Comparison of Drugs for the Reduction of Blood Pressure (Twenty Animals)

Initial B.P. z	Final B.P. y	Change $y_1^* = y - z$	Percentage $p = 100y/z$
Drug A ($x = -1$):			
135	90	−45	67
125	80	−45	64
125	100	−25	80
130	80	−50	62
105	80	−25	76
130	95	−35	73
140	90	−50	64
95	75	−20	79
110	85	−25	77
100	85	−15	85
Total: 1,195	860	−335	727
Drug B ($x = 1$):			
90	55	−35	61
135	80	−55	59
130	80	−50	62
115	70	−45	61
110	80	−30	73
140	95	−45	68
130	85	−45	65
95	70	−25	74
90	50	−40	56
105	70	−35	67
Total: 1,140	735	−405	646

may therefore be estimated by statistical analysis of y alone. For an experiment with only two treatments, analysis of variance is not essential, and calculations can be related to the t distribution; however, the greater generality of the analysis of variance makes it preferable for presentation here. I assume the method to be familiar to the reader. Table 2 summarizes this analysis.

TABLE 2 Analysis of Variance of y in Table 1

Adjustment for mean:		127,201	
	DF	SS	MS
Drugs	1	781	781
Error	18	2,193	121.8
Total	19	2,974	

TABLE 3   Analysis of Variance of y_1^* in Table 1

Adjustment for mean:		27,380	
	DF	SS	MS
Drugs	1	245	245
Error	18	2,325	129.2
Total	19	2,570	

The mean values of final blood pressure are 86.0 and 73.5. The variance of the difference between the means is

$$\text{Var}\,(\bar{y}_A - \bar{y}_B) = \sigma^2(\tfrac{1}{10} + \tfrac{1}{10}), \tag{1}$$

where σ^2, the variance per animal, is estimated with 18 DF (degrees of freedom) by the error mean square in Table 2. Hence the variance is taken as

$$\text{var}\,(\bar{y}_A - \bar{y}_B) = 24.36. \tag{2}$$

The estimated advantage for treatment B over treatment A, in respect of blood pressure, is therefore

$$\bar{y}_A - \bar{y}_B = 12.5 \pm 4.9. \tag{3}$$

Here and elsewhere the sign $\pm$ introduces the standard error.

Randomization ensures that any differences in the two groups of animals *before* treatment were solely due to chance. Therefore, an alternative estimator of the advantage for treatment B is obtainable from the compound variate y_1^*, the difference between final and initial blood pressure:

$$y_1^* = y - z. \tag{4}$$

Table 3 contains the corresponding analysis of variance. This leads to

$$\text{var}\,(\bar{y}_{1A}^* - \bar{y}_{1B}^*) = 25.84, \tag{5}$$

and $$\bar{y}_{1A}^* - \bar{y}_{1B}^* = 7.0 \pm 5.08. \tag{6}$$

Despite the intuitive idea that taking account of the chance differences in initial pressures should increase the precision of the estimate, in this instance the simple process of working with change in pressure has slightly *reduced* precision (*increased* variance and standard error).

Because randomization ensures that the expected value of $\bar{z}_A - \bar{z}_B$ is zero, *any* compound variate of the form

$$y^* = y - \beta z \tag{7}$$

will lead to valid estimation of the difference between the effects of the two drugs on blood pressure. The particular values $\beta = 0$ and $\beta = 1$ correspond to the variates y and y_1^* already examined. Evidently the precision of the estimated difference will be made greatest by so choosing β as to minimize the variance of y^*. This is equivalent to taking β as the regression coefficient (within groups of subjects treated alike) of y on z. The calculations required are those for a covariance analysis of y on z; Table 4 contains the first steps for this and some explanatory notes that refer to entries in Table 1.

TABLE 4   Analysis of Covariance of y and z in Table 1

Adjustments for means:		272,611	186,216	127,201
	DF	(z^2)	(yz)	(y^2)
Drugs	1	151	344	781
Error	18	5,463	2,665	2,193
Total	19	5,614	3,009	2,974

Notes on calculations:

analogously,

$(860 + 735)^2/20 = 127,201$;

$(1,195 + 1,140)(860 + 735)/20 = 186,216.$
$90^2 + 80^2 + 100^2 + \cdots + 50^2 + 70^2 - 127,201 = 2,974$;

analogously,

$135 \times 90 + 125 \times 80 + 125 \times 100 + \cdots + 90 \times 50 + 105 \times 70 - 186,216 = 3,009.$
$(860^2 + 735^2)/10 - 127,201 = 781$;

analogously,

$(1,195 \times 860 + 1,140 \times 735)/10 - 186,216 = 344.$
$2,974 - 781 = 2,193$;

analogously,

$3,009 - 344 = 2,665.$

The arithmetic for Table 4 is a simple extension of that required for Table 2: sums of squares for z are formed exactly as were those for y in Table 2, the y squares are incorporated into the new table, and a new column of sums of products for y and z is added. A simple rule enables the product column to be calculated: whatever manipulation involving squares of single values or of totals of y gives an entry in the (y^2) column, exactly the same process with products of corresponding y and z values or totals gives the corresponding entry in the (yz) column. Details are summarized in Table 4, and reference to Table 2 should make clear the operation of the rule (note that entries for sums of products, unlike sums of squares, may be negative, though in this example none is).

The optimal value of β is then estimated as the regression coefficient of y on z from the "error" line of Table 4:

$$b = \frac{2,665}{5,463} = 0.488. \tag{8}$$

Then, with b inserted for β,

$$\bar{y}_A^* = 86.0 - 0.488 \times 119.5 = 27.7,$$
$$\bar{y}_B^* = 73.5 - 0.488 \times 114.0 = 17.9. \tag{9}$$

The variance per observation appropriate to y^* is estimated from a "residual" sum of squares:

$$\text{sum of squares for } y - \frac{(\text{sum of products})^2}{\text{sum of squares for } z} = 2,193 - \frac{2,665^2}{5,463}$$
$$= 2,193 - 1,300$$
$$= 893.$$

The estimation of β by b removes 1 DF from this sum of squares, and therefore the variance estimate is

$$s^2 = 893/17 = 52.5 \tag{10}$$

with 17 DF. This is substantially smaller than the mean squares in Tables 2 and 3, indicating that the estimate of the difference between drugs now achieved is more precise than that from y or y_1^*. In assessing the variance, account must be taken of the fact that b is only an estimate of β. This adds a term to the variance, in the standard manner of regression calculations. Equation 1 is modified to

$$\text{Var}\,(\bar{y}_A^* - \bar{y}_B^*) = \sigma^2 \left(\frac{1}{10} + \frac{1}{10} + \frac{(\bar{z}_A - \bar{z}_B)^2}{\Sigma_{zz}} \right), \tag{11}$$

where Σ_{zz} is the error sum of squares for the analysis of variance of z. Substitution of s^2 for σ^2 gives the estimated variance,

$$\text{var}\,(\bar{y}_A^* - \bar{y}_B^*) = 52.5 \left(\frac{1}{10} + \frac{1}{10} + \frac{(119.5 - 114.0)^2}{5,463} \right),$$
$$= 10.79, \tag{12}$$

and therefore

$$\bar{y}_A^* - \bar{y}_B^* = 9.8 \pm 3.28. \tag{13}$$

Note that comparison between the drugs in terms of y^* has led to a much smaller error than did either y or y_1^*. The advantage is best measured by the ratio of variances. From Equations 2 and 3, the precision of the estimation of drug differences is increased by the factor

$$\frac{24.36}{10.79} = 2.26. \tag{14}$$

Thus the covariance analysis has led to an estimation as precise as one based on analyzing y alone for an experiment with twenty-two or twenty-three subjects on each drug instead of ten. To analyze y alone gives a valid comparison of the drugs but represents a substantial sacrifice of information.

The method extends easily so as to permit covariance adjustment for two or more concomitant variates simultaneously. The theory is simple, though the computations can be laborious. Perhaps I should add that the arguments I have used above are equivalent to the more familiar textbook presentation of covariance analysis, in terms of adjusting treatment means of y to equality in x. The approach here has some advantages in logical generalization.

4. Combination of variates

Provided that the allocation of treatments to subjects has been performed properly, in accordance with the design adopted for the experiment and totally independently of any concomitant variates, the expectation of any concomitant variate (or of any specified function of concomitant variates) is the same for all treatments. Consequently, such a variate or function of variates may be subtracted from each response without affecting the validity of estimation of a difference between treatments in respect of the response variate. If y is a response and z_1 and z_2 are two concomitants, analyses of such composite variates as

$$y - 3 \log z_2,$$
$$y + z_1^2 - z_2^2,$$
$$y - \beta_1 z_1 - \beta_2 z_2 \quad \text{for any fixed } \beta_1, \beta_2,$$
$$y - \beta_1(z_1 z_2) - \beta_2(z_1/z_2) \tag{15}$$

are valid alternatives to analysis of y itself, if interest lies in the extent to which the mean value of y depends upon treatments. Of course, in general no interest attaches to an adjustment unless prior knowledge or evidence from the data indicates that it will improve the precision of comparisons of responses.

Commonly a composite variate is further adjusted by a constant so as to keep the general mean equal to the mean of all values of y; Equation 7 might have been modified to

$$y^* = y - \beta(z - \bar{z}), \tag{16}$$

where $\bar{z}$ (equal to 116.75) is the mean of all twenty initial blood pressures. This has the merit of aiding comparability between alternatives. Thus one obtains for the blood pressure example the following as three alternative sets of estimates:

β	Variate	A	B	Difference
0	y	86.0	73.5	12.5 ± 4.9
1	y_1^*	83.3	76.3	7.0 ± 5.1
b	y^*	84.7	74.9	9.8 ± 3.3

The covariance procedure involves taking a function of z that includes arbitrary multipliers and then determining these so as to maximize precision (minimize variance). To use a function such as

$$y - \beta_1 z - \beta_2 z^2 \tag{17}$$

is permissible, z^2 then being used in calculations exactly as if it were a concomitant distinct from z, but this seldom gives a further advantage.

An investigator who obtained results such as columns z and y in Table 1 might choose to measure response by final blood pressure expressed as a percentage of initial, that is to say by

$$p = 100y/z. \tag{18}$$

This is a major change in the scale of measurement; it cannot be assessed relative to y, y_1^*, and y^* in terms of precision, and a different letter has been used in order to emphasize the change. No rule of science demands that the effect of a drug on blood pressure be measured in percentage terms or that adjustment for initial values be made in this way rather than by Equation 4 or Equation 7; equally, no rule forbids this, and the procedure is reasonable. It leads to

$$\bar{p}_A - \bar{p}_B = 8.1 \pm 3.1. \tag{19}$$

The contrast between Equations 18 and 7 highlights a distinction between the responsibilities of the biologist and of the statistician. Measurement of the comparison between treatments by the use of Equation 7 with an optimally chosen β, rather than by the use of y alone, is largely a statistician's decision: he needs to be satisfied that randomization ensured that z was independent of treatment and that the regression of y on z is close to linearity over the range of values that matters, but he is then entitled to choose the covariance procedure purely in order to maximize the precision of treatment comparisons in respect of blood pressure differences. On the other hand, choice of the scale of measurement for comparing treatments rests with the biologist, who is at liberty to insist on using p instead of y if he wishes; indeed, he could choose to work on some other scale, such as z/y or $(y/z)^{1/2}$, if he thought this biologically more relevant. Whatever scale is chosen, the possibility of continuing with a covariance on the concomitant z remains. I here neglect questions of normality of distribution, which are different in character and often unimportant.

5. Multivariate techniques

If the experiment has produced several response variates y_1, y_2, y_3, etc., several lines of action are open. If each variate is of intrinsic importance (for example, if each relates to the effects of treatments on a distinct organ or function of the whole animal treated), a series of separate statistical analyses is likely to be appropriate. If a specified compound of the responses is of paramount importance, statistical analysis of this alone may extract all or most of the information in the experiment; for example, the y's might be weights of a certain substance excreted in successive days after treatment, and the sum for the first week could then be a particularly suitable compound variate. If the experiment is primarily for detecting whether treatments manifest *any* differences, one may form a compound of the y's that uses arbitrary coefficients, such as

$$y^* = \alpha_1 y_1 + \alpha_2 y_2 + \alpha_3 y_3, \tag{20}$$

and then determine these multipliers so as to maximize the criterion used in assessing statistical significance. To this category belong techniques of *discriminant function analysis*. They can be useful in biological assay, in which responses are not of intrinsic interest but are solely part of the machinery for discriminating between effects of different doses, and in statistical procedures for disease diagnosis. If the aims of the experiment are less definite than any of these, various procedures of multivariate analysis (canonical variates, principal components, etc.) may be used as aids to exploration; they may persuade the numerical observations themselves to indicate compound responses that well summarize the information or that deserve further study.

To the biologist, and sometimes also to the statistician, the choice is confusing. Variates of class 2 must be taken fully into account (explicitly or implicitly), for they represent the treatments under study. To neglect any variates of class 3 is almost always unwise, for they are integral to the structure of the experiment. Moreover, there is little doubt about how these two classes should enter into the analysis, and in a well-planned experiment dealing with them is usually fairly easy. The difficulties and the computing labor arise mostly in connection with variates of classes 1 and 4. What combination of variates of class 1 is most relevant to the problems that face the biologist? How far is it appropriate to let the experiment itself estimate the optimal combination? Is it appropriate to incorporate into the analysis adjustments for the accidental inequalities in variates of class 4 and, if so, how is this best done? Table 5 summarizes recommendations. Computers make practicable many multivariate analyses that previously were intolerably laborious, and even in category

4 of Table 5 a great amount of mathematical theory exists, but greater experience of the practical implications of alternative methods grouped in category 4 is needed before clear advice can be given.

TABLE 5   Summary of Recommendations on Multivariate Analysis

1. Variate(s) y to be studied without modification:
     Separate analysis on each of $y_1, y_2, y_3, \ldots$ needed, but remembering that two or more may be measuring related aspects of the phenomena studied and may therefore be closely correlated.
2. Treatments to be compared with maximal precision in respect of variate(s) y:
     As in category 1, with addition of covariance on one or more of variates z for each of variates y.
3. No intrinsic interest in y; objective primarily to find a characteristic in which treatment differences are most evident:
     Discriminant functions, combined with covariance on concomitants. Particularly relevant to classificatory questions, statistically aided diagnosis of disease, and biological assay (Finney, 1964, pp. 355–364).
4. Interrelation of variates the primary object of study:
     Canonical analyses and other techniques.

6. Bioassay with covariance

Although consideration of precision must always be to the fore in the planning and analysis of bioassays, examples of the use of covariance analysis are difficult to find. The first published discussion appears to have been that of Bliss and Marks (1939), and other applications were reported about the same period (Bliss, 1940; Bliss and Rose, 1940; Fieller et al., 1939; Fieller, 1940). Doubtless, since then the method has been an accepted, though infrequently used, part of statistical practice in bioassay. I have shown one example elsewhere (Finney 1964), but here I have chosen a different one. In the strictest sense, indeed, this example is not a bioassay, since it is concerned with comparing the potency of one drug under three sets of conditions rather than with estimating the potencies of two drugs relative to that of a standard; however, the computations are of the same form and the data ideally suited to my purpose.

Guillemin and Sakiz (1963) describe an experiment in which doses of 0.3, 0.9, and 2.7 μg of luteinizing hormone (LH) were injected into rats. The rats were of three types: "normal" (N), injected with prolactin 90 minutes previously (P), and hypophysectomized after prolactin injection (H). The experiment will be regarded as an "assay" of the effects of P and H on the potency of the hormone relative to the potency for N animals. The experiment was conducted on two days, twenty-seven rats per day being assigned three to each of the nine combinations of dose and N, P, and H. There were some slight differences in other conditions on the two days, and hereafter the days will be regarded as blocks I and II of the experiment. (The experiment in fact also included rats not injected with prolactin that were hypophysectomized but, for reasons explained by Guillemin and Sakiz, these are here omitted.)

The response to be used for the assay was the ascorbic acid content of the left ovary of each rat. The weight of each ovary was also recorded; this is most unlikely to have been affected by the hormones and will be used as a concomitant. Table 6 summarizes the totals of these two

TABLE 6 Data from an Experiment on Luteinizing Hormone: Totals for Doses and Days*

		Total	
Type of Rat	Dose of LH, μg	Response y	Ovary weight z
Normal (N)	0.3	357.5	569.8
	0.9	302.9	619.1
	2.7	158.5	584.4
		818.9	1,773.3
Prolactin-injected (P)	0.3	356.2	578.6
	0.9	289.3	598.0
	2.7	106.5	494.6
		752.0	1,671.2
Hypophysectomized (H)	0.3	334.0	525.1
	0.9	249.2	574.6
	2.7	233.7	683.3
		816.9	1,783.0
Grand total		2,387.8	5,227.5
Day 1		966.5	1,758.1
Day 2		1,421.3	3,469.4

* From Guillemin and Sakiz (1963). Individual values are not available.

variates for the three doses of each preparation in the units (unstated). From these totals and from the original records for individual rats, Table 7 was constructed on essentially the same plan as Table 4. This is to say, an analysis of variance for the response y in the standard form for a bioassay has been extended so as to contain an exactly similar analysis for the concomitant z; an analysis of sums of products is made by exactly the rule stated for Table 4.

Implicit in the calculation of Table 7 is a set of treatment variates and a classification variate (days). The doses of LH (Table 6) were geometrically spaced with ratio 3; if the regression of response on log dose

TABLE 7   Analysis of Covariance for Experiment on Luteinizing Hormone (Table 6)

Adjustments for means:	DF	506,051.0 z^2	231,152.3 yz	105,585.0 y^2
Blocks (days)	1	54,232.4	14,412.9	3,830.4
Types	2	426.3	260.5	161.0
Linear dose L	1	219.0	−1,354.2	8,372.2
Quadratic dose Q	1	201.7	186.4	172.3
Types × L (parallelism)	2	2,472.3	1,537.7	962.0
Types × Q (differences of quadratics)	2	510.6	532.4	558.3
Treatments	8	3,829.9	1,162.8	10,225.8
Error	44	16,057.6	9,742.9	7,294.1
Total	53	74,119.9	25,318.6	21,350.3

is linear, as may be expected, the main variate used for dose (x_3, below) will have equal spacing. Table 8 shows one possible set of eight treatment variates corresponding to the analysis in Table 7; alternative definitions of the pairs (x_1, x_2), (x_5, x_6), and (x_7, x_8) are permissible, but those used here have been chosen for simplicity and close correspondence with later stages of the analysis. The classification variate is most easily taken as $u = -1$ for each of the twenty-seven rats on the first day and $u = 1$ for each on the second day.

The coefficients in Table 8 can be used in the construction of the treatment components of Table 7 — a little awkwardly, because the contrasts to which they correspond have deliberately not been chosen as mutually orthogonal. The special advantage of the definition of treatment

TABLE 8   A Set of Treatment Variates for the Experiment on Luteinizing Hormone

Type of rat	Dose of LH, μg	Types x_1	x_2	Doses x_3 (L)	x_4 (Q)	Types × L x_5	x_6	Types × Q x_7	x_8
N	0.3	−1	−1	−1	1	1	1	−1	−1
	0.9	−1	−1	0	−2	0	0	2	2
	2.7	−1	−1	1	1	−1	−1	−1	−1
P	0.3	1	0	−1	1	−1	0	1	0
	0.9	1	0	0	−2	0	0	−2	0
	2.7	1	0	1	1	1	0	1	0
H	0.3	0	1	−1	1	0	−1	0	1
	0.9	0	1	0	−2	0	0	0	−2
	2.7	0	1	1	1	0	1	0	1

and classification variates appears when an experiment is less symmetrical and an analysis like that in Table 7 cannot be constructed directly; this is discussed further in Section 7.

From Table 7 the analysis proceeds somewhat as it did from Table 3. The regression coefficient of y on z is estimated (error line) as

$$b = \frac{9{,}742.9}{16{,}057.6} = 0.6067, \tag{21}$$

and the variance per observation is estimated from the residual sum of squares,

$$7{,}294.1 - 9{,}742.9^2/16{,}057.6 = 1{,}382.6 \tag{22}$$

with $(44 - 1)$ DF. A first step before estimating relative potency is to check various aspects of assay validity. This is achieved by taking each of four lines of Table 7 in turn, adding to the error line, and forming a reduced sum of squares exactly as in Equation 22. For example, for Q one forms

$$(7{,}294.1 + 172.3) - [(9{,}742.9 + 186.4)^2/$$
$$(16{,}057.6 + 201.7)] = 1{,}402.7. \tag{23}$$

The difference between this and the error residual is then the appropriate sum of squares for Q after adjustment of y by linear regression on z. Table 9 summarizes the four results.

TABLE 9 Validity Tests for Assay Calculations in Experiment on Luteinizing Hormone (after Adjustment for Regression of y on z)

	DF	SS	MS
Types	2	1.8	0.9
Q	1	20.1	20.1
Types $\times$ L	2	6.1	3.0
Types $\times$ Q	2	97.2	48.6
Residual error	43	1,382.6	32.15

If any mean square in Table 9 substantially exceeded the error mean square, the validity of the experiment for assay calculations would be in doubt. The logic is essentially as for assay data without covariance. In fact, inspection of Table 9 suffices to show that only one mean square exceeds the error and this not significantly. Assay calculations will therefore be described by using as the adjusted response, y^*, the original y adjusted for its linear regression on z. The error mean square,

$$s^2 = 32.15, \tag{24}$$

is so much smaller than the unadjusted value (165.8, Table 7) that a great gain in precision is almost certain. The variance of the regression coefficient is estimated as

$$\text{var}\,(b) = \frac{s^2}{16,057.6}. \tag{25}$$

The divisor is taken from the error line of Table 7, and the expression is best left in this form for the present.

Consider the calculations for the potency of H relative to N. The difference between the total responses of the two types (in the usual terminology of bioassay, the "preparations difference") is easily seen to be the sum of $x_2 y$; from this or from additions and subtractions in Table 6, the difference (a difference between two sets of eighteen rats) is

$$816.9 - 818.9 = -2.0.$$

The corresponding result for z is

$$1,783.0 - 1,773.3 = 9.7.$$

In terms of a single rat the adjusted difference between types is

$$\bar{y}_H^* - \bar{y}_N^* = (-2.0 - 9.7b)/18$$
$$= -0.4381 \tag{26}$$

with variance estimated as

$$\text{var}\,(\bar{y}_H^* - \bar{y}_N^*) = s^2\left(\frac{1}{18} + \frac{1}{18}\right) + \left(\frac{9.7}{18}\right)^2 \text{var}\,(b)$$
$$= s^2\left(\frac{1}{9} + \frac{0.2904}{16,057.6}\right). \tag{27}$$

The total difference between high and low doses is the sum of $x_3 y$; in this way or directly from Table 6 the value is found as

$$498.7 - 1,047.7 = -549.0,$$

with the corresponding difference for z,

$$1,762.3 - 1,673.5 = 88.8.$$

Hence the increase in response per rat for unit increase in log dose[1] (using logarithms to base 3 and remembering that the differences just calculated are between sets of eighteen rats at doses two units apart) is

$$(-549.0 - 88.8b)/(18 \times 2) = -16.75 \tag{28}$$

---

[1] In standard bioassay calculations *this* is the quantity usually denoted by b, the regression coefficient of response on log dose. In order to avoid confusion, I have here avoided using any symbol for it.

with variance

$$\frac{s^2}{4}\left(\frac{1}{18}+\frac{1}{18}\right)+\left(\frac{88.8}{36}\right)^2 \text{var}(b) = s^2\left(\frac{1}{36}+\frac{6.084}{16,057.6}\right). \tag{29}$$

Although the unadjusted "preparations" and "slope" contrasts for the assay are orthogonal, the regression adjustments that give rise to Equations 26 and 28 both involve b and therefore introduce a covariance estimated by

$$\left(\frac{-9.7}{18}\right)\left(\frac{-88.8}{36}\right)\text{var}(b) = \frac{1.3293}{16,057.6}s^2. \tag{30}$$

Hence the logarithmic relative potency (base 3) is, from Equations 26 and 28,

$$M = \frac{-0.4381}{-16.75} = 0.0262, \tag{31}$$

and the variance-covariance matrix for numerator and denominator is, from Equations 27, 29, and 30,

$$\begin{pmatrix} 3.5728 & 0.0027 \\ 0.0027 & 0.9052 \end{pmatrix}. \tag{32}$$

In this example omission of the terms arising from var (b) would have made a negligible difference, but of course with other data these may be important. Calculation of fiducial limits for M then follows by the usual application of Fieller's theorem to the ratio. This gives, at probability 0.95,

$$g = \frac{2.015^2 \times 0.9052}{16.75^2} = 0.0131. \tag{33}$$

The limits then are (Finney, 1964, Section 2.5):

$$\begin{aligned} M_\text{L}, M_\text{U} &= [0.0262 - 0.0000 \\ &\quad \pm (2.015/16.75)(3.5733 - 0.0468)^{1/2}]/0.9869 \\ &= (0.0262 \pm 0.2259)/0.9869 \\ &= -0.2024, 0.2554. \end{aligned} \tag{34}$$

Values of M have been calculated with the aid of logarithms to base 3 and must be multiplied by 0.47712 in order to be converted to base 10. The antilogarithms then give the estimated potency of H relative to N as 1.029, with 0.95 limits at 0.801, 1.314; these are almost exactly the results published by Guillemin and Sakiz (1.029, 0.800, 1.324). Similar calculations can be made for the relative potency of P.

7. Treatment and classification variates

For those familiar with analysis of variance who never encounter problems of nonorthogonality, explicit introduction of treatment and classification variates is clumsy and unnecessary. Sometimes, however, restrictions on the material available compel a lack of complete symmetry in design; sometimes accidents during an experiment cause loss of observations and a consequent nonorthogonality. Although many such complications can be dealt with by standard devices (for example, "missing value" techniques), a general procedure based upon multiple regression can aid systematic computation.

The example in Section 3 is so simple that no amount of misfortune could cause the analysis to develop orthogonality difficulties. Nevertheless, it can serve as an illustration. With x as defined in Table 1, a matrix of sums of squares and products of y, z, and x can be formed (all for deviations about means). This is

$$
\begin{array}{cccc}
 & y & z & x \\
y & 2{,}974 & 3{,}009 & -125 \\
z & & 5{,}614 & -55 \\
x & & & 20
\end{array}
\tag{35}
$$

with 19 DF. Note that the matrix corresponds to the "total" line of a covariance analysis; no calculation or subtraction of items for particular sources of variation is required. Next the linear regression of y on z and x is formed, an entirely routine operation. The inverse matrix for z and x is

$$
\begin{array}{ccc}
 & z & x \\
z & 0.000183058 & 0.00050341 \\
x & & 0.0513844
\end{array}
\tag{36}
$$

Hence the regression coefficients are

$$
b_z = 3{,}009 \times 0.000183058 - 125 \times 0.00050341 = 0.48790,
$$
$$
b_x = 3{,}009 \times 0.00050341 - 125 \times 0.0513844 = -4.9083. \tag{37}
$$

The residual mean square for y (17 DF) is

$$
s^2 = (2{,}974 - 3{,}009 b_z + 125 b_x)/17 = 52.5, \tag{38}
$$

exactly as in Equation 10. By standard regression theory,

$$
\mathrm{var}\,(b_x) = 0.0513844 s^2 = 2.70 = 1.64^2. \tag{39}
$$

Now b_x is the increase in y per unit increase in x, after adjustment of both variates for z. But the difference between drugs B and A is 2 on the scale of x. Hence the estimated difference in blood pressure between the drugs is obtained by doubling b_x:

$$\bar{y}_B^* - \bar{y}_A^* = -9.8 \pm 3.28, \tag{40}$$

which agrees perfectly with Equation 13.

The two methods of calculation are algebraically the same, although arithmetical rounding may produce minor discrepancies. In this example the computational labor is possibly a little greater than for the covariance analysis described in Section 3. It has the advantage of requiring no statistical theory other than the widely known techniques of multiple regression: a great many human computers and electronic computers are able to perform these calculations yet do not have skill in covariance analysis. Some loss of speed may be a small price to pay for the gain in convenience. The method requires no modification of principle when the numbers of animals in the groups are unequal, or when there are additional concomitant variates. Classification variates (u) can be similarly incorporated.

The same kind of analysis could be made for the LH experiment in Section 6, using the one classification variate required to discriminate between the two blocks and the treatment variates in Table 8. The matrix is given as Table 10 (53 DF). This is used in calculation of the linear regression equation of y on u, z, and the eight x variates. The residual sum of squares (43 DF) will reproduce that found in Equation 22. Tests of significance of the partial regression coefficients corresponding to x_1, x_2, x_4, x_5, x_6, x_7, and x_8 are exactly equivalent to tests of assay validity by significance tests in Table 9. The regression coefficient on x_3 is the estimated increase in response per rat for unit increase in log dose. The regression coefficient on x_2 is one-half the estimated mean difference in response between H and N animals. These responses have been "adjusted" for u and z by the regression calculations, and the numerical values will be in agreement with Equations 28 and 26, respectively. Moreover, the inverse matrix used in the regression calculations immediately leads to the variance and covariance estimates for the two regression coefficients, quantities which will be in numerical agreement with Equations 27, 29, and 30. Potency calculations can then be completed exactly as in Equations 31 to 34.

Inspection of Table 10 exposes both the strength and the weakness of this method of conducting the calculations. The method is powerful, in that it can be applied to an experiment of complicated design without special concern for the use of orthogonal contrasts and without close familiarity with covariance analysis. No change in computing instructions would have been required even if the symmetry of the experiment had been ruined by accidental loss of records for several of the fifty-four

TABLE 10 Matrix of Sums of Squares and Products (53 DF) for Experiment with Luteinizing Hormone

y	u	z	x_1	x_2	x_3	x_4	x_5	x_6	x_7	x_8
21,350.3	454.8	25,318.6	−66.9	−2.0	−549.0	−136.4	−50.7	98.7	−26.1	159.1
	54	1,711.3	0	0	0	0	0	0	0	0
		74,119.9	−102.1	9.7	88.8	−147.6	−98.6	143.6	−38.8	143.2
			36	18	0	0	0	0	0	0
				36	0	0	0	0	0	0
					36	0	0	0	0	0
						108	0	0	0	0
							24	12	0	0
								24	0	0
									72	36
										72

rats. On the other hand, the regression calculations invoke general procedures for the inversion of a 10×10 matrix, despite the fact that many of the off-diagonal elements are zero (and more could have been, by redefinition of x_2, x_6, and x_8). In a much larger and more complicated experiment, the price paid in computing time for a matrix inversion that takes no account of the special pattern of the matrix might be important. Indeed, classical covariance analysis may be regarded as a way of using the simplicity of the pattern and restricting formal general inversion to the much smaller matrix produced by the concomitants alone (in both my examples, a 1×1 matrix). Accidental loss of records or other disturbances of orthogonality will reduce the proportion of zero or very small off-diagonal elements, and will make general regression methods relatively more attractive.

I do not believe that either method of computation should be advocated as universally the best. For the user who occasionally encounters assay data among many other statistical problems and for the experimenter whose material forces him to tolerate "missing values" or other distortions of symmetry and balance, the multiple-regression method described in this section has many merits. On the other hand, the man who must analyze many assays may be wiser to invest in special skills and special programming appropriate to covariance analysis for balanced designs. Most important of all, consultation between experimenter and statistician on the efficiency of designs and on the planning of new assays is likely to be more fruitful if related to the covariance analysis; my experience is that complete reliance upon very general regression methods distracts attention from the special merits of balance in experimental design and encourages the false notion that, because almost any set of data can be analyzed by a computer, balanced arrangement of treatments and classifications no longer matters!

A further objection to *indiscriminate* use of the regression method is that a large experiment requires inversion of a large matrix. This can permit the solution to accumulate large or even disastrous errors of numerical rounding. The danger is small when a balanced experiment produces a matrix with as many zero cells as Table 10 has, but it can increase when departures from balance or flaws in experimental design make the matrix more complicated. The skilled computer user can do much by organizing his method so as to minimize the risk and to warn, if trouble arises, but the problems of doing so are by no means trivial.

8. Summary

Two examples of covariance analysis are presented in numerical detail, one for a simple comparison of treatments and one for a bioassay.

With them is associated a formal account of different systems of variates appropriate to the responses, treatments, classifications, and concomitants of any experiment, a discussion of the logic of covariance, and a brief summary of the roles of different types of multivariate analysis.

The chapter ends with a description of an alternative computational procedure, in which standard multiple-regression calculations are used instead of the special devices of classical covariance. The advantages and disadvantages of the two methods of computation are discussed critically.

The chapter is purely expository, and makes no pretence at introducing new statistical theory or presenting the results of experiments.

Acknowledgment

I am indebted to Dr. R. Guillemin for making available unpublished details of his computations, which have helped the presentation of Sections 5 and 6.

APPENDIX

This addendum, prepared by the editors, contains some of the algebraic and numerical details.

Equations 1 and 2

In general, the variance of the difference between two independent means is estimated as

$$\text{var}\,(\bar{y}_A - \bar{y}_B) = s^2\left(\frac{1}{n_A} + \frac{1}{n_B}\right), \tag{A1}$$

where s^2 is the mean square error from the corresponding analysis of variance. Hence, for the data in Section 3

$$\text{var}\,(\bar{y}_A - \bar{y}_B) = 121.8(\tfrac{1}{10} + \tfrac{1}{10}) = 24.36.$$

Equations 8, 10, 21, 22, 24, and 25

If Σ_{zz}, Σ_{yz}, and Σ_{yy} denote the sums of squares in the error line of an analysis-of-covariance table, the covariance regression is estimated as

$$b = \Sigma_{yz}/\Sigma_{zz}. \tag{A2}$$

For the reduced variate $y^* = y - bz$ the variance per observation is obtained as

$$s^2 = (\Sigma_{yy} - \Sigma_{yz}^2/\Sigma_{zz})/(\text{DF} - 1). \tag{A3}$$

An estimate of the variance of the covariance regression b is obtained as

$$\text{var}\,(b) = s^2/\Sigma_{zz}. \tag{A4}$$

For the data in Sections 3 and 6 an application of Equations A2, A3, and A4 gives Table A1.

Equations 9, 11, 12, 26, and 27

The covariance adjusted difference in means and its variance obtain from

$$\bar{y}_A^* - \bar{y}_B^* = (\bar{y}_A - b\bar{z}_A) - (\bar{y}_B - b\bar{z}_B),$$
$$= (\bar{y}_A - \bar{y}_B) - b(\bar{z}_A - \bar{z}_B), \tag{A5}$$

so that

$$\text{var}\,(\bar{y}_A^* - \bar{y}_B^*) = \text{var}\,(\bar{y}_A - \bar{y}_B) + (\bar{z}_A - \bar{z}_B)^2\,\text{var}\,(b),$$

which from Equations A1 and A4 gives

$$\text{var}\,(\bar{y}_A^* - \bar{y}_B^*) = s^2\left(\frac{1}{n_A} + \frac{1}{n_B} + \frac{(\bar{z}_A - \bar{z}_B)^2}{\Sigma_{zz}}\right). \tag{A6}$$

Application to the two examples gives Table A2.

Table 7

The analysis of variance in Table 7 is an extension of the two-way classification discussed on pp. 37–40 with nine treatments (three types times three doses) and two groups (days), but here with three rats per group per treatment. The full analysis of variance would yield

Term	DF
Treatments	8
Groups (days)	1
Treatments × groups	8
Residual	36
Total	53

The analysis of variance in Table 7 has an error term in which the treatments × groups and the residual terms are pooled.

Following a format similar to that described on p. 64, the subdivision of the degrees of freedom for the treatments sum of squares is indicated in Table A3, and the calculation of the cross-product terms is shown. To obtain the entries in the z^2 and y^2 columns of Table 7, replace the cross-product figures at the foot of Table A3 with the appropriate squared value; for example, for linear regression the entry under y^2 in Table 7 is $-549.0^2/36 = 8{,}372.2$ and that under z^2 is $88.8^2/36 = 219.0$.

Equations 28, 29, and 30

The adjusted increase in response per rat for unit increase in log dose may, alternatively, be estimated by means of the regression contrast in

TABLE A1

Term	Section 3		Section 6	
	Blood pressure data	Text eq.	LH bioassay	Text eq.
Covariance regression b	$2{,}665/5{,}463 = 0.488$	(8)	$9{,}742.9/16{,}057.6 = 0.6067$	(21)
Residual variance s^2	$\dfrac{2{,}193 - 2{,}665^2/5{,}463}{18 - 1} = 52.5$	(10)	$\dfrac{7{,}294.1 - 9{,}742.9^2/16{,}057.6}{44 - 1} = 32.15$	(22), (24)
Estimated variance of covariance regression, $\mathrm{var}(b)$	$\dfrac{52.5}{5{,}463} = 0.0096$		$\dfrac{32.15}{16{,}057.6} = 0.0020$	(25)

TABLE A2

Term	Section 3		Section 6	
	Blood pressure data	Text eq.	LH bioassay	Text eq.
Adjusted differences in means (Equation A5)	$\bar{y}_A^* - \bar{y}_B^* = (86.0 - 73.5) - 0.488(119.5 - 114.0)$ $= 9.8$	(9)	$\bar{y}_H^* - \bar{y}_N^* = \dfrac{-2.0}{18} - 0.6067\,\dfrac{9.7}{18}$ $= -0.4381$	(26)
Estimated variance of adjusted difference in means (Equation A6)	$\mathrm{var}(\bar{y}_A^* - \bar{y}_B^*) = 52.5\left(\dfrac{1}{10} + \dfrac{1}{10} + \dfrac{(119.5 - 114.0)^2}{5{,}463}\right)$ $= 10.79$	(11), (12)	$\mathrm{var}(\bar{y}_H^* - \bar{y}_N^*) = s^2\left(\dfrac{1}{18} + \dfrac{1}{18} + \dfrac{(9.7/18)^2}{16{,}057.6}\right)$ $= 0.111129s^2$	(27)

TABLE A3 Work Table for Subdivision of Treatments Sum of Squares in Table 7

Term	Coefficients of contrast (dose, μg)			Divisor		Variate	Main-effect contrast*	Entries for calculation of interaction by type†		
	0.3	0.9	2.7	Main effect	Interaction by type			N	P	H
Linear regression	−1	0	1	$2 \times 18 = 36$	$2 \times 6 = 12$	y	$-549.0 = L_{y,r}$	−199.0	−249.7	−100.3
						z	$88.8 = L_{z,r}$	14.6	−84.0	158.2
Quadratic curvature	1	−2	1	$6 \times 18 = 108$	$6 \times 6 = 36$	y	−136.4	−89.8	−115.9	69.3
						z	−147.6	−84.0	−122.8	59.2
Dose totals										
y:	1,047.7	841.4	498.7							
z:	1,673.5	1,791.7	1,762.3							

Calculation of cross-product terms (yz):

Types: $[(818.9)(1,773.3) + (752.0)(1,671.2) + (816.9)(1,783.0)]/18 - 231,152.3 = 260.5.$

Linear regression: $(-549.0)(88.8)/36 = 1,354.2.$

Quadratic curvature: $(-136.4)(-147.6)/108 = 186.4.$

Linear regression × types: $[(-199.0)(14.6) + (-249.7)(-84.0) + (-100.3)(158.2)]/12 - (-1,354.2) = 1,537.7.$

Quadratic curvature × types: $[(-89.8)(-84.0) + (-1,159)(-122.8) + (69.3)(59.2)]/36 - 186.4 = 532.4.$

* Result of applying coefficients of contrast to dose totals at foot of table.

† Result of applying coefficients of contrast to dose totals by type in Table 6 (e.g., $-199.0 = (-1)(357.5) + (0)(302.9) + (1)(158.5)$).

Table A3. Denoting the value of the regression contrast for y by $L_{y,r}$, that for z by $L_{z,r}$, and the divisor by D_r gives as an estimate

(28) $\qquad \dfrac{L_{y,r} - bL_{z,r}}{D_r} = \dfrac{-549.0 - (0.6067)(88.8)}{36} = -16.75.$ $\qquad$ (A7)

The estimated variance of the adjusted increase in response per rat for unit increase in log dose is found to be

$$\frac{s^2}{D_r} + \left(\frac{L_{z,r}}{D_r}\right)^2 \text{var}(b) = \left[\frac{1}{D_r} + \left(\frac{L_{z,r}}{D_r}\right)^2 \frac{1}{\Sigma_{zz}}\right]s^2$$

(29) $$= \left[\frac{1}{36} + \left(\frac{88.8}{36}\right)^2 \frac{1}{16{,}057.6}\right]s^2$$

$$= 0.028157s^2. \qquad \text{(A8)}$$

Since both the adjusted mean difference in response (Equation A5) and the adjusted increase in response per rat for unit increase in log dose (Equation A7) both involve b, it may be seen that their covariance is given by

(30) $\qquad (\bar{z}_H - \bar{z}_N)\dfrac{L_{z,r}}{D_r}\text{var}(b) = \dfrac{(\bar{z}_H - \bar{z}_N)L_{z,r}}{D_r\Sigma_{zz}}s^2$

$$= \frac{(9.7/18)88.8}{36(16{,}057.6)}s^2 = 0.000083s^2. \qquad \text{(A9)}$$

Equations 31, 33, and 34

The logarithmic relative potency is expressed as

(31) $\qquad M = \dfrac{\text{adjusted difference in means}}{\substack{\text{estimated increase in response per rat} \\ \text{for unit increase in log dose}}}$

$$= \frac{\text{Equation A5}}{\text{Equation A7}} = \frac{-0.4381}{-16.75} = 0.0262. \qquad \text{(A10)}$$

For M denote the variance of the numerator by $v_{11}s^2$ (Equation A6), the variance of the denominator by $v_{22}s^2$ (Equation A8), and the co-variance of the numerator and denominator by $v_{12}s^2$ (Equation A9). Then application of Fieller's theorem to determine 95% confidence limits on M gives (Finney, 1964, p. 28):

(33) $\qquad g = \dfrac{t^2s^2v_{22}}{(\text{denom. of }M)^2} = \dfrac{(2.015)^2(32.15)(0.028157)}{16.75^2}$

$$= 0.0131. \qquad \text{(A11)}$$

$$(34) \quad M_L, M_U = \frac{1}{1-g} \left\{ M - g\frac{v_{12}}{v_{22}} \pm \frac{ts}{\text{denom. of } M} \right.$$

$$\left. \times \left[v_{11} - 2Mv_{12} + M^2v_{22} - g\left(v_{11} - \frac{v_{12}^2}{v_{22}}\right) \right]^{1/2} \right\}$$

$$= \frac{1}{0.9869} \left\{ 0.0262 - 0.0131\frac{0.000083}{0.028157} \right.$$

$$\pm \frac{(2.015)(5.67)}{16.75}\left[0.111129 - 2(0.0262)(0.000083) \right.$$

$$+ 0.0262^2(0.028157)$$

$$\left. \left. - 0.0131\left(0.111129 - \frac{0.000083^2}{0.028157}\right) \right]^{1/2} \right\}$$

$$= (0.0262 \pm 0.2259)/0.9869$$

$$= -0.2024, 0.2554. \qquad\qquad (A12)$$

DISCUSSION

SMITH   With regard to the use of a generalized regression program, I agree that it can cause some difficulties. However, a carefully written general regression program that handles both balanced and unbalanced designs will account for patterns in matrices. Thus, it will invert the orthogonal portion first and then deal with the nonorthogonal portion.

FINNEY   Your comment is valuable. Unfortunately, one cannot safely assume that every program advocated for this purpose contains these precautions.

MCHUGH   With regard to the choice of measurement scale (Equation 18), in what situation is the percentage of initial the response with a sound biological rationale?

HIRSCH   There would be as much disagreement among endocrinologists about the appropriate way to measure the response as among statisticians about the method of analysis.

FINNEY   To use the percentage change rather than the absolute change implies a different question, but a question that commonly will have qualitatively the same answer. It is for the experimenter to say what question he will ask, although discussion with the statistician may often be helpful.

BORTH   Does not the population distribution of the parameter have some bearing on the choice of measurement scale? For example, suppose the y's are not normally distributed and the p's are.

FINNEY   I do not think a statistician *ought* to say, "It is easier for me to deal with a variate that is normally distributed, and therefore I choose p for analysis." Should he not, as Cochran said (p. 76), look for the analytical techniques appropriate to the scale on which the experimenter presents his results? The argument is tempting, because almost all of us are incompetent in dealing with a variate that is not normally distributed, but I believe the criterion for choice ought to be different.

LOWENSTEIN   For one faced with the problem of whether to do an analysis in absolute change, percent of y/z or z/y, I'd like to suggest the following: Compute the mean, standard deviation, and coefficient of variation (standard deviation divided by mean) for each alternative response scale, and then choose the scale that yields the lowest coefficient of variation.

FINNEY   In my view, this is sometimes excellent but sometimes inappropriate. If one's primary object is to show that treatments had differential effects on the animals, then I agree with you. You are suggesting a kind of discriminant technique, seeking a combination of variates that is most successful in detecting a difference. This applies also in deciding a suitable response metameter for bioassay. On the other hand, if one wishes to discuss the extent to which a particular property of the animals has been affected by treatments, one does not answer the question by analyzing a different variate that manifests proportionately greater effects. If one is interested in whether a particular drug affects the uterine weight of rats, it is no answer to discover effects on the angle of curl in the tail that are larger relative to their standard errors! Your proposal is less extreme.

RINARD   What is the consequence of nonnormality on F tests performed in an analysis of variance? Is one any more likely to be led into either rejecting a null hypothesis that is, in fact, true (Type I error) or failing to reject a null hypothesis that is, in fact, false (Type II error)?

FINNEY   It is impossible to assert any general effect in any one direction unless one knows rather more about the nature of nonnormality. Furthermore, my concern has been with estimating means and minimizing variances, not with tests of significance and Types I and II errors.

FORTIER   Regarding the use of covariance in bioassay, I should like to ask about the relative advantages of computing confidence limits on log potency from the adjusted treatment effects and the covariance-corrected error variance or from so-called "reduced" variances. Both procedures are described by Bliss (1952, pp. 532–533).

FINNEY The procedure that I described is not exactly the same as Bliss's computations from adjusted totals. Bliss explicitly neglected sampling variation in the regression coefficient. My formulæ, Equations 27, 29, and 30, take account of the variance of b. This makes my computations somewhat longer than Bliss's, but the results are then algebraically the same as those that he obtained from his second method, using reduced variances. Thus, Bliss's reduced-variance method and the one I have described should be identical with the accuracy of the arithmetic, whereas Bliss's first method is only an approximation. I think that the logic underlying the analysis is clearer in my method, and that is why I used it here, but it may necessitate a little more arithmetical labor than would reduced variances.

CHAPTER EIGHT

Obtaining Maximal Information from Bioassays

C. W. EMMENS

This chapter deals with the purposes for which biological assays are conducted, the different requirements that accompany different purposes, the sources of error and their control, and methods of exploring assay techniques. Attention will be confined to those assays applicable to endocrine research, omitting the more statistical aspects, which are considered in Chapters 4, 5, and 6.

1. Purposes of bioassay

Standardization

The standardization of preparations for use in research and clinical investigation or in treatment requires a high degree of accuracy and may demand repeated assays until predetermined limits of error are reached. Familiar examples are the standardization of commercial batches of such substances as insulin or the establishment of a new standard preparation. The greatest accuracy is required when contributions are being made toward the setting up of an international standard, when it is usual for assays to be conducted in laboratories scattered throughout the world so that a broad base is secured for making decisions.

A substance intended to serve as a standard or to receive wide circulation for clinical use naturally is prepared with all possible care and with the expectation that it will be homogeneous. However, occasions have arisen in which, because many assays were performed, heterogeneity was demonstrable. An example is given in Tables 1 and 2. These tables concern the setting up of an international standard of human chorionic gonadotropin (HCG), for which a number of preparations were offered. Since none was available in sufficient quantity, it was proposed that the final standard preparation be formed by mixing all those found suitable. Assays were performed by various methods in thirty-two laboratories, to ascertain the properties and relative potencies of the preparations.

TABLE 1   Intermethod and Intramethod Variances and Variance
Ratios of Estimates of the Potency of Each Preparation*

Preparation, PU no.	Type of variance,† method	DF	MS	Variance ratio‡	P
1	B	4	0.0872	0.90	< 0.95
	W	21	0.0787		
2	B	4	0.0240	1.22	< 0.95
	W	41	0.0292		
3	B	4	0.0469	1.09	< 0.95
	W	40	0.0511		
4	B	4	0.0168	8.26	> 0.95
	W	39	0.1391		
8	B	4	0.0375	2.19	< 0.95
	W	26	0.0820		
10	B	4	0.0364	1.22	< 0.95
	W	19	0.0445		

* Data of Emmens (1939a).   ‡ W ÷ B.
† B, between; W, within.

An undiluted sample of pregnancy urine, PU 5, was used as a tem-
porary standard preparation for the assay of the rest. Table 1 compares
the variances between and within the different test methods used,
irrespective of the laboratory in which the assays were carried out. These
variances are the mean squares for log estimates of relative potency, of
which 216 were available. It will be seen that the intermethod variation
approximated the intramethod variation in the case of 4 of the 6 preparations compared with PU 5. It was twice as large in another case, and 8
times as large in the case of PU 4, the last being statistically significant.
Thus, with that particular preparation the different test methods showed
closer agreement than could be expected from the distribution of results
within methods.

The explanation emerges upon examination of those estimates which
were made by different test methods but by the same person or laboratory with the same or similar animals (Table 2). The variances in this
sample tend to be smaller than in the complete data, although in no
single case is the difference significant. This follows because those
estimates which contributed an intralaboratory correlation to the estimate
of variance have been sorted out. In all cases the variance between
laboratories is greater than that within them and is significantly so for all
except PU 2. With the exception of this substance the greater part of the
variance of all estimates turns out to be, as expected, due to inter-
laboratory differences. Note that the estimates for PU 2 do not show this

TABLE 2 Interlaboratory and Intralaboratory Variances and Variance Ratios of Estimates of the Potency of Preparations Assayed by More Than One Method by the Same Laboratory*

Preparation, PU no	General MS	DF	Type of variance,† laboratories	DF	MS	Variance ratio	P
1	0.06000	12	B	4	0.12125	4.13	>0.950
			W	8	0.02937		
2	0.02626	27	B	10	0.03000	1.25	<0.950
			W	17	0.02406		
3	0.03912	25	B	9	0.06344	2.53	≈0.950
			W	16	0.02504		
4	0.09921	24	B	9	0.20677	5.96	>0.990
			W	15	0.03469		
8	0.08607	15	B	6	0.19133	39.78	>0.999
			W	9	0.00481		
10	0.01889	9	B	2	0.06450	10.93	>0.990
			W	7	0.00590		

* Data of Emmens (1939a).
† B, between; W, within.

phenomenon and that the others show it in varying degrees. This points strongly to the conclusion that the variation among estimates based on the same and different test methods in different laboratories is not necessarily greater than that among estimates based on different methods in the same laboratory. It is noteworthy that PU 2 was the only other undiluted extract being compared with the undiluted PU 5 as standard. Thus, there was evidence that those preparations which were diluted with inert material had not been diluted in a homogeneous manner prior to testing. PU 8 and PU 10 show significantly depressed intralaboratory differences relative to the rest and may give an exaggerated impression for this reason. However, PU 4, with more degrees of freedom for within-laboratory estimates, once more shows up as heterogeneous. After discussing this matter the manufacturers of PU 4 were inclined to agree that the mixing might not have been perfect. This preparation was not included in the eventual standard. Those which were included were carefully remixed beforehand.

This is a rather interesting example of bioassay revealing inequalities in preparations that might have been expected to be homogeneous.

Establishment of norms

In either laboratory or clinical experiments it may be necessary to establish the normal range of results to decide whether a particular sample or group of samples is abnormal. Many individual samples will be needed, and the extent of their variation will determine the assay accuracy required. If there is wide variation between samples, there is little point in determining their individual potencies with great accuracy.

Passing to material that does not have the status of a pure or semi-purified standard, one may also expect methods of assay to affect the results. A situation in which it does is shown in Table 3, where HCG is again the subject of investigation. HCG dissolved in saline, compared with HCG dissolved in serum or plasma, does not always give the expected mean potency ratio of 100%. The uterine weight test in rats yields approximately twice the potency expected and seen in other tests (upper half of the table). It is also apparent that the potency ratio is affected by the concentration of serum used in the tests (lower half of the table). Thus, care must be taken to compare like with like as strictly as possible. Any assumption inherent in comparisons made otherwise must be carefully examined.

TABLE 3   Comparison of Potency of HCG Dissolved in Saline with That Dissolved in Serum or Plasma by Various Assay Methods*

Method	Serum concn., % v/v	Mean potency ratio,†	Fiducial limits, % (P = 0.95)	Bibliog. ref.
Total prostatic wt. (intact rats)	100	106	84–132	Diczfalusy and Loraine (1955)
Seminal vesicle wt. (intact rats)	100	114	80–199	Diczfalusy and Loraine (1955)
Ventral prostatic wt. (hypophy-sectomized rats)	100	117	75–192	Diczfalusy and Loraine (1955)
Uterine wt. (intact rats)	100	190	160–230	Diczfalusy and Loraine (1955)
Expulsion of spermatozoa (*Rana esculenta*)	50 100	30 20	10–60 7–30	Salvatierra and Torres (1952)
Expulsion of spermatozoa (*Bufo viridis*)	100	170	150–190	Lunenfeld et al. (1957)
Ovarian hyperæmia (intact rats)	10 25–100	100 decreasing to 30% as serum concn. increased	not stated not stated	Albert and Berkson (1951)
	35 70 100	90 100 70	60–100 90–110 50–90	Borth, Lunenfeld and de Watteville (1957)

* After Borth et al. (1957), from Loraine (1957).
† The potency of HCG in 0.9% saline is assumed to be 100%.

Changes in individuals

Bioassay is often used to follow the changes in individuals resulting from treatment, the natural consequences of age or growth, or the effects of various rhythms. A reasonably high accuracy of assay will usually be necessary but, if the changes are large, the need for this decreases. Again, one method of assay may reveal changes that another does not.

An interesting example is given in Tables 4 and 5 and in Figure 1.

If HCG is injected into immature female mice, it increases their uterine weight by increasing ovarian steroid production. In intact mice tests conducted in the morning and afternoon of the same day show no difference in response to graded doses of HCG. However, if the mice are hypophysectomized immediately prior to injection, the response in the morning is less than that in the afternoon, four to five times the amount of hormone being necessary in the earlier part of the day (Table 4). In mice artificially subjected to a reversed light cycle and hypophysectomized before injection a reversal of this phenomenon occurs, the higher dose being required in the afternoon instead of in the morning (Figure 1). The analysis of variance is shown in Table 5.

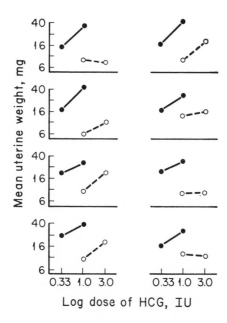

FIGURE 1   Uterine weights (mg) after HCG in mice from normal (left) and re-versed (right) light cycles after injection at four times during the day: (a) 5 A.M., (b) 8 A.M., (c) 5 P.M., (d) 8 P.M., (●) intact mice, (○) hypophysectomized mice. From Bindon and Lamond (1966).

TABLE 4* Effect of Circadian Rhythm on Responsiveness to Injected Gonadotropin

Mean uterine weights (mg ± standard error of the mean) of mice, in groups of six, injected with HCG morning or afternoon. Hypophysectomized mice were injected a few minutes after removal of pituitary gland.

	9–11 A.M., dose (IU)		
	0.33	1.0	3.0
Intact mice	15.3 ± 0.8	31.3 ± 2.3	36.2 ± 1.7
Hypophysectomized mice	7.5 ± 0.2	7.2 ± 0.3	16.9 ± 4.4
	3–5 P.M., dose (IU)		
	0.33	1.0	3.0
Intact mice	14.9 ± 0.9	37.7 ± 3.6	39.2 ± 2.1
Hypophysectomized mice	7.9 ± 0.8	20.6 ± 4.8	24.3 ± 4.9

Effective doses (IU) of HCG, calculated from results above, adjusted for body weight differences. Figures in parentheses are 95% limits of error.

	9–11 A.M.	3–5 P.M.
Intact	0.23 (0.17–0.31)	0.26 (0.21–0.33)
Hypophysectomized mice	2.64 (1.68–4.13)	0.58 (0.48–0.69)

* From Lamond and Bindon (1966).

The test reveals the following:

1. The participation of the animal's own pituitary gland in the response to injection of HCG.

2. The existence of a circadian rhythm that is light-dependent and the need for strict control of any assay based upon this technique. Not only is it essential to inject the standard and the unknown as nearly simultaneously as possible, but also it is essential to confine the injection period to a narrow time band if large errors of estimate are to be avoided.

Table 6 illustrates a similar circadian rhythm in blood levels of 17-hydroxycorticosteroids in normal young men. The early-morning levels are at least twice those seen by early afternoon. In this instance the time of sampling is important in comparing the hormone levels in different patients and in establishing norms. Many surveys have been made without attention to time of day or relationship to sleeping, eating, rest, or exercise — all factors now known to affect the level of many endocrine secretions.

TABLE 5   Analyses of Variance of Effect of HCG in Intact and Hypophysectomized Mice That Were on Reversed Light Cycles and Injected Twice per Day*

Source of variation	DF	MS
Hypophysectomized mice:		
Light treatment (L), normal versus reversed	1	2,689†
Time of injection (T), 9 to 10 A.M. vs. 3 to 4 P.M.	1	150
Dose		
Linear (D_L)	1	13,257†
Quadratic (D_Q)	1	230
Interactions		
$L \times T$	1	7,320†
$L \times D_L$	1	2,015‡
$L \times D_Q$	1	2,093‡
Remainder	4	289
Error	60	196.3
Intact mice:		
Light treatment, normal versus reversed	1	828‡
Time of injection, 9 to 10 A.M. vs. 3 to 4 P.M.	1	269
Dose	2	10,328†
Remainder	7	134
Error	46	95.0

* From Bindon and Lamond (1966).
† $P < 0.001$.
‡ $0.01 < P < 0.05$.

2. Sources of error

Sampling

Sampling from patients may be liable to other sources of error, in that duplicate samples taken at the same time may not, in fact, contain the same amount of active material. Adequate replication is often omitted at this stage and is sometimes difficult to obtain. Whenever possible, the true accuracy of bioassays should be determined by replicate sampling from the same initial source.

Treatment of samples

Treatment of samples, such as extraction and purification before use in assay, is liable to introduce further errors. With careful standardization

TABLE 6   Endogenous   Levels   of
Free 17-Hydroxycorticosteroids in
Three Normal Young Men During
the Forenoon*

	Level, μg/(100 ml)		
Time	I	II	III
8 A.M.	11.4	17.6	12.6
9 A.M.	10.4	15.0	—
10 A.M.	5.4	13.2	10.2
12 NOON	5.2	6.8	5.0
2 P.M.	6.0	7.8	3.4

* From Samuels et al. (1957).

of procedures these additional errors should be small, but they should also be checked. Chemistry is not always the exact science that it is sometimes assumed to be, and quite large differences in yield may follow small or even undetected changes in reagents or technique.

The assay itself

Every procedural detail in the performance of an assay may contribute to error. It is not even safe to assume that injection by one person is equivalent to injection by another. Table 7 shows a test of the activity of estradiol given intravaginally to ovariectomized mice and measured by vaginal smears. Portions of the same test solutions in which the total dose of estradiol was dissolved in 0.01 or 0.005 ml of saline solution were placed in the vagina by two different operators. Thereafter the assay was performed by one person alone, so that the only nonrandom source of variation was the placing of the test material at the site of action. It will be seen that a large difference in response occurred between operators

TABLE 7   Scores for Groups of 20 Mice Injected with 2 ×
0.005 ml or 2 × 0.01 ml of Test Solutions of Estradiol-3:17β
by Two Different Operators (Each Mouse Contributes a Potential Score of 2 to the Total, One for Each of Two Smears)*

Total dose of estradiol, μg × 10^{-4}	Volume of each injection			
	Operator I		Operator II	
	0.01 ml	0.005 ml	0.01 ml	0.005 ml
0.8	4	21	29	22
4.0	5	13	34	36
20.0	18	34	36	39
100.0	25	36	36	39

* From Emmens and Martin (1963).

when 0.01 ml of solution was used; a considerably smaller difference occurred with 0.005 ml. It so happens that 0.01, small though it may seem, is a sufficiently large volume for leakage to occur from the castrate mouse vagina if great care is not taken at the time of application. It is much safer to use 0.005 ml. Operator I, although taking all possible care, was less skilled than operator II, and a high proportion of the active material presumably was lost. As it seemed unlikely that the accidental leakage would be uniform, it was expected and found that operator II's results not only differed from those of operator I but were more reproducible. In the particular test shown in Table 7 operator II is working toward the top of the dose–response line throughout. This was necessary in order to reach it with 0.01 ml in the hands of operator I.

Reading and interpreting results

Objective measurements of results, such as the weight of an organ or the percentage of blood sugar, should not in themselves provide any very great source of variation. This may occur, however, if the operator is not skillful in dissection, in bleeding, in chemical manipulations, or even in the reading of the end point. Only meticulous care and knowledge of the characteristic errors of such tests can guide those concerned with biological assay in assessing their results. Where the reading of results is more subjective, as in the scoring of vaginal smears or the reading of agglutination tests, care should be taken to avoid bias resulting from prior knowledge of the expected outcome. In all instances it is best not to know the treatment that a group of animals has received until after all measurements are made. In cases of subjective judgment this becomes virtually a necessity. However, it seems rather uncommon for the laboratory worker to take this precaution.

Replication is therefore necessary to determine the various errors that may occur at different stages in the preparation of material and in its use in assays. Initially, duplicate samples should be processed and the various steps repeated from beginning to end of the assay. Only by such methods can the most rational way of conducting an assay, particularly of clinical material, be determined.

3. Exploring assay techniques

Factorial designs

Whenever possible, it pays to explore techniques of assay factorially. Contrary to expectation, animal experiments exhibit interactions between main effects less often than do experiments in such fields as agriculture and chemistry. This will be seen in the few examples quoted below.

A diagrammatic representation of the kind of factorial experiment that may be used in exploring the possibilities of an assay is shown in Figure 2 (experiment no. 1 of Claringbold and Lamond, 1957). In this experiment the response of the mouse uterus to gonadotropin (GA fraction of the urine of pregnant women) was being explored with treatment groups consisting of four mice each. Immature mice were allocated to cages at random, after which the whole cage was treated as an experimental unit. Three factors were investigated, each at three levels, giving a total of twenty-seven treatment groups. Doses were administered over three time periods: 72, 48, and 24 hours. Each dose was partitioned three ways into increasing, equal, or decreasing increments, and three different dose levels, of 4, 12, and 36 μg, were administered. The dependence of

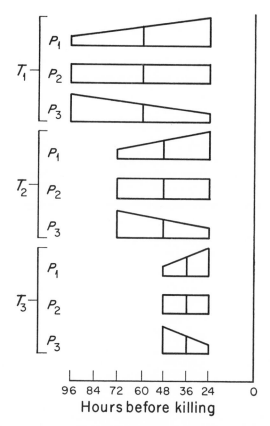

FIGURE 2 Diagrammatic representation of treatments. The abscissæ indicate the time T over which the injections were made. The ordinates represent the proportion P of the total dose given at each injection. Doses at three levels were given for each of the treatment combinations 4, 12, and 36 μg. From Claringbold and Lamond (1957).

variance on the response level necessitated a logarithmic transformation of the response. Covariance correction for body weight of animals was also used, which explains the dropping of a degree of freedom in the analysis of variance in Table 8.

The results (Table 8) show that three equal doses gave a greater response than either a decreasing or increasing series. Administraton over the shortest period gave the highest response. The slope of log dose versus log response increased as more of the dose was given in the first injection and was linear over all treatment combinations. Further exploration resulted in the administration of one injection of gonado-tropin 32 to 44 hours before killing the animals, since it was eventually found that the shortest time base possible, a combining of all doses into one, was optimal. Table 8 also reveals a linear relationship between length of time base and response and a linear relationship between dose level and response. The significant quadratic term under "Partition" in Table 8 simply indicates that three equal doses gave the highest response.

TABLE 8   Analysis of Variance of Results in Figure 2*

Source of variation	DF	MS
Time base	2	
Linear	1	2,532.3†
Quadratic	1	176.0
Partition	2	
Linear (P_L)	1	93.4
Quadratic	1	1,768.2‡
Levels	2	
Linear (L_L)	1	40,375.3†
Quadratic	1	210.0
Interactions	20	
$P_L \times L_L$	1	1,575.5§
Remainder	19	134.9
Error mean square	77	236.5

* The interactions listed as "remainder" were tested separately and, on being found not significant, were pooled to save space. The degrees of freedom of the error mean square are reduced by 4 owing to three missing values and one degree of freedom per covariance correction.

† $P < 0.001$.

‡ $0.01 \leq P \leq 0.001$.

§ $0.05 \leq P \leq 0.01$.

Only one out of twenty degrees of freedom for interaction shows significance at the 5% level, as would be expected by chance.

Table 9 illustrates the application of factorial technique at an early stage in the development of an assay with immature mice. The causes of death after hypophysectomy of weanling mice were being investigated. It was suspected that the technique of anæsthesia, the use of mice too soon after weaning, the air temperature at which they were kept after operation, and the withholding of glucose therapy might all contribute

TABLE 9   Surviving Hypophysectomized Immature Albino Mice*

	Treatments†			No. of surviving mice		
Anæsthetics	Days weaned	Air temp., °F	0.3 ml. glucose, I.P.	24 hr	48 hr	72 hr‡
Avertin (0.01 ml/g)	0	78	+	4	1	1 (1)
			−	5	4	3 (2)
		87	+	2	2	2 (2)
			−	5	4	3 (2)
	7	78	+	9	7	7 (4)
			−	7	7	7 (6)
		87	+	7	7	7 (2)
			−	8	8	7 (4)
Avertin (0.005 ml/g) plus ether	0	78	+	9	6	6 (5)
			−	9	7	6 (5)
		87	+	9	9	8 (7)
			−	10	10	10 (8)
	7	78	+	10	9	9 (8)
			−	9	9	9 (5)
		87	+	10	10	10 (7)
			−	9	9	9 (6)

Analysis of variance (completely hypophysectomized survivors):

Source of variation	DF	MS
Anæsthetics	1	1,853§
No. of days weaned	1	251
Air temperature	1	11
Glucose therapy	1	13
Interaction	11	84
Error variance	∞	82.1

* From Lamond and Emmens (1959).

† Ten mice per group.

‡ Figures in parentheses are completely hypophysectomized survivors.

§ $P < 0.001$.

to mortality. The analysis of variance at the bottom of Table 9 clearly implicated the technique of anæsthesia. The number of completely hypophysectomized survivors in groups of ten mice was used as the response, and the analysis was performed with the angular transformation.

Graded versus quantal responses

It is usually advisable to employ graded responses, such as body weight, organ weight, percentage of blood sugar, or any measure that can be quantitatively expressed, rather than quantal responses. It also pays to employ semiquantal responses, if these are possible, instead of completely quantal responses. The allotment of responses into grades 1, 2, 3, and 4, for example, will usually be superior to a purely quantal measurement. The weighting factors used in calculations with quantal responses by the probit technique illustrate that a graded response gives, on the average, about twice the information of a quantal response. In practice the use of graded responses is usually more valuable than this would indicate, since they can normally be measured over a wider range than quantal responses, without a high probability of running into extremes.

It is sometimes possible to transform what would otherwise be a quantal response into a graded response. Thus, when graded doses above the 100% level are administered so that all of the animals die, the quantal response of death or survival may be replaced with the time elapsing between injection and death. The quantal response of a positive or negative vaginal-smear result may be replaced with degree of response or with a biochemical measurement, such as triphenyltetrazolium reduction in the organ (Martin, 1960).

Quantal responses in groups of animals are preferable to a series of single observations at many different dose levels, as is commonplace in immunology. Some of the earlier immunoassays were so performed as to yield a series of pluses and minuses, only those tubes adjacent to the crossover point being informative. Such observations are better replaced with two or more groups within which the subjects receive identical treatment and therefore provide a typical quantal assay.

Interanimal and intra-animal measurements

Observations derived serially from the same animal may be four to six times as precise as observations made simultaneously upon different animals. Where it is impossible to repeat observations on the same animal, the use of littermates or sometimes of genetically homogeneous material is helpful.

Table 10 illustrates some of the gains realized from within-animal or within-litter comparisons and from the use of graded rather than quantal responses. In the assay of estrogenic hormone by the vaginal-smear

TABLE 10   Examples from Bioassay of Gain from Using Within-Animal or Within-Litter Comparisons and of Using Graded Rather than Quantal Response*

Type of assay		Comparable limits of error, % ($P = 0.99$)
Chorionic gonadotropin:	graded, within-litters	80–125
	graded, random animals	65–155
Serum gonadotropin:	graded, within-litters	90–111
	graded, random animals	80–125
Estrogenic hormone:	quantal, random animals	78–128
	quantal, within-animal	88–115
	graded, random animals	89–114

* From Emmens (1960).

technique a within-animal quantal response gave almost as accurate an assay as a graded response with different animals used simultaneously. The possibility of a within-animal quantal response with estrogenic hormones and insulin, when the same animals could be used again, had occurred to a number of workers. However, prior to the investigations of Claringbold (1956) the best attempts seem to have involved the use of small groups of animals as units in the assay.

The twin-crossover test for the assay of insulin provides a nice example of the use of an intra-animal technique for minimizing variability. In a typical twin-crossover test groups of animals are used on two successive days. The high dose of the standard, the low dose of the unknown, the low dose of the standard, and the high dose of the unknown are administered to different groups in all four possible ways. In Table 11 the results of a test with three rabbits per group are shown; these are expressed as the percentage reduction in blood sugar after the injection of insulin. The within-group variances s_Y^2 for the sum of the responses of individual animals and for their differences s_y^2 are determined as shown. In general, comparisons that can be built up from differences in response within animals have a lower variance than those that are built up from the sums of such responses. In other words, variation within animals is less than that between animals. The higher variance is associated with interaction; the lower variance, with main effects, such as doses, substances, and days. It may be noted that in the particular example shown the s_Y^2 of 733.1 compared with the s_y^2 of only 47.0 gives an unusually high ratio.

In the assay of a substance such as insulin it is important to measure differences between substances and the slope of the combined dose-response lines as precisely as possible. The precision is based on within-

TABLE 11   Twin-Crossover Test on Rabbits*

Group	Rabbit no.	Day 1†		Day 2†		Sum Y	Diff. y
1	1	S_2	14	U_1	10	24	4
	2	(0.5 u)	40	(0.25 u)	22	62	18
	3		33		36	69	−3
			87		68	155	19
2	4	S_1	26	U_2	48	74	−22
	5	(0.25 u)	4	(0.5 u)	14	18	−10
	6		13		30	43	−17
			43		92	135	−49
3	7	U_2	10	S_1	12	22	−2
	8	(0.5 u)	45	(0.25 u)	40	85	5
	9		29		26	55	3
			84		78	162	6
4	10	U_1	26	S_2	28	54	−2
	11	(0.25 u)	32	(0.5 u)	39	71	−7
	12		8		16	24	−8
			66		83	149	−17

Within-groups variance:

For sum, $s_Y^2 = 733.1$ For difference, $s_y^2 = 43.5$

$$1/w = 1/n_1 + 1/n_2 + 1/n_3 + 1/n_4 = \tfrac{4}{3}$$
$$1/W = -1/n_1 + 1/n_2 + 1/n_3 - 1/n_4 = 0$$

* Results are percent reduction in blood sugar after injection.

† S, standard; U, unknown; u, unit.

animal variation. It is assumed that the standard and unknown preparations have the same slope. This assumption (parallelism) can be verified, but only at a lower level of precision, that is, one involving the between-animal variation. Details of the arrangement of the results of a twin-crossover test for computing are shown in Table 12.

TABLE 12   Twin-Crossover Test Rearranged for Computing

Group no.	No. of animals*	Mean response				Sum Y	Diff. y
1	3	S_2	29.00	U_1	22.67	51.67	6.33
2	3	S_1	14.33	U_2	30.67	45.00	−16.33
3	3	S_1	26.00	U_2	28.00	54.00	−2.00
4	3	S_2	27.67	U_1	22.00	49.67	5.67
						Total:	−6.33

* This need not be constant for this type of computation.

The details of the computation needed are as follows.

Departure from parallelism of substance is measured by:

$$Y_1 - Y_2 - Y_3 + Y_4, \quad \text{with variance } s_Y^2/w$$
$$= 51.67 - 45.00 - 54.00 + 49.67, \quad \text{with variance } 733.1 \times \tfrac{4}{3}$$
$$= 2.34 \pm 31.3 \text{ approx.}; \quad \text{not significant.}$$

Calculations of M and fiducial limits:

$$M = I \sum y/(-y_1 + y_2 + y_3 - y_4), \quad I = \log \text{ dose interval}$$
$$= (0.3010)(-6.33)/(-30.33)$$
$$= 0.06282$$

$$\text{Potency ratio} = \text{antilog}_{10} M = 1.156$$

Limits are given by:

(i) $F = 5.32$ for 1 and $(\sum n_i - 4)$ DF at 5% probability

(ii) $U^2 = (-y_1 + y_2 + y_3 - y_4)^2 - Fs_y^2/w$
$$= (-30.33)^2 - 5.32 \times 43.5 \times \tfrac{4}{3}$$
$$= 919.91 - 308.56$$
$$= 611.35, \quad \text{since positive, real limits exist.}$$

(iii) $UT = (-y_1 + y_2 + y_3 - y_4) \sum y - Fs_y^2/W, \quad T = \sum y$
$$= (-30.33)(-6.33) - 0$$
$$= 191.99$$

(iv)   Limits are the roots of:
$$U^2 m^2 - 2UTIm + T^2 I^2 = 0, \quad \text{solving for } m$$
$$611.35 m^2 - 2 \times 191.99 \times 0.3010 m + (-6.33)^2 \times 0.3010^2 = 0$$
$$611.35 m^2 - 115.58 m + 3.6303 = 0$$
$$m^2 - 0.18906 m + 0.0059382 = 0$$
$$(m - 0.09453)^2 - 0.09453^2 = -0.0059382$$
$$m - 0.09453 = \pm 0.05475$$
$$m = 0.09453 \pm 0.05475 = 0.03978 \text{ and } 0.14928$$
$$\text{Antilog}_{10} m = 1.096 \text{ and } 1.410$$

In Table 13 the comparisons for the analysis of variance of such a test are given, illustrating the association of main effects with the smaller error variance and of first-order interactions with the larger one.

TABLE 13 Orthogonal Comparisons for the Factorial Analysis of the Twin-Crossover Test

Comparison	Coefficients of comparison*								Sum that variance relates to
Group:†	1		2		3		4		
Day:‡	1	2	1	2	1	2	1	2	
Substance:	S_1	U_2	S_2	U_1	U_1	S_2	U_2	S_1	
Days	+1	−1	+1	−1	+1	−1	+1	−1	s_y^2
Substances	+1	−1	+1	−1	−1	+1	−1	+1	s_y^2
Doses	+1	−1	−1	+1	+1	−1	−1	+1	s_y^2
Day × sub.	+1	+1	+1	+1	−1	−1	−1	−1	s_Y^2
Day × dose	+1	+1	−1	−1	+1	+1	−1	−1	s_Y^2
Sub. × dose	+1	+1	−1	−1	−1	−1	+1	+1	s_Y^2
Day × sub. × dose	+1	−1	−1	+1	−1	+1	+1	−1	s_y^2

* Comparisons that can be built up from differences *within* groups have the lower variance, associated with s_y^2, and these are the important ones in the table.

† "Group" can be same operators, animals, flasks, instruments, etc.

‡ "Day" can be two separate occasions, members of a litter, etc.

Intra-animal quantal assays

An example of an intra-animal quantal assay introduced by Claringbold (1956) is given in Table 14. This was an assay of estrogenic hormone in mice by the vaginal-smear technique. It was repeated on four separate occasions with twenty-four animals, so that each group had all possible doses of standard and unknown in a series of Latin squares, the design of the assay being 2 × 2. Each animal having been standardized beforehand by the staircase, or up-and-down, procedure (see Chapter 11), its approximate level of sensitivity was known. The doses of the standard and the unknown were in constant ratio but scaled to individual sensitivity. This procedure avoids areas of 0 or 100% response. In the assay under discussion no animal responded negatively, and only one responded positively throughout.

To perform an analysis by the probit or even by the angular transformation with such an assay would be tedious; in a twin-crossover or similar test it would be impossible. Instead of attempting this Claringbold utilized a direct analysis of variance of the crude score 0 or 1, which is presented in Table 15. The results are, to say the least, pleasing. They illustrate that the sensitivity of the different animals was so accurately located that there were no significant differences between them in the analysis (not that this would matter). The only significant difference was between standard and unknown, with an error term approximately a

Table 14   Results Obtained in Four-Point Crossover Assay with Quantal Responses*

Latin square	Mouse No.	Mean sensit., 10^{-4} μg	Tests 1st	2nd	3rd	4th	Responses S_L	S_H	U_L	U_H
I	1	4	S_L	S_H	U_L	U_H	0	1	0	1
	2	2	U_L	S_L	U_H	S_H	0	1	1	1
	3	8	U_H	U_L	S_H	S_L	0	1	0	1
	4	23	S_H	U_H	S_L	U_L	0	1	1	0
II	5	8	S_H	U_H	S_L	U_L	0	1	0	1
	6	6	U_L	S_H	U_H	S_L	0	1	0	1
	7	4	U_H	S_L	U_L	S_H	0	0	1	1
	8	4	S_L	U_L	S_H	U_H	0	1	0	1
III	9	3	U_H	S_H	S_L	U_L	0	0	0	1
	10	11	S_H	U_H	U_L	S_L	0	1	0	1
	11	3	S_L	U_L	S_H	U_H	0	1	1	1
	12	11	U_L	S_L	U_H	S_H	0	1	1	1
IV	13	8	U_H	S_H	S_L	U_L	0	1	0	1
	14	16	U_L	S_L	S_H	U_H	1	1	1	1
	15	4	S_L	U_H	U_L	S_H	0	1	0	1
	16	8	S_H	U_L	U_H	S_L	0	0	1	1
V	17	3	U_L	S_L	U_H	S_H	0	1	0	1
	18	23	U_H	U_L	S_H	S_L	0	1	1	1
	19	1	S_H	U_H	S_L	U_L	0	1	0	1
	20	23	S_L	S_H	U_L	U_H	0	1	1	1
VI	21	6	S_L	U_H	S_H	U_L	1	1	1	1
	22	1	U_H	S_H	U_L	S_L	0	0	1	1
	23	3	U_L	S_L	S_H	S_H	0	1	0	1
	24	11	S_H	U_L	S_L	U_H	0	1	0	1

* From Claringbold (1956).

Table 15   Analysis of Variance of Data in Table 14*

Source of variation	DF	MS
Animals	23	0.12
Times	3	0.05
Slope	1	0.38†
Preparations	1	1.50‡
Parallelism	1	0.38
Error	66	0.138

* From Claringbold (1956).
† $P < 0.001$.
‡ $P < 0.01$.

quarter of that normally encountered in quantal assays by the vaginal-smear technique. Further assays of a similar design confirm that this is a regular finding. To those who may be shocked by the use of the crude response without transformation it may be pointed out that, if desired, the results from an analysis such as that presented in Table 15 may be used as the entering approximation to probits or angles. In such cases it has never been found necessary to perform a further cycle of iteration. The results of zero-one analysis do not differ substantially from those found by more orthodox methods. Nevertheless, it is not recommended for the analysis of straightforward quantal assays when the numbers of groups and the total number of observations are small.

4. General recommendations

In summary, it is best to keep an assay as simple as possible after once having decided on a particular technique, to keep it balanced both in numbers of animals per group and in the dose ratio of standard and unknown, to make within-animals observations whenever possible, and to employ graded rather than quantal responses.

To this it should be added that accuracy is rarely improved by expressing results in a complicated manner. It does not follow that an organ weight expressed as a percentage of body weight or a fall in blood sugar expressed as a percentage of the initial blood sugar level is necessarily superior. Whenever possible, covariance techniques should be employed to determine the optimal relationship. In the assay of insulin quoted above the percentage reduction in blood sugar was used merely because these were the figures available for analysis. In the fully developed assay several measurements were made of blood sugar levels after injection; their mean was expressed as a percentage reduction from the initial level and corrected by covariance for the initial level. It was subsequently shown that a single determination of blood sugar level two hours after injection could be employed without knowledge of any other measurements. The value of more complicated procedures should never be assumed, since it depends on correlations between measurements. A sum or difference of two uncorrelated variables has, for instance, a variance equal to the added variances of the two.

In large-scale assays, particularly those which extend over a period of some time, some animals may die or some observations may be lost, disturbing the initial balance. There are techniques for adjusting for missing values. However, it is often easier for the experimenter to include one or two extra animals per group and to reject results at random from those groups whose eventual number is greater than the smallest. With only a little extra practical work this method yields an unbiased, balanced experiment so long as animals do not die because of treatment effects (the latter can be examined in several ways). With the use of computers it is, of course, less necessary to rely on such precautions, just as it is less necessary to worry about complicated analyses. However, if a computer is not available, the bioassayist will find it easier to anticipate trouble than to deal with it afterwards.

DISCUSSION

ARMITAGE   I have a comment on Table 14. I have recently been analyzing a number of similar sets of data in which the individual responses were zeros and ones. I have used a generalization of the usual probit or logistic model in which there is more than one independent variable, with dummy variables, as employed in Chapter 7 (p. 180). General computer programs are available for the procedure. I have always found that the results of this sort of analysis are very much the same as one would obtain by analyzing zeros and ones. I suspect that the reason for this is that in my examples the average number of zeros is about half the total number of observations. It is likely that most of the observations are at factor combinations for which the probability of a 1 is neither very low nor very high. I suspect, however, that in other circumstances there might be quite a difference between the assumptions of constant variance and additivity on the zero-one scale, which were made in Table 14, and the corresponding assumptions on the logit or probit scales. I cannot, however, produce examples to back up that assertion.

EMMENS   I entirely agree. I should perhaps have added that I would not advocate using the zero-one techniques in the following circumstances: when samples are small, as is the case in ordinary assay, and when banks of 0 and 100% are obtained. Claringbold and his colleagues (1953) have put forward laboratory techniques by which one avoids the latter. This involves fitting results into what we define as the region of useful information, using, for example, parallelogram designs.

DIXON   Cochran (1954) pointed out that analysis of variance of zero-one data yields essentially what the chi-square techniques produce. He also stressed what was stated concerning the importance of the fractions' being near 50%. The speaker indicated that Claringbold succeeded in designing his experiments so that the number of zeros and ones came out sufficiently balanced for a good analysis. The up-and-down procedure is designed specifically for that purpose.

Are there instances in which quantal response would result in a better analysis than a graded response?

EMMENS   I certainly haven't found it in my own experience, nor can I recall an instance in the literature in which this was shown to be the case.

SMITH   When I look at an analysis like that set out in Table 15 I am concerned by the fact that significance tests are performed. I look at the degrees of freedom and visualize an F statistic with one degree of freedom in the numerator and sixty-six in the denominator. From the point of view of design and significance testing one could substantially reduce the degrees of freedom in error without radically changing the critical value for an F statistic. I question whether such an elaborate design with so many degrees of freedom allocated to the error term is actually an efficient way of doing such experimentation.

EMMENS   A fair comment on behalf of the author would be that at this stage he was more interested in demonstrating what sort of error occurred. This was a new technique, and his method consisted of first exploring the use of quantal responses in this particular type of test. He was more concerned with an adequate estimation of the error term than with anything else.

RODBARD   When faced with an array of quantal data like that in Table 14, might one consider the use of nonparametric tests? These techniques may be more powerful, especially when the underlying assumptions of the analysis of variance are violated.

FINNEY   This experiment was an *assay*. The major objective was once again an estimate of the potency, and for adequate precision high replication was required. This gave rise to the large number of degrees of freedom for error. Nonparametric tests might be relevant to the examination of parallelism and the difference between preparations but not to the major purpose, which is estimation.

SMITH   I understand that in this case the sixty-six degrees of freedom were needed for estimation of the error variance. However, when does the estimate of variance become critical with respect to degrees of freedom?

FINNEY   Because this was an exploration of a new statistical technique, many degrees of freedom were wanted in the error. But this is not my point; in the general use of this statistical technique for analyzing bioassays I do not think it important. What was important was replication for ensuring that the means for the different treatments (doses) had a large value of n in forming a σ^2/n. Consequently (but incidentally) this gives a large number of degrees of freedom for estimating error. I agree completely with Dr. Smith that, in the general design of experiments, to have as many as sixty error degrees of freedom is extravagant. I would try to keep down to something like twenty; I would expect to transfer, by suitable factorial design, many degrees of freedom to the estimation of useful contrasts among treatments, hoping in doing this not to sacrifice the overall replication.

ARMITAGE   There is another way of looking at the mean square on sixty-six degrees of freedom. It provides a test of the adequacy of the model, since there is a theoretical error term here. The variance of any one observation is pq, where p is the estimated probability of a 1. I suspect that, if one estimated this probability for all of the observations and averaged the values of pq, the result would not be very different from the value 0.138. This is equivalent to what happens in the use of a probit or logistic model, in which one has effectively an infinite number of degrees of freedom for the theoretical variance, and the sixty-six degrees of freedom again tests the adequacy of the model.

EMMENS   In my more ponderous and unadjusted 8×8 Latin square, referred to on p. 17, I found that the error term was about what was expected, if one obtained it within a homogeneous group such as one of the Latin squares. If the error term was derived from the entire experiment, there was heterogeneity, and the error term was inflated to approximately twice what was expected.

BANGHAM   To reopen the subject of obtaining maximal information from bioassays: how should one deal with a mass of assay data in which half the assays may be invalid for one reason or another? It seems a pity to throw away a large body of data simply on these grounds.

EMMENS   One cannot make general remarks without having the data. If I had collaborative assays, and some missing assays would seriously interfere with an easy interpretation of the whole lot, I would not discard any results very willingly. If I had a set of assays gathered from here and there, I would not hesitate to throw a few out, for what seemed to be adequate reasons.

BANGHAM   That is a point that makes me feel uncomfortable, because assays discarded on grounds of statistical invalidity may be the very ones that distinguish the dissimilarity we should be taking note of. Although there is a convention that one use so-called valid assays to derive a potency figure, it may be that one should really use the invalid ones.

CHAPTER NINE

Nonparametric Statistics

I. RICHARD SAVAGE

1. Introduction

The purpose of this chapter[1] is to consider how the need for nonparametric procedures arises by using an endocrinological example. Section 2 concerns the analysis of data from matched observations, and Section 3 contains an introduction to the nonparametric comparison of two samples.

The data are taken from an experiment reported by Kaneto et al. (1967) concerning the effect of vagal nerve stimulation on insulin secretion. The subjects were twenty-seven mongrel dogs with body weights varying from 8.1 to 17.7 kg. The radical differences in their weights show clearly that the experimental material is very heterogeneous. The animals were divided into four groups in some manner not specified, and the experiment was conducted.

In analyzing their data the investigators did not utilize the t or F statistics but elected to employ a very simple approach: they used the Wilcoxon signed-rank procedure, which is discussed below. I shall work through some of the methods they chose and indicate why their approach seems reasonable, considering the nature of their experimental material. When one is confronted with poor material, a natural question is, Why do the experiment? The answer is that one may be able to extract a modicum of information notwithstanding and that it may be exceedingly difficult to do a good experiment. The alternative to the performance of an experiment with deficiencies may be no experiment at all.

2. Data from matched samples

The data from the first group of seven dogs are reproduced in Table 1. It was important to compare the amount of immunoreactive

---

[1] The viewpoint taken herein is compatible with the frequentist conception of the foundations of statistics, which stresses tests of significance. My own viewpoint is the Bayesian, in which subjective probability distributions are assigned to the population parameters of the statistical model. Both viewpoints raise similar questions but provide different answers. To those interested in exploring the Bayesian position I recommend papers by Edwards et al. (1963) and Mosteller and Tukey (1968).

TABLE 1   Effect of Stimulating the Dog's Left Cervical Vagus on Blood Levels of Immunoreactive Insulin and Sugar*

Expt. no.	F_1	F_2	\multicolumn{5}{c}{Time, min†}				
			0	5	10	30	60
Immunoreactive insulin, µU/ml:							
			\multicolumn{5}{c}{*Pancreatic venous plasma*}				
1	290	350	700	480	840	580	910
2	140	200	260	130	90	100	130
3	190	240	680	250	200	90	160
4	170	290	640	310	270	360	370
5	60	90	460	280	300	180	310
6	320	370	1,550	1,450	840	560	440
7	310	240	410	280	300	430	—
Mean ± SD:	211 ± 90	254 ± 88	671 ± 389	454 ± 417	405 ± 282	328 ± 164	386 ± 257
p:‡			<0.05	>0.05	>0.05	>0.05	>0.05
			\multicolumn{5}{c}{*Femoral venous plasma*}				
1	45	38	30	45	36	34	33
2	5	4	5	5	7	4	7
3	15	16	22	18	11	11	17
4	27	23	29	26	24	39	29
5	21	22	33	27	22	23	20
6	27	27	83	90	44	32	30
7	41	38	47	44	38	65	64
Mean ± SD:	25.8 ± 12.9	24.0 ± 11.1	35.5 ± 22.6	36.4 ± 25.4	26.0 ± 12.9	29.7 ± 18.5	28.5 ± 16.6
p:‡			>0.05	<0.05	>0.05	>0.05	>0.05

Blood sugar, mg/(100 ml):

Pancreatic venous plasma

1	143	146	138	133	134	130	113
2	106	106	99	106	98	107	109
3	107	111	101	109	103	99	116
4	121	127	134	128	131	129	111
5	123	117	130	115	128	124	128
6	95	91	97	101	103	98	94
7	129	132	132	128	122	137	136
Mean ± SD:	117.7 ± 14.5	118.5 ± 16.8	118.7 ± 17.2	117.1 ± 11.5	117.0 ± 14.0	117.7 ± 14.8	115.2 ± 12.5
p:‡			>0.05	>0.05	>0.05	>0.05	>0.05

Femoral venous plasma

1	129	136	140	131	122	130	134
2	96	98	89	95	91	89	100
3	102	94	103	102	103	100	105
4	113	123	121	125	124	133	121
5	121	123	130	125	125	126	117
6	102	99	113	118	116	113	95
7	126	129	131	131	130	133	134
Mean ± SD:	112.7 ± 10.7	114.5 ± 15.8	118.1 ± 16.4	118.1 ± 13.2	115.8 ± 12.9	117.7 ± 16.2	115.1 ± 14.5
p:‡			>0.05	>0.05	>0.05	>0.05	>0.05

* Data from Kaneto et al. (1967).
† F_1 and F_2, prestimulation values before and after sectioning of vagus nerve, respectively.
‡ The p values refer to F_2 prestimulation versus poststimulation values when the Wilcoxon signed-rank test is applied.

insulin just before the stimulation of the left vagus nerve (F_2) with the amount measured immediately after stimulation (0). A natural hypothesis would be that stimulation of the vagus nerve increases the blood level of immunoreactive insulin. This seems to be borne out by the data, in that all of the seven differences were positive. A frequently used test of significance, such as the t test, would examine the null hypothesis that the treatment had no effect — that is, that the means of the underlying populations were equal. It would be based upon the assumption that the samples had been taken from an underlying normal population.

An alternative to the mean as a measure of location, or central tendency, of a population is the median. The median of a population is the middle observation: half the values in the population exceed it, and half fall short of it. Of a population that is normally distributed (in fact, of any population that is symmetric) the mean and median are identical. However, if the distribution is skewed, the median may constitute a more descriptive average than the mean. If the data are such that it seems wiser to avoid specifying the distribution from which one is sampling, the median is a reasonable measure of central tendency. Null hypotheses regarding the medians of underlying populations are the concern of this section.

The authors avoided using a t test for their comparison. Let us endeavor to see why:

1. A prerequisite of the use of the t test is that there be random sampling from the underlying population. The dogs in this experiment can hardly be considered to constitute a random sample from a well-defined population.

2. A further prerequisite of t-test use, especially with small sample sizes, is that the underlying population be normally distributed. There are two indications that the data do not arise from a normal population. The first is the coarse appearance of the measurements, which for immunoreactive insulin extend from 60 to 1,550. The second is the similarity in magnitude of the standard deviations and the means. If measurements are normally distributed, the existence of standard deviations that approximate the mean in magnitude implies the existence of a substantial proportion of negative measurements. Since in this case the quantity being measured must be positive, the assumption of a normal population is not warranted.

The first point, that these are not random samples from some underlying population, is the more important argument against the use of t procedures.

In the first test of significance to be considered here one calculates the difference in each pair of matched observations (for example, 0 min and

F_2). These differences are (1) 350 (or 700 − 350), (2) 60, (3) 440, (4) 350, (5) 370, (6) 1,180, and (7) 170. First we shall consider only the signs, plus and minus, of the observed differences.

If vagal nerve stimulation had no effect on response, each difference would result entirely from random errors of measurement. These random errors should have a median of zero, so that plus and minus signs are equally likely. The differences observed yield 7 plus signs out of 7. Assuming that the observations of each animal were independently determined (which appears to be the case), the chance of obtaining all 7 plus signs when plus and minus signs are equally likely is the same as the chance of 7 heads with a fair coin tossed 7 times. This probability is $(1/2)^7 = 1/128$, which is, indeed, small. Hence, one might reasonably reject the null hypothesis of no stimulus effect.

The procedure described above[2] is an application of the *sign test*. The algebraic sign of the difference was the only aspect of the data used in conducting the test. Further, a one-sided sign test was employed. This is appropriate to these data, since one would not regard the stimulus as possibly reducing the level of immunoreactive insulin. A two-sided test would have considered the possibility of either 0 or 7 plus signs. The corresponding chance is $2(1/2)^7 = 1/64$ which, again, is small. Hence a two-sided sign test would also have rejected the null hypothesis of no effect of stimulation.

In general, the sign test consists of determining the chance, when the null hypothesis of equally likely plus and minus signs prevails, of results at least as extreme as those observed. Hence, the binomial distribution with $p = 1/2$ is used. If n observations yield x positive differences, this chance (one-tail) is

$$\sum_{r=x}^{n} \frac{n!}{r!\,(n-r)!} \left(\frac{1}{2}\right)^n$$

A two-tailed probability is obtained by doubling this. For example, if 6 positive differences are observed, one calculates for the one-sided sign test the probability of either 6 or 7 plus signs, that is, $7(1/2)^7 + (1/2)^7 = 8(1/2)^7 = 1/16$. When the conventional 5% significance level is adopted, the calculated chance exceeds 5%, so one would accept the null hypothesis of no effect. The only assumption necessary for performing the sign test is that the observations of the individual dogs are independent.

A nonparametric method that utilizes more of the data than the sign is the *Wilcoxon signed rank* procedure. In Table 1 for immunoreactive insulin the comparison of 5 minutes with F_2 yields the following

[2] Most of this discussion concerns hypothesis-testing. The word *procedure* is used to suggest that other forms of inference, such as confidence intervals or multiple decisions, could be used.

differences: (1) 130, (2) −70, (3) 10, (4) 20, (5) 190, (6) 1,080, (7) 40.
Ignoring the signs, one ranks the numbers from high to low, assigning 1
to the lowest (dog 3 with 10) and 7 to the highest (dog 5 with 190). One
then replaces each value with its rank but now takes the sign into consideration. For example, the rank of 4 for dog 2 is replaced with the
signed rank −4. The signed rank for the observations then are (1) 5,
(2) −4, (3) 1, (4) 2, (5) 6, (6) 7, (7) 3. The sum of the positive signed
ranks is called the *Wilcoxon statistic*, which in this case is 24.

A first question is, What assignment of signs yields this or larger
values of the Wilcoxon statistic? All 7 such possibilities are exhibited in
Table 2. When the null hypothesis of no stimulus effect is true, there is a
total of $2^7 = 128$ equally likely assignments of the algebraic signs, the
same number as that obtained with the sign procedure. Seven such
assignments yield results at least as extreme as the observed Wilcoxon
statistic of 24. Hence, the attained level of significance is 7/128 (note that,
had the sign test been used, the attained significance level would have
been 8/128).

The Wilcoxon procedure requires the assumption that the population
distribution is symmetric, an assumption that is not required when the
sign test is used. This assumption is always satisfied when the treatment
(vagal nerve stimulation in our case) has no effect whatsoever on response.
However, it is conceivable that the treatment alters the shape of the
population distribution without altering the median level of response. In
such situation the sign test is appropriate whereas the Wilcoxon procedure
is not.

Details on the use of the Wilcoxon procedures and relevant probability
tables are available in Siegel (1956) and Snedecor and Cochran (1967,
pp. 128–129, 555).

An important question is which procedure — the sign, the Wilcoxon,
or the *t* test — should be used in a given experimental situation. When

TABLE 2   List of All Possible Assignments of Signs to the Ranks
of 7 Observations Yielding a Wilcoxon Statistic of 24 or more

Rank							Sum of positive
1	2	3	4	5	6	7	signed ranks
+	+	+	+	+	+	+	28
−	+	+	+	+	+	+	27
+	−	+	+	+	+	+	26
+	+	−	+	+	+	+	25
+	+	+	−	+	+	+	24
−	−	+	+	+	+	+	25
−	+	−	+	+	+	+	24

the assumptions for the t procedure are met, it should be used. If the choice is between the Wilcoxon and sign procedures, when both are applicable, the Wilcoxon procedure should be used. These rules will reduce the possibility of Type I errors, yield shorter confidence intervals, and provide greater power (ability to reject alternative hypotheses). To achieve the desired power for some specific alternative hypothesis the t test, when applicable, requires roughly 65% of the observations required by the sign test and 95% of those required by the Wilcoxon test.

The latter point indicates that there is little to be lost by employing the Wilcoxon procedure, even when the t procedure is applicable. The chief advantages of nonparametric methods such as the Wilcoxon procedure are that they are easy to apply (when the sample size is not too large) and that their use imposes minimal demands upon the experimental conditions. This should not suggest that the Wilcoxon procedure can invariably be employed with impunity. It has its disadvantages. A Wilcoxon-like procedure for confidence intervals and point estimation is difficult to apply. With large samples the Wilcoxon calculations are cumbersome. Finally, Wilcoxon-like procedures have not been adequately developed for the performance of analyses in complicated experimental situations.

The data in the lower parts of Table 1 can be handled in a similar manner. As an alternative, one could use averages in making the basic comparison, that is, $(0 \text{ min} + 5 \text{ min})/2 - (F_1 + F_2)/2$. Averages would yield greater power than would the single observations that were employed. It should also be noted that the several tests of significance performed in Table 1 suggest the possibility of a procedure by multiple comparisons (see Chapter 3) or one by simultaneous hypothesis-testing (Miller, 1966). A further possibility, arising from the dependencies between the observations within a line (since each line of the table corresponds to a dog), is to employ a multivariate procedure (Bradley, 1967).

3. Data from two independent samples

In this section we consider the Wilcoxon procedure appropriate to the comparison of two independent samples, also called the *Mann-Whitney test*. Analogous to Table 1, Table 3 presents results for a second group of seven dogs in which the right vagus nerve was stimulated. Let us consider the question whether the change in level of immunoreactive insulin, resulting from vagal nerve stimulation, differs between the right and left cervical vagus (this question was not considered by Kaneto and his colleagues and is treated here for illustrative purposes only).

TABLE 3   Effect of Stimulation of the Right Cervical Vagus in Dogs on Pancreatic Venous Plasma Level of Immuno-reactive Insulin (μU/ml)*

Expt. no.	F_1	F_2	Time, min†				
			0	5	10	30	60
8	20	60	80	90	80	—	170
9	440	230	1,010	330	650	200	760
10	200	140	830	200	200	240	670
11	90	100	190	230	220	100	100
12	450	550	1,610	1,610	470	590	930
13	190	100	200	130	120	170	200
14	160	120	210	150	120	110	160
Mean ± SD:	221 ± 152	185 ± 156	590 ± 533	391 ± 502	265 ± 198	235 ± 166	425 ± 320
p:‡			<0.05	<0.05	>0.05	>0.05	<0.05

* Data from Kaneto et al. (1967).

† F_1 and F_2, prestimulation values before and after sectioning of vagus nerve, respectively.

‡ The p values refer to F_2 prestimulation versus poststimulation values when the Wilcoxon signed-rank test is applied.

As in the previous section, we shall consider the difference in the level of immunoreactive insulin at 0 minutes and F_2. The null hypothesis is that the differences (0 min $- F_2$) for the left nerve in Table 1 and those for the right nerve in Table 3 are from the same population.

The differences are shown in Table 4. The two samples of seven observations each are combined into one group of fourteen, and all fourteen observations are ranked from low to high. The Wilcoxon statistic, W, is defined as the sum of the ranks in the second sample (right nerve stimulation) and in this case is $W = 49$ (of course, W could be alternatively defined as the sum of the ranks in the first sample, left nerve stimulation).

When the null hypothesis is true, the probabilities of possible values of W can be computed by combinatorial methods in a manner similar to that employed in Section 2 with paired samples. However, the process is considerably more involved. Tables giving critical values and further details on methodology are available in Siegel (1956, p. 271), Snedecor and Cochran (1967, p. 555), and Bliss (1967, p. 521). For the data at hand such tables are not necessary. When the null hypothesis is true, the average value of W is

$$7 \times \text{average rank of an observation} = 7 \times 7.5 = 52.5$$

The observed $W = 49$ is so close to the expected 52.5 that, clearly, the results must not be statistically significant.

It should be emphasized that use of the Wilcoxon procedures requires that, when the null hypothesis is true, all the observations form a random

TABLE 4 Illustration of Wilcoxon Two-Sample Test Applied to Differences in Immunoreactive Insulin of Pancreatic Venous Plasma at Times 0 and F_2, Comparing 7 Dogs with Left (Table 1) and 7 Dogs with Right (Table 3) Vagus Nerve Stimulation

Left nerve stimulation		Right nerve stimulation	
Difference $0 - F_2$, $\mu U/ml$	Rank in combined sample	Difference $0 - F_2$, $\mu U/ml$	Rank in combined sample
350	8	20	1
60	2	780	12
440	10	690	11
350	7	90	4
370	9	1,060	13
1,180	14	100	5
170	6	90	3
Sum of ranks:	56		49

sample or that two experimental conditions yield two random samples from the same population. The Wilcoxon procedure does not, however, require the assumption of an underlying normal population. It is particularly effective in tests of significance in which the alternative hypothesis corresponds to one population that is being shifted away from another.

4. Discussion

A common procedure in statistics has been to estimate, and to test hypotheses about, the means and variances of a population assumed to have some known form, such as the normal distribution. The equation for the normal frequency distribution contains two parameters,[3] the mean and the standard deviation. A more recent development is methods that are applicable to a wide variety of distributions, including those in which the form of the distribution cannot be simply specified by one or several parameters. Since such methods are independent of the form of the distribution, they are called nonparametric.

Nevertheless, although *distributions* may not be parameterized, one may be interested in determining certain parameters of the population (such as the median). For making inferences about such parameters one seeks a procedure that has desirable properties (such as a specified Type I error) for all possible frequency distributions.

Experience has shown that the t and other procedures designed for use with normal error distributions are "robust," that is, insensitive to departures from their underlying assumptions. Even when samplings are from nonnormal frequency distributions, these procedures often provide approximately the same protection that would obtain were the distribution normal. Selection of the appropriate statistical analysis thus requires experience with both statistical methods and a variety of types of experimental data. For the data in Table 1, I found the need for nonparametric methods compelling.

If accurate measurements are made within a carefully designed experiment involving random sampling, procedures based upon a normal frequency distribution (or some other appropriate parametric assumption) are, as a rule, preferable to nonparametric procedures.

Bibliographical notes

Siegel (1956) presents the standard methodology for nonparametric methods; his book has been critically reviewed by Savage

---

[3] A parameter is defined as "an arbitrary constant or variable in a mathematical expression which distinguishes various specific cases" (James and James, 1959).

(1957). Mosteller and Tukey (1968) present an expository critical approach. Savage (1968) surveys the field of nonparametric statistics. Bradley (1967) reviews current work on sequential and multivariate nonparametric procedures. Miller (1966) reviews multiple-comparisons aspects of nonparametric procedures.

DISCUSSION

MOSTELLER   First, do you mean to say that the need for non-parametric methods stems from an inability to handle many parameters? Second, might it not have been appropriate to analyze these data by taking logarithms of each of the observations and applying standard techniques? Third, with regard to the Wilcoxon test, I see two opposing positions. On the one hand, I think of it as a good way to allow some weights for larger differences. On the other hand, I say to myself, as Dixon does when he's thinking about Winsorizing, "Why should I let a wild observation contribute more than its fair share to the analysis?" This dilemma must be something you have faced.

SAVAGE   First, the need for nonparametric statistics stems from our inability in some situations to characterize in a simple way the type of population that we are sampling. That is, we are not willing to say that the population is normal, and we do not happen to know what the mean and variance are. We wish to allow greater latitude. Nonparametric methods enable us to ignore many unspecified parameters, most of which will play a nuisance role (parameters in which we have no real interest, but which clutter up the analysis). For example, when the t test is applied to means of normal distributions, the standard deviation is of little interest, and it is a nuisance parameter.

It is important to emphasize that the nonparametric statistician is concerned with parameters. The median is an important one that often arises. Kruskal (1958) and Goodman and Kruskal (1954, 1959, 1963) have several interesting interpretations of the parameters that arise in non-parametric correlation analysis and contingency tables. The hypotheses discussed for the first data of Tables 1 and 3 (immunoreactive insulin) were that the median responses were not increased by electrical stimulation. In the two-sample Wilcoxon procedure the natural parameter was the probability that the response of the left vagus nerve was greater than that of the right. Is this a meaningful probability in this study?

Second, to take logarithms with a view to making the data amenable to standard procedures based upon the normal distribution is a logical suggestion. However, this entails some assumptions about the homogeneity of the original observations.

A related question is, "What if I had known that the experimenter had randomized in the formation of the groups and in the assignment to the groups, so that fourteen animals were randomly selected from twenty-eight and then randomly assigned to the two groups? Might one then use the Wilcoxon procedure?" The answer is "Yes." If the experimenter employs randomization, it ensures that the conditions for applying the Wilcoxon procedure are obtained, provided that there is no difference between treatments. Consequently, a valid test of significance can be performed. If one has done the randomization, one will actually have a test at the 0.05 level or whatever level is preferred. With proper randomization one could take the original data (that is, not go to ranks) and compute a t statistic as a result of the randomization. This t statistic will roughly follow the t distribution, whether or not the data came from a normal population. A careful reading of Fisher (1966, p. 45) indicates that he uses the t and F distributions as approximations to the distributions created by the experimenter's randomization in forming his groups. They were not used because of the assumption that errors are normally distributed. If randomization had been performed, I would still have reservations about using the Wilcoxon two-sample procedure or the t statistic. One cannot generalize beyond the experimental data unless one is actually dealing with a random sample from some population.

Third, with regard to the wild observation and the weight in the Wilcoxon test, I cannot give a good answer.

One topic I did not discuss is nonparametric estimation. As was mentioned earlier, such procedures as Winsorizing are robust, having less effect due to the tail or erratic observations. An extreme form of neglect of deviations is the use of the median. There is another, related to the quality of the data: that is, sometimes there are no data. For instance, it is not unusual in psychobiological experiments to be able to say only that this observation is larger than that, there being no method of measuring the differences. In such case one may have merely the equivalent of the algebraic signs of differences or, if one can intercompare all of the observations, the signed ranks. Thus, there are situations in which thickness of tails of distributions and large observations are not the problem. One is forced to contend with the ranks, which are the basic data.

FINNEY   I was interested in the experiment discussed, because one of my colleagues in Edinburgh recently drew my attention to a logically similar experimental situation. In that experiment twelve human subjects provided urine samples at thirty-minute intervals for several hours. After the first four samples a certain drug was administered, and subsequent observations were used in discussion of whether or not a particular constituent of the urine was affected by the drug. The important, but neglected, feature that I want to mention is that all subjects began at 8 A.M., and all received the drug at 10 A.M. Thus, a test such as has been described was based on a comparison of the 10:30 A.M. and 9:30 A.M. determinations for each subject. Now, irrespective of whether a rank test, a sign test, or a parametric test is used, the danger is that any difference may have nothing whatsoever to do with the drug but may constitute a manifestation of a diurnal cycle in the property under observation. This does not necessarily apply to the data cited in the speaker's example; however, there is the possibility that all dogs in the experiment were started at the same hour of the day (not necessarily all on the same day) and that a diurnal cycle or some unintended signal by a laboratory assistant affected the observations.

Such an experiment cannot give statistical evidence on this point unless control subjects receiving a dummy or placebo treatment have been included. This, in turn, would reintroduce problems of randomization that the speaker sought to avoid. Perhaps one should note that the difference between columns "F_1" and "F_2" is almost significant by a Wilcoxon test, suggesting that a systematic change may have been occurring during the preliminary period. I want to emphasize that in some circumstances a valid statistical *analysis* can be irrelevant because of a fault of design.

EMMENS To comment on the physiology, the vagus is a nerve that differs in structure on the right and left sides. Usually one side, not always the same, unfortunately, contains more sympathetic fibers. These are opposite in effect, generally speaking, to those of the parasympathetic nervous system. There is, indeed, good reason to look at what happens in left vagus stimulation as against right. This should be done with the same animal. I'm fairly certain, since I know the experimenter, that he did not stimulate seven dogs at the same time; he probably stimulated one dog at a time, one in the morning and one in the afternoon. It seems logical to take a dog and do a left and right vagal stimulation and use a control according to some reasonable plan. In other words, I should have expected a within-animal sequence of operations, not a between-animal one at all.

CHAPTER TEN

Continuous-Variable Experimentation*

HARRY SMITH, JR.

1. Introduction

This chapter is concerned with the controlled experimental approach when a single continuous response variable is to be represented by a linear combination of a set of continuous controllable variables believed to affect the response. For example, Claringbold (1955a) showed the relationship of percentage of positive vaginal smears of spayed albino mice to estrone dosage and amount of bovine plasma albumin. The percentage of positive vaginal smears represents a continuous response variable (also referred to as the dependent variable), and estrone dosage and amount of bovine plasma albumin represent two continuous controlled variables (also referred to as the independent variables).

Some of the more efficient designs for a mathematical model are examined. In general, an efficient design is one that provides mutually independent estimates of the parameters of the model, permits a separate determination of the variation due to lack of fit of the model and that due to random, or pure, error, and simultaneously conserves the total amount of experimental effort. A simple linear model with one independent variable is considered in Section 2; an illustration appears in Section 3. The extension to the simple case of two controllable variables and an example are described in Section 4. Some designs for fitting a complete quadratic model for two independent variables are examined in Section 5; for three independent variables, in Section 6. Finally, Section 7 contains an example of an unbalanced (nonorthogonal) design, for which a computer program was used to fit a quadratic model.

2. A simple linear-regression model

The simple linear-regression model states that a response y is related to a controllable variable x by the equation

$$y = \alpha + \beta x + \varepsilon$$

* This research was supported by a grant from the National Institutes of Health, 5 T01 GM 00038, to the Department of Biostatistics, University of North Carolina.

where α is the intercept, β the slope of the line, and ε a random-error component.

The method of least squares is one by which estimates of the unknown parameters α and β may be obtained. Assuming that the variance of the random-error component is constant over the range of applicability of the linear model, the method of least squares determines those values of α and β which minimize

$$\sum_1^n (y - \alpha - \beta x)^2$$

where n is the number of observed sample points. Differentiating with respect to α and β and setting the derivatives equal to zero yields the two equations

$$n\alpha + (\textstyle\sum x)\beta = \textstyle\sum y$$
$$(\textstyle\sum x)\alpha + (\textstyle\sum x^2)\beta = \textstyle\sum xy$$

which are called the *normal equations*.

It is well known that after substitution of a and b, to denote estimates of α and β, the solution of the normal equations yields the estimates

$$b = \frac{\sum xy - (\sum x)(\sum y)/n}{\sum x^2 - (\sum x)^2/n} = \frac{[xy]}{[x^2]} \qquad \text{and} \qquad a = \bar{y} - bx$$

The corresponding analysis of variance is also well known and is

Term	DF	SS	MS
Regression (due to b)	1	$[xy]^2/[x^2]$	$[xy]^2/[x^2]$
Residual	$n-2$	$[y^2] - [xy]^2/[x^2]$	s^2
Total:	$n-1$	$[y^2]$	

On the further assumption that the random errors are normally distributed with mean zero one can test for the significance of the slope with the F ratio of mean square regression divided by mean square residual. The variance of the predicted mean response $\hat{y}$ for some particular value of x, say x_k, is given by

$$\{1/n + (x_k - \bar{x})^2/[x^2]\}s^2$$

The solution of the normal equations can be simplified by first making a simple linear transformation of the x variable to a u variable, where u is defined as

$$u = (x - \bar{x})/c$$

The c is a constant chosen to simplify the arithmetic. Then, by considering the model

$$y = \alpha' + \beta'u + \varepsilon$$

it will be seen that the normal equations (since $\sum u = 0$) are

$$n\alpha' + 0 = \sum y$$
$$0 + (\sum u^2)\beta' = \sum uy$$

This gives as estimates of α' and β'

$$a' = \bar{y} \quad \text{and} \quad b' = \sum uy / \sum u^2$$

The model can, of course, easily be expressed in terms of the original x units:

$$y = \bar{y} + b'u = \bar{y} + b'(x - \bar{x})/c$$

In placing the experimental points along the x axis (or along the u axis) it is often desirable to minimize the variance of the estimate of slope, that is, minimize $\sigma^2 / \sum (x - \bar{x})^2$, by making $\sum (x - \bar{x})^2$ or $\sum u^2$ as large as possible. This can be done by choosing values of x or u at the extremes of the range over which the linear model is applicable.

3. Example of a simple linear-regression model

A linear-regression model was fitted for the percent impurities in a chemical batch process (y) against the temperature at which the batch was processed (x). Five experimental points were determined, as indicated in Table 1. It was most convenient to transform temperature to the u variable:

$$u = (x - 220)/10$$

The estimates a' and b' are then

$$a' = \bar{y} = 45/5 = 9 \quad \text{and} \quad b' = \sum uy / \sum u^2 = 30/10 = 3$$

giving the fitted regression equation

$$y = 9 + 3u = 9 + 3(x - 220)/10 = -57 + 0.3x$$

The analysis of variance is presented in the lower half of Table 1.

Since the experiment lacks replication at any of the experimental design points, the residual mean square error 12 is an estimate of both random, or pure, error and any error arising from the use of a wrong model. However, the plotting of individual residuals is a useful device in

TABLE 1 Simple Linear-Regression Model Fitting Percent Impurities in Chemical Batch Process against the Temperature at Which the Batch was Processed

Data:

Temp. x, °F	Transformed variate u	Percent impurities y	Predicted response $\hat{y}$	Residual $y - \hat{y}$
200	−2	6	3	3
210	−1	5	6	−1
220	0	5	9	−4
230	1	11	12	−1
240	2	18	15	3

Calculations:

$$\sum u = 0, \quad \sum u^2 = 10, \quad \sum uy = 30, \quad \sum y = 45, \quad \sum y^2 = 531$$

Analysis of variance:

Term	DF	SS	MS	F
Total	5	531		
Correction for mean	1	$45^2/5 = 405$		
Total (corrected)	4	126		
Regression (due to b)	1	$30^2/10 = 90$	90	7.5
Residual	3	36	12	

providing guidelines concerning the adequacy of the model. The individual residuals, $y - \hat{y}$, are shown in the upper half of Table 1. The systematic pattern in the residuals is indicative that a more suitable model should have been used (in this case a quadratic model in u or, correspondingly, in x).

It is wiser to provide an original design that enables the experimenter to test for the inadequacy or lack of fit of the model he has chosen. In the example given above the experimenter needs to provide a design that will enable him to obtain the following: (a) an unbiased estimate of random, or pure, error and (b) an estimate of the lack of fit of the linear model; that is, to have in the design space enough different x or u values to obtain an estimate of an additional parameter, say β_2, for the model, $y = \alpha + \beta_1 x + \beta_2 x^2 + \varepsilon$.

The random-error estimate is obtained by replicating experimental runs, and the lack-of-fit term is obtained by choosing at least three different x values (usually equally spaced).

Hence, the five experimental points would be better placed if there were two replicates each at 200°F and 240°F and one at 220°F. The resulting breakdown of the degree of freedom for the analysis of variance then would be

Term	DF
Total (corrected)	4
Regression	1
Residual	3
Lack of fit	1
Pure error	2

The random-error term has 2 DF, one from each of the two replications at the extreme levels. The lack-of-fit term with 1 DF shows whether the linear model is adequate or whether the model should be

$$y = \alpha + \beta_1 x + \beta_2 x^2 + \varepsilon$$

that is, whether there is quadratic curvature. Hence, with this design it is possible to segregate variation due to random error from that due to lack of fit of the linear model. It should be noted that this example is only an illustration of the partitioning of the residual sum of squares; one would require more degrees of freedom in practice.

4. A linear-regression model with two independent variables

Let us now consider design aspects of a linear model containing two independent, or controllable, variables, namely

$$y = \alpha + \beta_1 x_1 + \beta_2 x_2 + \varepsilon$$

As before, it is more convenient to consider the transformed, or centered, variables,

$$u_1 = (x_1 - \bar{x}_1)/c_1 \quad \text{and} \quad u_2 = (x_2 - \bar{x}_2)/c_2$$

and the model,

$$y = \alpha' + \beta_1' u_{1'} + \beta_2' u_2 + \varepsilon$$

The method of least squares requires a determination of the values of α', β_1', and β_2' that minimize

$$\sum_1^n (y - \alpha' - \beta_1' u_1 - \beta_2' u)^2$$

yielding the normal equations

$$
\begin{aligned}
n\alpha' + 0 \quad\quad + 0 \quad\quad\quad &= \sum y \\
0 + (\sum u_1^2)\beta_1' \;+ (\sum u_1 u_2)\beta_2' &= \sum u_1 y \\
0 + (\sum u_1 u_2)\beta_1' + (\sum u_2^2)\beta_2' \;\; &= \sum u_2 y
\end{aligned}
$$

By selecting a balanced set of the initial points (x_1, x_2) or the transformed points (u_1, u_2) the normal equations can be further simplified. For example, consider the balanced set of four points shown in the left half of Figure 1. The design is balanced in that the levels of one factor occur at each level of the other factor. When

$$c_1 = (x_{1H} - x_{1L})/2 \qquad \text{and} \qquad c_2 = (x_{2H} - x_{2L})/2$$

are chosen, the u values for the four points are as shown in Table 2, where the values of u_1^2, u_2^2, and u_1u_2 have also been calculated; the subscripts H and L refer to high and low values. Since this balanced design gives $\sum u_1 u_2 = 0$, the normal equations for this design (see Table 2) simplify to

$$4\alpha' + 0 + 0 = \sum y$$
$$0 + 4\beta_1' + 0 = \sum u_1 y$$
$$0 + 0 + 4\beta_2' = \sum u_2 y$$

In other words, this balanced design yields mutually independent estimates of α', β_1', and β_2' as

$$a' = \sum y/4, \qquad b_1' = \sum u_1 y/4, \qquad b_2' = \sum u_2 y/4$$

One can, of course, transform back to the original x units with appropriate substitution for u_1 and u_2. Had we chosen an unbalanced design, such as that shown in the right half of Figure 1 (that is, the four points form a parallelogram rather than a rectangle), the normal equations would not simplify as they did for the balanced design, and it would not be possible to obtain the mutually independent estimates b_1' and b_2'.

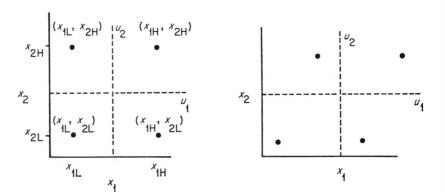

FIGURE 1   Balanced (left) and unbalanced (right) four-point designs.

TABLE 2 Transformation of Design in Upper Half of Figure 1 to Variates u_1 and u_2

Exptl. point	Original variate		Transformed variate*				
	x_1	x_2	u_1	u_2	u_1^2	u_2^2	$u_1 u_2$
1	x_{1L}	x_{2L}	-1	-1	$+1$	$+1$	$+1$
2	x_{1L}	x_{2H}	-1	$+1$	$+1$	$+1$	-1
3	x_{1H}	x_{2L}	$+1$	-1	$+1$	$+1$	-1
4	x_{1H}	x_{2H}	$+1$	$+1$	$+1$	$+1$	$+1$
		Total:	0	0	4	4	0

* Here $u_1 = (2x_1 - x_{1L} - x_{1H})/(x_{1H} - x_{1L})$ and $u_2 = (2x_2 - x_{2L} - x_{2H})/(x_{2H} - x_{2L})$.

If now for the balanced design k replications are obtained at each of the four experimental points in Figure 1, and if the total of the responses at each point is denoted by T_y, then the estimates of the parameters α', β_1', and β_2' become

$$a' = \frac{\sum y}{4k}, \qquad b_1' = \frac{\sum u_1 T_y}{4k}, \qquad b_2' = \frac{\sum u_2 T_y}{4k}$$

The corresponding analysis of variance is

Source of variation	DF	SS
Total	$4k$	$\sum y^2$
Due to a	1	$C_m = (\sum y)^2/(4k)$
Total (corrected)	$4k - 1$	$\sum y^2 - C_m$
Regression on u_1	1	$(\sum u_1 T_y)^2/(4k)$
Regression on u_2	1	$(\sum u_2 T_y)^2/(4k)$
Residual	$4(k-1)+1$	By subtraction
Lack of fit	1	By subtraction
Pure error	$4(k - 1)$	$\sum_i \sum_j (y_{ij} - \bar{y}_i)^2$

Table 3 illustrates this procedure; it gives responses for two replications at each of four points corresponding to the two controllable variables temperature and pressure. The fitted regression equation is as follows,

$$y = 8.250 + 3.850\left(\frac{x_1 - 70}{10}\right) + 4.775\left(\frac{x_2 - 110}{10}\right)$$
$$= -71.225 + 0.3850x_1 + 0.4775x_2$$

and the analysis of variance is shown in the bottom part of Table 3. It should be noted that the experimental design and the analysis of variance correspond with a 2^2 factorial in a completely randomized design, each

TABLE 3   Fitting of Linear-Regression Model with Two
Independent Variables

Data:				Transformed variables		
	Temp.	Pressure	Response			Response
	x_1	x_2	y	u_1	u_2	total T_y
	60	100	1.0	-1	-1	2.7
	60	100	1.7			
	60	120	7.0	-1	$+1$	14.9
	60	120	7.9			
	80	100	6.0	$+1$	-1	11.2
	80	100	5.2			
	80	120	18.0	$+1$	$+1$	37.2
	80	120	19.2			

Calculations:

$\sum y = 66.0, \quad \sum y^2 = 870.98, \quad \sum T_y^2 = 2.7^2 + 14.9^2 + 11.2^2 + 37.2^2 = 1{,}738.58$

$\sum u_1 T_y = 2.7 - 14.9 + 11.2 + 37.2 = 30.8, \quad b_1' = \sum u_1 T_y / 4k = 30.8/8 = 3.850$

$\sum u_2 T_y = -2.7 + 14.9 - 11.2 + 37.2 = 38.2, \quad b_2' = \sum u_2 T_y / 4k = 38.2/8 = 4.775$

$$a' = \sum y/4k = 66.0/8 = 8.250$$

Analysis of variance:

Term	DF	SS	MS	F
Total (corrected)	7	$870.98 - 544.50 = 326.480$		
Regression on u_1	1	$30.8^2/8 = 118.580$	118.580	
Regression on u_2	1	$38.2^2/8 = 182.405$	182.405	
Residual error	5	25.495	5.099	
Lack of fit	1	23.805	23.805	56.34
Pure error	4	1.690	0.4225	

group having two replicates (see pp. 10 and 44). The regression terms on u_1 and u_2 correspond to the main effects, and the lack-of-fit term corresponds to interaction. Since in this numerical example the interaction, or lack of fit, was significant, the simple linear model does not adequately describe the data.

With two independent variables we have thus far considered uniform replication at each of the design points. However, as with one independent variable, if common variance prevails throughout the experimental region, then replication could be performed anywhere. In this instance it may be preferable to replicate at the center of the experimental region for the following reasons: (a) such replication permits an examination for curvature, that is, a comparison of the mean response at the center with the mean of the responses at the extremities, and (b) an experiment is often designed with a known, controlled point as the center. Returning to this known position enables the experimenter to determine whether an extraneous variable has caused some shift in the general response during the time of the experiment.

5. A quadratic-regression model with two independent variables

Although the linear model provides an adequate fit in many instances, one is often interested in examining quadratic terms, too. With two independent, or controllable, variables the model with quadratic effects is

$$y = \alpha' + \beta_1' u_1 + \beta_2' u_2 + \beta_{11}' u_1^2 + \beta_{22}' u_2^2 + \beta_{12}' u_1 u_2 + \varepsilon$$

where we have again converted the original x_1 and x_2 variables into the more convenient u_1 and u_2. There are six parameters in this model.

Geometrically, the linear model of the preceding section generated a plane in the three dimensions y, u_1, and u_2. This model in three dimensions generates a quadratic surface relating response y to the two independent variables u_1 and u_2. The exploration of various response relationships in more than two dimensions is generally called *response surface* analysis. Note that if there are more than two independent variables, we cannot graphically depict the response surface. For example, with three independent variables u_1, u_2, and u_3 and a response variable y we have a four-dimensional situation. Although we cannot visualize the surface, we can, as mathematicians often do, conceptually consider surfaces existing in a hypothetical world of four or more dimensions.

For the three-dimensional quadratic response surface under consideration, let us consider several experimental designs, that is, various combinations of points (u_1, u_2), which permit estimation of the six parameters in the model. It is clear that the previous four-point, or 2^2, factorial design will be inadequate, since the number of parameters requiring estimation exceeds the number of experimental points.

A 3^2 factorial design

The natural analogue of the 2^2 factorial design is a balanced design in which each of the two controllable variables occurs at *three* equally spaced levels, and in which nine (3×3) possibilities or combinations of one factor with the other are considered. Such a design is shown in Table 4. The nine points of the design are listed with the calculations necessary to determine the normal equations. In order further to simplify the normal equations it is more convenient to substitute $u_1^2 - \overline{u_1^2}$ for u_1^2

TABLE 4   The 3^2 Factorial Design

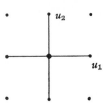

Design points and calculations:

	Design points		Calculations				
	u_1	u_2	$u_1 u_2$	u_1^2	u_2^2	$u_1^2 - 6/9$	$u_2^2 - 6/9$
	-1	-1	1	1	1	$3/9$	$3/9$
	-1	0	0	1	0	$3/9$	$-6/9$
	-1	1	-1	1	1	$3/9$	$3/9$
	0	-1	0	0	1	$-6/9$	$3/9$
	0	0	0	0	0	$-6/9$	$-6/9$
	0	1	0	0	1	$-6/9$	$3/9$
	1	-1	-1	1	1	$3/9$	$3/9$
	1	0	0	1	0	$3/9$	$-6/9$
	1	1	1	1	1	$3/9$	$3/9$
Total:	0	0	0	6	6	0	0
Mean:	0	0	0	$6/9$	$6/9$	0	0
SS:	6	6	4	6	6	2	2

Normal equations:

$$
\begin{aligned}
9\alpha'' + 0 + 0 + 0 + 0 + 0 &= \sum y \\
0 + 6\beta_1' + 0 + 0 + 0 + 0 &= \sum u_1 y \\
0 + 0 + 6\beta_2' + 0 + 0 + 0 &= \sum u_2 y \\
0 + 0 + 0 + 4\beta_{12}' + 0 + 0 &= \sum u_1 u_2 y \\
0 + 0 + 0 + 0 + 2\beta_{11}' + 0 &= \sum (u_1^2 - 6/9) y \\
0 + 0 + 0 + 0 + 0 + 2\beta_{22}' &= \sum (u_2^2 - 6/9) y
\end{aligned}
$$

Properties:

Number of experiments	9
Number of points	9
Degrees of freedom	
Lack of fit	3
Pure error	0

and $u_2^2 - \overline{u_2^2}$ for u_2^2 (note that $\overline{u_i^2}$ denotes the mean of the squares of u_i and *not* the squared mean of u_i). This entails fitting a model,

$$
y = \alpha'' + \beta_1' u_1 + \beta_2' u_2 + \beta_{11}'(u_1^2 - \overline{u_1^2})
$$
$$
+ \beta_{22}'(u_2^2 - \overline{u_2^2}) + \beta_{12}' u_1 u_2 + \varepsilon
$$

The normal equations for fitting this model are shown in the lower part of Table 4. Note that the estimates of the parameters are, as in the case of the balanced design of Section 4, mutually independent.

With mutually independent estimates the variance of a predicted mean $\hat{y}$ for specified values of u_1 and u_2 (or x_1 and x_2) is obtained simply by adding together the variances corresponding to each parameter in the model. The estimated variance of each parameter in the model is of the form

$$s^2/(\text{coefficient in normal equations})$$

For example,

$$\text{var } (a'') = s^2/9, \qquad \text{var } (b_1') = \text{var } (b_2') = s^2/6, \qquad \text{etc.}$$

Hence, for specified u_1 and u_2 the variance of a predicted mean $\hat{y}$ is

$$\text{var } (\hat{y}) = \left(\frac{1}{9} + \frac{u_1^2}{6} + \frac{u_2^2}{6} + \frac{(u_1^2 - 6/9)^2}{2} + \frac{(u_2^2 - 6/9)^2}{2} + \frac{u_1^2 u_2^2}{4}\right)s^2$$

Note that this variance will differ at the different points of the design. For example,

when $u_1 = 0$ and $u_2 = 0$,

$$\text{var } (\hat{y}) = \left(\frac{1}{9} + \frac{36/81}{2} + \frac{36/81}{2}\right)s^2 = 5s^2/9$$

when $u_1 = 1$ and $u_2 = 1$,

$$\text{var } (\hat{y}) = \left(\frac{1}{9} + \frac{1}{6} + \frac{1}{6} + \frac{9/81}{2} + \frac{9/81}{2} + \frac{1}{4}\right)s^2 = 29s^2/36$$

With six parameters to be determined and nine points in the design, this leaves 3 DF for the lack-of-fit term. Only by replication at the points in the design can degrees of freedom be secured for the determination of pure error. To preserve the balance and to allow mutually independent estimates of the parameters, equal replications at each of the nine point is required. With k such replicates one obtains $9(k - 1)$ DF for pure error.

A pentagon design

An alternative design for investigating the quadratic described above is the pentagon design. This design is illustrated in the left-hand portion of Figure 2 and has the nice property that the variance of a $\hat{y}$ for chosen u_1 and u_2 is the same at each point of the design. The design has six different experimental points; five are at a distance $\sqrt{2}$ from the origin

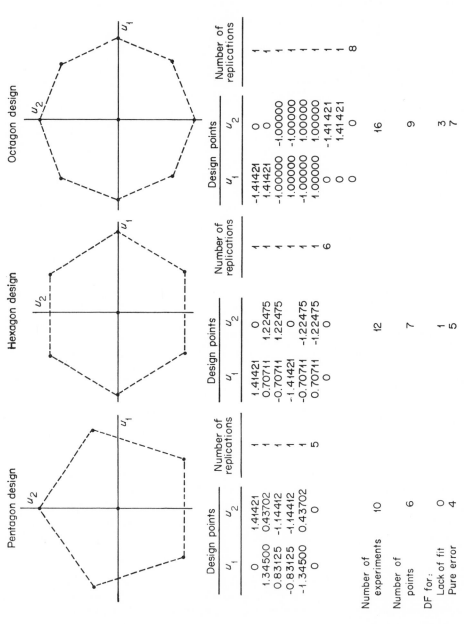

FIGURE 2   The pentagon, hexagon, and octagon designs for fitting a quadratic response surface with two independent variables

and form a pentagon, and one is at the origin with five replications. The variance of a $\hat{y}$ for chosen u_1 and u_2 is

$$\frac{s^2}{5} [1 + (u_1^2 + u_2^2)^2]$$

which can be seen to be equivalent for all points of the design.

Six parameters and six different experimental points unfortunately leave no degrees of freedom for testing for lack of fit of the model; however, the five replicate observations at the origin do provide 4 DF for pure error.

Other polygon designs

A hexagon design (middle part of Figure 2) has seven different experimental points, six of them at a distance $\sqrt{2}$ from the origin and forming a hexagon and one with six replications at the origin. The design provides 1 DF for determining lack of fit and 5 DF for pure error.

Analogously, an octagon design (right-hand part of Figure 2) has nine different experimental points, eight of them at a distance $\sqrt{2}$ from the origin and forming an octagon, and one with eight replications at the origin. The design provides 3 DF for lack of fit and 7 DF for pure error.

Although not shown, the normal equations for each of these designs can easily be obtained, and they provide mutually independent estimates of the six parameters in the model. There is a corresponding analysis of variance with each design, and one can easily determine the variance of $\hat{y}$ for chosen u_1 and u_2. Like the pentagon design, the hexagon and octagon designs have the property of equal variance for $\hat{y}$ at each point in the design.

6. Response surface designs with three independent variables

With three independent variables u_1, u_2, and u_3 the quadratic model contains ten parameters and is

$$y = \alpha' + \beta_1' u_1 + \beta_2' u_2 + \beta_3' u_3 + \beta_{11}' u_1^2 + \beta_{22}' u_2^2 + \beta_{33}' u_3^2 + \beta_{12}' u_1 u_2 + \beta_{13}' u_1 u_3 + \beta_{23}' u_2 u_3 + \varepsilon$$

Table 5 gives the pertinent characteristics of several possible three-variable balanced designs, the 3^3 factorial, the icosahedron, the central composite, and the three-level maximum (three-level max). The normal equations for each can easily be calculated and will yield mutually independent estimates of the ten parameters in the model. The 3^3 factorial and central composite designs do not permit estimation of a

TABLE 5 Designs for Fitting a Quadratic Response Surface with Three Independent Variables

3³ Factorial			Icosahedron			Central composite			Three-level max		
u_1	u_2	u_3	u_1	u_2	u_3	u_1	u_2	u_3	u_1	u_2	u_3
-1	-1	-1	1.41421	0	0.70711	-1	-1	-1	-1	-1	0
0	-1	-1	0.43702	1.34500	0.70711	1	-1	-1	1	-1	0
1	-1	-1	0.43702	-1.34500	0.70711	-1	1	-1	-1	1	0
-1	0	-1	-1.14412	0.83125	0.70711	1	1	-1	1	1	0
0	0	-1	-1.14412	-0.83125	0.70711	-1	-1	1	-1	0	-1
1	0	-1	-1.41421	0	-0.70711	1	-1	1	1	0	-1
-1	1	-1	-0.43702	1.34500	-0.70711	-1	1	1	-1	0	1
0	1	-1	-0.43702	-1.34500	-0.70711	1	1	1	1	0	1
1	1	-1	1.14412	0.83125	-0.70711	-1.21541	0	0	0	-1	-1
-1	-1	0	1.14412	-0.83125	-0.70711	1.21541	0	0	0	1	-1
0	-1	0	0	0	1.58114	0	-1.21541	0	0	-1	1
1	-1	0	0	0	-1.58114	0	1.21541	0	0	1	1
-1	0	0	0	0	0	0	0	-1.21541	0	0	0
0	0	0				0	0	1.21541			
1	0	0				0	0	0			
-1	1	0									
0	1	0									
1	1	0									
-1	-1	1									
0	-1	1									
1	-1	1									
-1	0	1									
0	0	1									
1	0	1									
-1	1	1									
0	1	1									
1	1	1									

(The first 8 rows of the Central composite design are marked "2³ fact."; the upper rows of the Three-level max design are marked "Three 2² fact.")

	3³ Factorial	Icosahedron	Central composite	Three-level max
No. of expts.:	27	20	15	16
No. of points:	27	13	15	13
Deg. freedom — Lack of fit	17	3	5	3
Pure error	0	7	0	3

separate residual-error term unless replication is provided at each of the points of the designs. The estimates of residual error with the three-level max and the icosahedron designs are obtained entirely by replication at the origin.

The icosahedron design is the three-dimensional analogue of the pentagon design of the preceding section. The central composite design consists of a 2^3 factorial design augmented with a point at the origin and points farther along the u_1, u_2, and u_3 axes. Finally, the three-level max design consists of three 2^2 factorial designs (one each for u_1 versus u_2, u_1 versus u_3, and u_2 versus u_3) augmented with four replications at the origin.

Of the four designs listed, the three-level max has the most generally useful properties. The icosahedron design has many advantages, but requires greater experimental effort. Both the three-level max and the icosahedron designs provide estimates of variation due to lack of fit and to random error. The 3^3 factorial design requires the greatest total experimental effort, extravagantly allots 17 DF for lack of fit, and fails to produce any degrees of freedom for pure error. Minimal replication of two observations at each point of the 3^3 design would require a doubling of the experimental effort. The central composite design also fails to provide degrees of freedom for pure error. However, the design provides estimates of all the parameters, allows 5 DF for lack of fit and, in comparison with the 3^3 factorial design, requires roughly half the total amount of experimental effort.

The designs discussed for obtaining quadratic response surfaces are just a few of many potential designs available to the experimenter. The optimal choice of a design will depend on additional experimental items, such as the cost of experimental effort, time, and manpower. The necessary elements of each design for the determination of such items have been given in each discussion. A suitable inspection of Table 5 will assist an experimenter in producing an optimal design for three independent variables. A similar table can be prepared for designs with two, four, five, or any other number of independent variables.

7. A quadratic response surface for an unbalanced design

Thus far our discussion has centered on orthogonal, or balanced, experimental designs. Quite often an experiment for one reason or another is nonorthogonal, or unbalanced. In such case one must be careful in interpreting the estimates of the coefficients of a resulting model, because these estimates will not be mutually independent. Even though this is true, often the model can be very useful for predictive purposes.

Let us consider an example described by Goldin et al. (1956), which

demonstrates the creation of a response surface plot with the use of unbalanced data. The investigation consisted of several experiments on the
treatment of leukemia in hybrid male mice nine to twelve weeks old.
The particular experiment of interest is one in which the treatment for
leukemia began on the eighth day. Five different dose frequencies (x_1)
and several different dose levels (x_2) were tested in order to determine
which combination maximized the median survival time (y) of the mice.
The raw data are shown in Table 6.

TABLE 6   Raw Data for Unbalanced Experiment on Survival of
Leukemia-Implanted Mice as a Function of Dose Frequency and
Dose Level*

Observation no.	Median survival time y	Dose frequency per day x_1	Dose level x_2, mg/kg
1	18	2	0.086
2	21	2	0.14
3	25	2	0.24
4	17	2	0.40
5	15	2	0.67
6	16	2	1.12
7	13	1	0.14
8	14	1	0.24
9	15	1	0.40
10	31	1	0.67
11	28	1	1.12
12	20	1	1.86
13	12	0.5	0.67
14	12	0.5	1.12
15	28	0.5	1.86
16	26	0.5	3.10
17	25	0.5	5.20
18	20	0.5	8.65
19	18	0.5	14.4
20	18	0.5	24.0
21	10	0.333	1.86
22	15	0.333	3.10
23	18	0.333	5.20
24	20	0.333	8.65
25	18	0.333	14.4
26	18	0.333	24.0
27	15	0.250	5.20
28	12	0.250	8.65
29	12	0.250	14.4
30	12	0.250	24.0

* From Goldin et al. (1956).

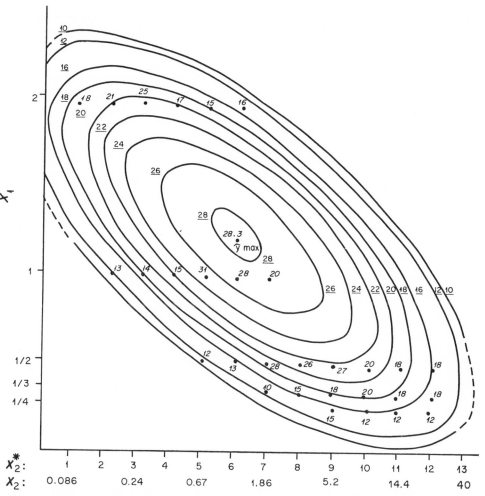

FIGURE 3 Response surface fitted to the data in Table 6 with the use of log dose level and log frequency. The underlined numbers are the response surface values obtained from fitting the model. The x_2^* values are logarithms of x_2 to the base 1.67.

Inspection of the data reveals that the experiment was unbalanced, since not all combinations of x_1 and x_2 were made. The reason for this is that a balanced experiment could not be performed: the drug, if given in too small a dose per day, would not retard the death of the mouse, because of the rapid growth of the tumor, whereas, if given in too large a dose per day, it would produce death due to toxicity.

Let us assume that the experimenter desired to fit a complete quadratic model, like that of Section 5, to the data; that is,

$$y = \alpha + \beta_1 x_1 + \beta_2 x_2 + \beta_{12} x_1 x_2 + \beta_{11} x_1^2 + \beta_{22} x_2^2 + \varepsilon$$

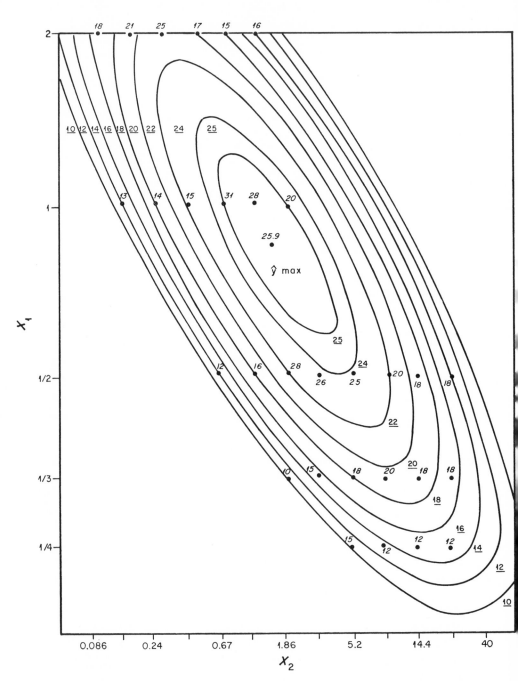

FIGURE 4   Response surface fitted to the data in Table 6 with the use of log dose level and log dose frequency.

TABLE 7 Predicted and Actual Responses and Their Differences (Both Absolute and Standardized) for the Response Surface in Figure 4

y, actual	y calculated from fitted response surface	Residual, actual-calculated	Standardized differences*
18	16.3305	+1.6695	+0.47
21	19.3605	+1.63955	+0.46
25	20.6878	+4.31223	+1.21
17	20.3125	−3.31245	−0.93
15	18.2345	−3.23449	−0.91
16	14.4539	+1.54611	+0.43
13	12.4213	+0.578658	+0.16
14	18.3143	−4.31428	−1.21
15	22.5046	−7.50459	−2.11
31	24.9923	+6.00774	+1.69
28	25.7773	+2.22271	+0.63
20	24.8597	−4.85968	−1.37
12	12.5780	−0.5780	−0.16
16	17.9287	−1.9287	−0.54
28	21.5767	+6.42328	+1.81
26	23.5221	+2.4779	+0.70
25	23.7648	+1.23516	+0.35
20	22.3049	−2.30494	−0.65
18	19.1424	−1.1424	−0.32
18	14.2772	+3.7228	+1.05
10	10.5372	−0.537166	−0.15
15	15.197	−0.196996	−0.06
18	18.1542	−0.154187	−0.04
20	19.4087	+0.591257	+0.17
18	18.9606	−0.960647	−0.27
18	16.8099	+1.19008	+0.33
15	10.4411	+4.55887	+1.28
12	13.5469	−1.54686	−0.44
12	14.95	−2.94996	−0.83
12	14.6504	−2.65041	−0.74

* Residual per standard deviation of residuals.

If the model fits reasonably well, a prediction of the combination of dose frequency and dose level that maximizes median survival can be made.

The reader is warned against using an available computer routine for fitting the response surface by multiple regression without first carefully inspecting the data. In this case using the data shown in the table would lead to a distorted contour picture. Instead, inspection of the data indicates that the dose levels of the drug are equally spaced on a logarithmic scale to the base 1.67. Making this transformation on x_2 and fitting the complete quadratic model to the data, one obtains Figure 3. However, note that on each of the lines corresponding to the number of doses per day the observed maximum $\hat{y}$ is to the left of the indicated maximum on the response surface. This indicates that the number of doses per day might also be linearized by a logarithmic transformation.

This new model was fitted, and the result is shown in Figure 4. The response surface is much improved. The fitted model is

$$y = -167.71987 + 83.17275x_1^* + 23.84667x_2^*$$
$$- 4.56563x_1^*x_2^* - 9.58599x_1^{*2} - 0.851319x_2^{*2}$$

where $x_1^* = 1.44269 \log_e x_1 + 3$ and $x_2^* = 1.94246 \log_e x_2 + 5.77212$.

The maximum $\hat{y}$ occurs at $x_1 = 0.855$ and $x_2 = 1.504$. Hence we should predict that the drug ought to be administered in doses of 1.504 mg/kg and 0.855 times a day. That is, of course, a *best* point estimate if we assume that the model provides a suitable fit. The maximum, shown in Figure 4, yields a predicted median survival time of 25.9.

The analysis of variance for this fit is as follows:

Term	DF	SS	MS	F	P
Regression	5	541.59	108.318	8.57	< 0.05
Residual error	24	303.21	12.73375		
Total:	29	844.80			

The residuals after fitting of the model are shown in Table 7. By carefully examining them one can determine where the model fits well and where it fits poorly. There is an indication that even a larger median survival time is possible. The residuals at the larger observed median survival times are all positive. It would be interesting to go further and determine by additional experimentation whether an improvement could be made for predicting the maximal median survival rate by a different model reflecting the apparent ridge line in Figure 4.

Additional information concerning the response surface designs mentioned in this chapter, plus many other designs, is given by Hill and Hunter (1966).

DISCUSSION

MOSTELLER   In Figure 3 could not one have traced a free-hand fit for each of those lines? What is the advantage of fitting a response surface? Second, in designing experiments we know that there are many symmetries that seem good to use. However, with the rise of the computer and the possibility of exploring every possible design we might expect to find designs that, if outrageous in shape, are nevertheless spectacularly good. Has this, in fact, come to pass, or is symmetry so binding that it cannot really be violated?

SMITH Your suggestion that several separate lines be made at each day's dosage level is exactly what the authors did. I have merely rephrased the problem as follows: "Is there any way that I can interpolate in this space for different times of the day and different dosages to obtain a predicted optimum?" This leads directly to the fitting of a response surface model. I was trying to determine the possibilities for interpolation. This is facilitated by the ellipsoid that was obtained.

With respect to the conjecture concerning outrageous designs, the analysis of the unbalanced-data problem is relevant. If one is trying to estimate independent effects of variables, one is compelled to use a balanced design, since with an unbalanced design the estimates of the parameters in the model are conditional not only upon the design space but also upon the intercorrelations of the independent variables. However, if one desires merely to predict the response surface and is not concerned with the role of individual variables, then the design makes little difference. One can usually construct a good predictive model; it may be a fifth-degree polynomial, but it will do a good job of prediction within the range of these data. However, if one intends to make inferences concerning points outside this range, there is greater security if the equation is derived from an underlying model. With the balanced design one at least approaches this position. Although the wrong variables may have been employed, or the equation may be nonlinear, at least one possesses a body of objective evidence. To feed unbalanced data into a computer and to utilize for prediction whatever equation results is exceedingly dangerous.

ARMITAGE The speaker discussed a design that looked like a 2×2 factorial squashed sideways and said that this should not be condemned as nonfactorial, because it could be made so by suitable transformation. This may be a more apposite remark in the present context than he realized, because for some years Professor Emmens and his colleagues have made very good use of this design, which they call, for obvious reasons, a parallelogram design.

SMITH The parallelogram design is a balanced design in a transformed space. However, one must be sure that it is reasonable to work in a transformed space.

COLTON Would you please comment on experimental designs for the fitting of nonlinear response surfaces?

SMITH Very little work has been done on the determination of optimal experimental designs for the fitting of nonlinear models. However, if the nonlinear model is specified, a careful examination of the iterative equations for determining the parameter estimates might reveal various designs that would be optimal for specific constraints.

BROWN   Would you please comment on the interpretation made from the residuals in Table 7?

SMITH   The residuals were standardized by dividing each by the square root of the mean square error. Employing the idea of control charts, that most of the standardized residuals should be within ± 2, one sees that the fit is good, much better than one would have expected with a squared multiple correlation coefficient of 64%. The trouble is that the location at which the residuals are large is exactly where the model should be improved. I am still dissatisfied with this model.

COCHRAN   From your experience in industry would you say that industrial experimenters have anything to teach biological experimenters? My impression is that if one likes industrial experimenters, one describes them as more daring than biological experimenters; if one dislikes them, one calls them rash. They deplore unnecessary replication, they never seem to randomize (at least not those I talk to), and they are willing to risk confusion between aliases in fractional factorials. Nevertheless, I assume that this is all being done for a worthy cause, in the interests of high efficiency.

SMITH   The industrial experimenter *has* to be innovative, fast-moving, and daring. The environment is profit-motivated, and results must be obtained at minimal costs. Thus, no unnecessary replication is employed, and randomization is used sparingly, usually when it entails no additional cost. A typical example of this minimal experimentation is saturated factorials in the optimization of a manufacturing process. In this case one is trying to find an operating position where one obtains a maximal yield for the least cost. The experimenter usually proceeds without replication, using any of the several available strategies. However, there are some outstanding exceptions. A pharmaceutical firm that is considering marketing a drug must do long and careful preliminary experimentation. Here the principles of replication and randomization are used constantly. Thus, one finds both conservative and daring experiments done within the same firm.

CHAPTER ELEVEN

Quantal-Response Variable Experimentation: The Up-and-Down Method

W. J. DIXON

1. Introduction

The purpose of this chapter is to present the up-and-down method and to illustrate its use in the design and analysis of quantal-response experiments and quantitative assays. In many circumstances the up-and-down method enjoys an advantage over the traditional fixed-sample-size methods in that it can provide a more simple and direct approach to experimentation.

The up-and-down method was first proposed by Dixon and Mood (1948). Recent further progress made in this method by Dixon (1965) is the basis of the present discussion.

2. The up-and-down method

The up-and-down method is applicable to the estimation of an LD_{50} or of an ED_{50} in a quantal-response situation (see Chapter 5). It should be remembered that measured responses can be rendered quantal by the establishment of cutoff points. An example with endocrinological data is given in Section 6.

To employ the up-and-down method one selects prior to the experiment a series of doses (test levels or dilutions), a starting dose, and a nominal sample size (this is defined later). The dose levels are so chosen as to be equally spaced on a log scale. The experiment consists of a series of trials in which the dose at a given trial is determined by the response result of the previous trial. If there is no response in a trial, the dose for the subsequent trialis raised one level; if there is a response, the dose for the subsequent trial is lowered one level.

A sample up-and-down series is shown in Table 1. The first trial consisted of a starting log dose of 0.903 administered to an animal. The O denotes that no response occurred. Hence, on the second trial the log dose was raised one level, to 1.204. The second animal exhibited a

TABLE 1   Example of a Test
Series with the Up-and-Down
Method*

Log dose	Results of tests			
1.204	X			
0.903	O	X	X	
0.602			O	O
0.301				
0				

* For this series OXXOXO the
estimate of $\log \mathrm{ED}_{50}$ is $0.602 +$
$0.831(0.301) = 0.852$.

response (denoted by X), so that the log dose for the third animal was
lowered one level, back to 0.903. The sequence proceeds in this up-and-
down manner until what is called the nominal sample size is reached.

The *nominal* sample size N of an up-and-down sequence of trials is a
count of the number of trials, beginning with the first pair of responses
that are unlike. For example, in the sequence of trial results OOOXOX
the nominal sample size is 4. For the sequence in Table 1 the nominal
sample size is 6, corresponding to the total number of trials (in Table 4
all the sequences in the body of the table are of nominal sample size 5,
although the total number of trials varies from 5 to 8).

Although the similar responses preceding the first pair of changed
responses are not used in determining the nominal sample size, they are
used in arriving at the estimate of the ED_{50}. The ED_{50} estimate is
obtained by means of Table 2 for nominal sample sizes 1 through 6. The
columns of Table 2 refer to the number of similar responses that precede determination of the nominal sample size. If the final dose level
in an up-and-down sequence is denoted by x_f, the log dose interval by
d, and the relevant entry in Table 2 by k, the estimate of $\log \mathrm{ED}_{50}$ is

$$\log \mathrm{ED}_{50} = x_f + kd \tag{1}$$

The calculation of $\log \mathrm{ED}_{50}$ for the sequence in Table 1 is shown at the
foot of the table (for the sequences in Tables 4 and 6 the reader may
verify with the use of Table 2 and Equation 1 the $\log \mathrm{ED}_{50}$ estimates
presented).

For nominal sample sizes greater than 6 the $\log \mathrm{ED}_{50}$ estimate is

$$(\textstyle\sum x_i + dA)/N \tag{2}$$

where the x_i's refer to the log dose levels among the N nominal sample
size trials, and where A is obtained from Table 3 and depends on the

TABLE 2 Values of k for Estimating the ED_{50} with Equation 1 for Nominal Sample Size 6 or Less (If the Table is Entered from the Foot, the Sign of k is Reversed)

N	Second part of series	\multicolumn{4}{c}{k for test series whose first part is}					Standard error of LD_{50}
		O	OO	OOO	OOOO		
2	X	−0.500	−0.388	−0.378	−0.377	O	0.88σ
3	XO	0.842	0.890	0.894	0.894	OX	0.76σ
	XX	−0.178	0.000	0.026	0.028	OO	
4	XOO	0.299	0.314	0.315	0.315	OXX	0.67σ
	XOX	−0.500	−0.439	−0.432	−0.432	OXO	
	XXO	1.000	1.122	1.139	1.140	OOX	
	XXX	0.194	0.449	0.500	0.506	OOO	
5	XOOO	−0.157	−0.154	−0.154	−0.154	OXXX	0.61σ
	XOOX	−0.878	−0.861	−0.860	−0.860	OXXO	
	XOXO	0.701	0.737	0.741	0.741	OXOX	
	XOXX	0.084	0.169	0.181	0.182	OXOO	
	XXOO	0.305	0.372	0.380	0.381	OOXX	
	XXOX	−0.305	−0.169	−0.144	−0.142	OOXO	
	XXXO	1.288	1.500	1.544	1.549	OOOX	
	XXXX	0.555	0.897	0.985	1.000^{+1}	OOOO	
6	XOOOO	−0.547	−0.547	−0.547	−0.547	OXXXX	0.56σ
	XOOOX	−1.250	−1.247	−1.246	−1.246	OXXXO	
	XOOXO	0.372	0.380	0.381	0.381	OXXOX	
	XOOXX	−0.169	−0.144	−0.142	−0.142	OXXOO	
	XOXOO	0.022	0.039	0.040	0.040	OXOXX	
	XOXOX	−0.500	−0.458	−0.453	−0.453	OXOXO	
	XOXXO	1.169	1.237	1.247	1.248	OXOOX	
	XOXXX	0.611	0.732	0.756	0.758	OXOOO	
	XXOOO	−0.296	−0.266	−0.263	−0.263	OOXXX	
	XXOOX	−0.831	−0.763	−0.753	−0.752	OOXXO	
	XXOXO	0.831	0.935	0.952	0.954	OOXOX	
	XXOXX	0.296	0.463	0.500	0.504^{+1}	OOXOO	
	XXXOO	0.500	0.648	0.678	0.681	OOOXX	
	XXXOX	−0.043	0.187	0.244	0.252^{+1}	OOOXO	
	XXXXO	1.603	1.917	2.000	2.014^{+1}	OOOOX	
	XXXXX	0.893	1.329	1.465	1.496^{+1}	OOOOO	
		X	XX	XXX	XXXX	Second part of series
		\multicolumn{4}{c}{$-k$ for series whose first part is}				

number of initial like responses and on the difference in the cumulative number of X's and O's that comprise the nominal sample size N. However, a sequence of trials with $N > 6$ is generally not recommended. It is preferable to run several small sequences of no more than 5 or 6. These can be most profitably accomplished by exploring several design

TABLE 3   Values of A for Estimating the ED_{50} with Equation 2 for Nominal Sample Size of 6 or More. N_O and N_X Refer to the Number of O's and X's That Comprise the Nominal Sample Size N. If the Table is Entered from the Foot, the Sign of A is Reversed.

| | A when first part of entire test series is | | | | |
$N_o - N_x$	O	OO	OOO	OOOO	OOOOO
5	10.8	10.8	10.8	10.8	10.8
4	7.72	7.72	7.72	7.72	7.72
3	5.22	5.25	5.25	5.25	5.25
2	3.20	3.30	3.30	3.30	3.30
1	1.53	1.69	1.70	1.70	1.70
0	0	0.44	0.48	0.48	0.48
−1	−1.55	−1.00	0.10	0.10	0.10
−2	−3.30	−2.16	−1.94	−1.92	−1.92
−3	−5.22	−3.45	−3.06	−3.00	−3.00
−4	−7.55	−5.07	−4.19	−4.03	−3.99
−5	−10.3	−6.8	−5.5	−5.1	−5.0
$N_x - N_o$	X	XX	XXX	XXXX	XXXXX
	$-A$ when first part of entire test series is				

variables, that is, by running several small sequences under differing experimental conditions.

The sampling error of the estimates in Equations 1 and 2 is evaluated in Dixon (1965). The mean square error of the estimate is remarkably independent of the starting level x_0 and is roughly approximated by $2\sigma^2/N$, where σ is the standard deviation of the underlying distribution of tolerances.

The low dependence on starting level is a substantial improvement over earlier work. The original up-and-down procedure presented by Dixon and Mood (1948) was based on asymptotic theory (that is, large-sample-size results). The mean square error of the ED_{50} estimate depended on the starting log dose x_0 and became increasingly large as $x_0 - \mu$ increased (μ is the true ED_{50}, or the mean of the underlying tolerance distribution). This presented difficulties in combining estimates having different standard errors. Brownlee et al. (1953) investigated this problem and provided an estimate whose mean square error depended less on x_0.

Although the up-and-down method fails to provide a direct estimate of σ^2, this is not a disadvantage. When a long up-and-down sequence of trials is collected, the sequence can be subdivided into a set of smaller sequences, each giving an estimate of the ED_{50}. Precision can then be obtained from the variation among the estimates from each of the smaller sequences. More often additional variables will be considered and, as indicated above, small up-and-down sequences can be collected under varying conditions, such as within a factorial design arrangement. The experimental error appropriate to the design will then yield an estimate of precision; see "Concomitant Variables" (Section 3) and Section 5. The fact that the mean square error of the up-and-down estimate for $N > 3$ is approximately constant is what facilitates this exploration of various design variables with small up-and-down sequences. For some uses the mean square error for $N = 3$ is sufficiently constant; for others the investigator will wish to take 4, 5, or 6 in the sequence.

3. Design considerations

Many considerations are necessary for the performance of an assay or the estimation of a dose–response curve.

Response

The up-and-down method is directly applicable to quantal-response experiments in which the end point is some event such as death, toxicity or shock. However, even with measured responses for the determination of thresholds the up-and-down method may be suitable; see Sections 6 and 7.

Prior information

Often preliminary assays are made before very much is known about the particular substance or hormone being assayed. The trials frequently will be sufficient to reveal the range of variation of doses over which measurable responses will occur. The up-and-down method requires only the knowledge of reasonable step sizes for the dose. The design rapidly moves testing to the neighborhood of median response and distributes subsequent testing in that neighborhood. If more extensive prior information is available, starting levels can be chosen with less error, and the step size can be optimized. In any case, one can avoid the disappointment of performing many tests in which no responses or all responses occur or in which graded responses occur far from the region of linear log-dose–response.

In some cases the region of response has been well investigated and is known, the response is linearly related to the log dose, and the measurements are well behaved (that is, they are normally distributed with no outliers) and can easily and quickly be determined. Here the up-and-down design will produce increased efficiency through proper placement of the tests. One will probably wish to use the standard regression techniques, in which the resulting estimates will have maximal efficiency, and one can obtain good estimates of this efficiency. However, moderate failures in the assumptions underlying the standard techniques may result in a greater efficiency with the up-and-down estimates. Experience with the actual conditions that prevail will be necessary to determine whether one estimate is better than the other.

Response distribution

It is widely assumed in bioassay that the distribution of response is either normal (usually after a logarithmic transformation) or logistic. The up-and-down design concentrates testing in regions that reduce the dependence on the distributional assumption. The assumption for the estimates in this chapter is normality of distribution. The results would differ very little if the assumption were that of logistic distribution. In fact, the estimates presented are almost distribution-free.

Concomitant variables

What are the feasible doses, routes of administration, and laboratory conditions? The estimation of a dose–response curve requiring a large number of animals under the same conditions can be very expensive and might necessitate a great amount of effort. Any possibility that the research design would cover other variables may allow the researcher to obtain much more information with the same number of animals. For instance, including the preconditioning variables, the researcher may wish to assay a substance with different routes of administration, in the presence of various sensitizing drugs, with different types of previous training, or with different previous feeding schedules. Other laboratory variables are different technicians and different methods of handling or housing the animals. Emmens in Chapter 8 has presented examples indicating sizable effects due to variations in laboratory conditions. The up-and-down method of collecting the data is particularly suited to exploration of these types of variable.

4. Designing up-and-down experiments

To plan an up-and-down experiment one needs to specify the starting log dose, the log dose spacing, and the nominal sample size. Obviously, it is advantageous to choose a starting dose as close to the ED_{50} as possible. The farther the starting dose is from the ED_{50}, the greater is the likelihood of a substantial string of similar responses prior to commencement of the nominal sample size count. Hence, for a specified nominal sample size a poorly located starting dose can result in increased experimental effort, in that a substantial total number of trials may be required.

The log dose levels should be equally spaced at, ideally, intervals of σ, the standard deviation of the underlying distribution of tolerances. However, a choice of spacing between $2\sigma/3$ and $3\sigma/2$ provides reasonably good estimates.

It is desirable to have nominal sample sizes of 3, 4, 5, or 6. This is because the mean square error of the up-and-down estimate for these nominal sample sizes is virtually independent of the starting dose and is relatively unaffected by the choice of log dose spacing within the interval indicated above (Dixon, 1965). The approximate homogeneity of variance permits the use of standard statistical designs (for example, randomized blocks, Latin squares) with application of the usual analysis of variance that accompanies these designs for exploring the concomitant variables discussed in the preceding section.

5. An example: assay of ryanodine

An example in which two design variables were simultaneously explored with several small sequences of up-and-down trials is an assay of ryanodine in mice conducted by Dr. Donald J. Jenden (Department of Pharmacology, University of California at Los Angeles) and described by Dixon (1965):

Ryanodine was administered intravenously to male mice in volume 0.1 to 0.2 ml in saline. The end point was considered to be the time of last visible movement. Four cut-off points with equal spacing in log time, 64, 96, 144, and 216 seconds were chosen for observing the status of the animal. Dosage was computed by body weight and a randomized block experiment with body weight as the blocking variable was used to obtain information on the validity of the use of the body weight basis for dosage.

Three levels of weight were used, yielding a 4×3 (times $\times$ weight) factorial arrangement (pp. 61–66). The design and results are shown in the top half of Table 4. For each of the twelve cells in the table the up-and-down sequence is indicated along with the final dose and the estimated LD_{50}. For each sequence the log dose interval was $d = 1$ and the nominal sample size was 5. The starting doses varied from one sequence to another.

The resulting LD_{50} estimates can now be summarized in an analysis of variance following the format on pp. 39 and 65. By means of orthogonal polynomials the sum of squares for weight (2 DF, degrees of freedom) can be partitioned into a linear and quadratic term and that for cutoff times (3 DF) into a linear, quadratic, and cubic term on log time (see p. 57). The analysis of variance is displayed in the bottom half of Table 4 and reveals a remarkable concentration of variability in the linear effect on log cutoff time.

TABLE 4   An Up-and-Down Experiment with Ryanodine in Mice

Design and results:

	Time to cutoff point, sec			
Weight, g	64	96	144	216
18–20				
Tests	OOOXXOX	OOOOXXOX	OOXXOO	XXOXXO
x_f	2.000	−0.107	−3.213	−7.213
k	−0.144	−0.142	0.372	0.861
Est.	1.856	−0.249	−2.841	−6.352
21–23				
Tests	OOOXOXX	OXXXX	XOXXX	XXOXOX
x_f	4.000	−1.107	−5.213	−6.213
k	0.181	0.555	0.157	−0.737
Est.	4.181	−0.552	−5.056	−6.950
24–26				
Tests	XXXOXXO	XXOXXO	OXXOX	OXOXX
x_f	1.000	−3.107	−4.213	−6.213
k	0.860	0.861	−0.305	0.084
Est.	1.860	−2.246	−4.518	−6.129

Analysis of variance:

Term	DF	SS	MS	F
Log time to cutoff	3	140.382		
Linear	1	139.086	139.086	114.10 ($P < 0.001$)
Quadratic	1	1.286	1.286	1.05
Cubic	1	0.010	0.010	0.01
Weight	2	1.630		
Linear	1	1.485	1.485	1.22
Quadratic	1	0.145	0.145	0.12
Interaction (time × weight) (individual degrees of freedom 0.021, 1.902, 0.014, 4.159, 0.877, 0.338)	6	7.311	1.219	
Total:	11	149.323		

The mean square interaction in the analysis of variance provides an estimate of the standard error of the LD_{50} of $\sqrt{1.219} = 1.10$. The last column of Table 2 shows that the standard error of the log LD_{50} with nominal sample size 5 is 0.61σ. Hence, σ, the standard deviation of the underlying tolerance distribution, is estimated as

$$1.10/0.61 = 1.81$$

As a result of this experiment the procedure was simplified by observing time to death with respect to fixed cutoff points.

When there are few degrees of freedom, as in this analysis, and one wishes to perform multiple tests of significance, it is instructive to employ a half-normal plot (Daniel, 1959) to check for uniformity among the single-degree-of-freedom sums of squares; see Figure 1. Homogeneous single-degree-of-freedom sums of squares will appear as an approximately straight line on half-normal paper. It is easy to see from the plot that only the one factor is present in these data.

In the ryanodine experiment it would have been difficult to choose fixed doses to cover the great differences in response without having many cases of 0 or 100% response. There was no loss of time in using a design requiring serial tests, since in this experiment the tests were necessarily sequential. The measurement of actual time to death is difficult, and sometimes death does not occur. The up-and-down technique avoids these problems. In general, the up-and-down design is advantageous if one knows the response range but not the corresponding dose range.

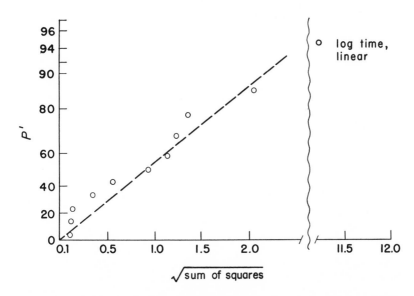

FIGURE 1   Half-normal plot of the eleven 1 DF sums of squares in the lower half of Table 4. On a sheet of arithmetic probability paper, where P denotes the probability scale, the portion below $P = 50\%$ is deleted. For $P > 50\%$ each value of P is replaced with $P' = 2P - 100$. The eleven 1 DF sums of squares are ranked from low to high. For each sum of squares, where i denotes its rank order ($i = 1, \ldots, 11$), the point is plotted with an abscissa equal to the square root of the sum of the squares and an ordinate equal to $P' = (i - 0.5)/11$.

6. Another example: a mouse uterine-weight assay

Data on mouse uterine weights for PM(B), a human menopausal gonadotropin, were kindly generated by Dr. Janet W. McArthur to provide an endocrinological example for this paper.

Preliminary data consisting of the uterine weights of forty mice (ten mice in each of four groups, doses of 0.02, 0.04, and 0.08 mg and saline) were analyzed and are shown in Table 5. An up-and-down experiment was planned on the basis of these data. The doses were specified to be at intervals of $\sqrt{2}$, or approximately 0.15 on the log scale. Four cutoff weights were chosen: 12, 16, 22, and 30 mg. For each cutoff weight an up-and-down sequence was conducted, to achieve a nominal sample size of 5. For example, with the cutoff weight of 12 mg a uterus that weighed more than 12 mg was classified "response." The mice were treated in sequence, the dose for each mouse being determined by the response of the previous mouse, as indicated in Section 2. The starting doses were determined from the preliminary information in Table 5. The results of the up-and-down trials and the actual uterine weights are shown in Table 6.

TABLE 5   Uterine Weights of Mice Treated with PM(B) or Saline

		PM(B)	
	Saline	0.02 mg	0.04 mg	0.08 mg
---	---	---	---	---
	6.4	14.2	21.8	39.6
	7.6	10.6	27.6	39.4
	8.2	12.4	16.0	30.4
	8.4	14.2	27.6	32.2
	6.8	16.2	16.0	45.8
	16.6	12.0	19.2	47.8
	9.4	10.6	17.4	28.8
	6.6	12.8	20.4	28.8
	7.2	12.4	23.0	47.8
	6.0	16.2	22.8	40.4
Mean:	8.3	13.2	21.2	38.1

Through the use of standard linear-regression methodology the regression of log ED_{50} on log weight was determined as

$$\log ED_{50} = -2.423 + 0.882 \text{ (log weight)}$$

In predicting log dose from log organ weight one can be concerned about the possible loss of accuracy resulting from the use of cutoff points rather than the actual weights in this relation. The more orthodox scheme for dose prediction would involve a predetermined number of

TABLE 6 Results of Up-and-Down Experiments with PM(B) on Uterine Weights of Mice

Cutoff wt., mg	Dose, mg	Log dose	1	2	3	4	5	6	7	Est. of log ED$_{50}$
			\multicolumn{7}{c}{Results of successive trials}	
12	0.040	−1.40		X		X		X		−1.474
	0.028	−1.55	O		O		O			
Actual wt., mg:			8.8	13.4	7.4	13.4	6.6	18.2		
16	0.057	−1.25			X					−1.408
	0.040	−1.40		O		X		X		
	0.028	−1.55	O				O		O	
Actual wt., mg:			5.6	15.6	17.2	18.6	12.0	16.8	7.8	
22	0.080	−1.10			X				O	−1.138
	0.057	−1.25		O		X		O		
	0.040	−1.40	O				O			
Actual wt., mg:			10.0	18.0	32.3	23.4	9.0	18.4	7.6	
30	0.080	−1.10		X		X		X		−1.173
	0.057	−1.25	O		O		O			
Actual wt., mg:			18.8	44.8	15.0	32.8	8.4	35.6		

animals tested at a set of predetermined doses. The linear regression of the log organ weight on log dose would be determined and, for a given log organ weight, the log dose would be predicted from this regression line.

To illustrate the standard procedure, the data in Table 6 were analyzed as if they came from a fixed-sample-size experiment (preselected dose levels and predetermined number of mice per dose level). The logarithms of the actual weights in Table 6 were calculated, and the data were grouped by dose, as is shown in the top half of Table 7. The design conforms to a one-way classification; the analysis of variance is shown in the bottom half of the table with the between-dose term (3 DF) subdivided into a regression on log dose term (1 DF) and a scatter term (2 DF); see pp. 54–59. The regression line for log organ weight on log dose is

$$\text{log organ weight} = 2.613 + 1.088 \text{ (log dose)}$$

Solving for log dose gives the resulting prediction relation:

$$\text{log dose} = -2.401 + 0.919 \text{ (log organ weight)}$$

Note that in Table 6 the value 0.88 in the highest dose group (0.080 mg) appears to be an outlier. The data could be further refined by Winsorization (see pp. 49 and 58 and Dixon and Tukey, 1968) to yield

$$\text{log dose} = -2.449 + 0.760 \text{ log weight}$$

TABLE 7 Analysis of the Actual-Weight Data in Table 6, Pre-selected Doses and Number of Animals per Group Assumed

Data:

Dose, mg	0.028	0.040	0.057	0.080
x = log dose	−1.55	−1.40	−1.25	−1.10
$u = (2x + 2.65)/0.15$	−3	−1	1	3

	y = log uterine weight			
	0.75	0.95	0.92	0.88
	0.82	1.00	1.18	1.51
	0.87	1.13	1.24	1.52
	0.89	1.13	1.26	1.55
	0.94	1.19	1.26	1.65
	1.08	1.23	1.27	
		1.26	1.37	
		1.27		

n_t (no. of observations)	6	8	7	5	$N = 26$
T_t (response totals)	5.35	9.16	8.50	7.11	$T = 30.12$
$\bar{y}_t$ (response means)	0.892	1.145	1.214	1.422	

Analysis of variance:

Term	DF	SS	MS	F
Between doses	3	0.7976		
Regression on log dose	1	0.7552	0.7552	25.16 ($P < 0.001$)
Scatter	2	0.0424	0.0212	0.71
Within doses	22	0.6605	0.03002	
Total:	25	1.4581		

In this example Winsorization also reduces the variance about the regression by a factor of 3. This is greater than the loss of efficiency in the use of an all-or-none response in place of a measurement response. Therefore, for the data at hand increased efficiency results from gathering the data according to the up-and-down rule. The effect of outliers and the nonnormal character of the data approximately offset the theoretical loss in information from using the all-or-none results in place of the actual measurements in the statistical analysis (assuming the standard analysis is used to relate log weight to log dose and no further "dry-cleaning" of the data such as that provided by Winsorization is used).

Hence, it appears reasonable to use the simpler method, to record, that is, only whether or not the weight exceeds the cutoff weight.

7. Discussion

The collection of data by the up-and-down procedure has several advantages over the more orthodox scheme. First, the assay could proceed without one's knowing precisely what doses would provide the appropriate range of response; that is, the data are more or less automatically gathered in the "right" region. Animals are not tested out of the range of interest. By contrast, the standard procedure can be wasteful of test material.

Second, the up-and-down technique is particularly suited to the situation in which there is no satisfactory response measurement or, in the extreme, in which only an all-or-none response is available. The data will then be gathered in a manner that permits the estimate, as given above, disregarding any actual measurement results. Even when graded responses are available, the measurements obtained may have many outliers or indeterminate extreme values or may generally come from a long-tailed distribution, so that the all-or-none estimates will yield a smaller variance than will estimates derived by orthodox regression procedures.

An additional factor, which is probably smaller, but which is in favor of the up-and-down method, is that the analysis procedure minimizes the sum of squares on log dose rather than on response, which is in the desired direction for bioassay prediction. The computations are simpler, and the interpretation follows the widely known and used regression analysis.

In summary, greater efficiency can result from the up-and-down design for obtaining data, since it provides for a better placement of tests and a predictable standard error of estimate for a given number of trials.

If the up-and-down estimate is used for analyzing the data, one also obtains a direct estimate of the predicting regression and an analysis that is independent of outliers or indeterminate extreme measurements and is relatively unaffected by lack of normality of distribution; further, one is able to form a quick judgment of the outcome.

Comments on the literature

An analogous sequential procedure for determining the ED_{50} is the Robbins-Monro method of stochastic approximation. With this method the spacing between successive log doses narrows as the testing continues. The theoretical basis of the method derives from Robbins and Monro (1951), its statistical properties have been investigated by Wetherill (1963) and Cochran and Davis (1965), and its application to toxicity testing has been exemplified by Hawkins (1964). In the short series of trials that have been the concern of this paper it appears that little would have been gained by using the Robbins-Monro method in place of the up-and-down procedure.

An application of the up-and-down procedure in a fairly long series of trials has been described by Rümke (1959). Rümke mentioned the lack of a method of obtaining confidence intervals for the LD_{50} estimate in the up-and-down procedure. However, by taking his data and breaking the long series into several small subseries with nominal sample sizes of 6 or less, suitable confidence intervals can be obtained with the methods described in this chapter.

Finally, Claringbold (1955b) has illustrated the use of the up-and-down method in an endocrinological experimental setting.

DISCUSSION

MOSTELLER   Is it true for the maximum-likelihood estimate that the sequence after, say, the first two observations does not matter provided that one had the same frequencies of X's and O's at each level in various series? If after OX one observed XOOX, would one get the same estimate as with OXXO?

DIXON   Yes. Moreover, I should like to comment on the nonparametric aspects. If it is assumed that the underlying distribution is symmetrical with a single mode, and if the responses (O's and X's) also satisfy that condition, this estimate is distribution-free (that is, independent of the form of the distribution). Therefore the table of maximum-likelihood estimates based on the normal-distribution assumption will, in certain instances, be the same, whatever the distributional assumption. Thus the result may or may not be nonparametric (distribution-free), depending on the particular configuration of responses.

MOSTELLER   I was interested in the regression line that went the other way: the regression of log dose on log organ weight. Looking at dosage data, I wonder what ways we have of obtaining that regression line from data collected in the usual manner.

DIXON   Choosing the data entirely at fixed doses and determining a sample size at each dose can produce a greater bias in the estimation of that regression line than can collecting the data with the up-and-down technique. The bias resulting from inability to guess correctly the starting point for the dose series is partly removed with the up-and-down method. In addition, with the usual regression calculated from fixed doses one is minimizing the sum of squares in essentially the wrong direction for the prediction of log dose from log organ weight.

FINNEY   I was interested in, and surprised by, what the speaker said about estimation from the regression line. An interesting recent claim (Krutchkoff, 1967) is that in a standard dose–response situation the estimation of an x that will, on an average, give a specified y is better obtained by a calculation of the regression of x on y than by that of y on x. I cannot easily believe this, although the arithmetic of the particular example presented seems correct. I do not fully appreciate the speaker's argument that with data of the conventional form the ordinary regression procedure is wrong. However, I think there is much to be said for his claim that the up-and-down approach enables one to place the doses in a better manner for obtaining a precise estimate. Of course, if one has obtained results from the up-and-down procedure, to take the regression of the four critical doses on the uterine weights is the correct way to estimate the appropriate critical dose for any other uterine weight.

One point worried me. Suppose that the distribution of uterine weight for fixed dose really is normal; then, *if* uterine weights have been measured but are subsequently used only to classify the uteri as greater or less than specified values, information appears to be sacrificed. Of course, as has been indicated, there may be economic advantages in not having to weigh, and merely grading, each uterus as greater or less than a stated figure. But if weights are available, if distributions are normal, and if the up-and-down procedure is used, what information is lost, and what becomes of it?

DIXON   I should like to reiterate that, when the data are normal, there is a loss in precision. In the examples I presented, including Dr. McArthur's experiment, the data were nonnormal to the extent that the standard errors were actually more than twice what one would obtain with normal data. In a strictly normal situation the up-and-down estimate has an asymptotic variance of $2\sigma^2/N$, compared to a mean having a variance of σ^2/N. This is the disadvantage that you referred to as a sacrifice of information. With data from a normal distribution one might say that one is throwing away roughly half of the information. In the analysis of Dr. McArthur's data the degree of nonnormality effectively doubles the variance of the mean. Winsorization (see pp. 49 and 58) is a procedure that may help to recoup some of this loss in the traditional estimating situation. Even with Winsorization it appears to be difficult to reduce the variance of the mean below twice its appropriate value, which is the level obtained with the up-and-down procedure. It is essentially a conflict between nonnormality and the supposed loss of information by using the up-and-down technique. In Dr. McArthur's data the standard errors were less in the up-and-down method than they were on the assumption of normality and with the use of the standard method.

EMMENS   What is the danger of the up-and-down procedure when, as in the case of Dr. McArthur's data, the test must have taken days or even weeks to complete? Diurnal and other rhythms might inflate the error to such a degree that other possible advantages would be lost.

DIXON   I have two answers to that. (1) If sufficient tests can be done at one time, one can estimate the variation over longer periods of time, so long as a single sequence may be considered to be homogeneous with respect to such variation. There can be some advantages in having tests spaced. (2) If one knows the possible variations, one can, for example, do a test with an animal at eight o'clock in the morning every third day. One may actually have less variation than if the animals are all tested in one morning, some at eight, some at nine, and some at ten o'clock. Thus, it is a matter of design. Each technique has its particular advantages in certain circumstances.

MOSTELLER   Will you comment on the reliability of estimates based on particular patterns? I take it that the error variance is averaged across all possible patterns that may occur. I presume that if one had a nominal case of $N = 6$ in which a starting OX was followed by OOOO rather than by an alternating sequence, OXOX, the estimate would be less reliable.

DIXON   Yes. The mean square error curve is an average of the error curves for each result. Its flatness is surprising, since the individual curves have large variations. These would be of great interest to users of the method. The experimenter also would be interested in the probability that each of these sequences would occur, because an unlikely sequence could be an indication of faulty procedure or some inconsistency among animals.

ALBERT   I should like an explanation of Winsorization.

DIXON   To Winsorize, one replaces the two extreme values (one at each end) with the values of their closest neighbors. This obviously reduces the variance. The appropriate changes in the distribution are given by Dixon and Tukey (1968).

RINARD   How can an experimenter determine when to apply the Winsorization technique?

DIXON   Well-documented objective rules are not available. A technique that I can recommend is as follows. If there is a substantial reduction in the confidence limits with Winsorization, one may conclude that the distribution is not normal. If the data were normally distributed, there would be an increase in the length of a confidence interval, since Winsorization "throws information away." The confidence limits for Dr. McArthur's data shrank to less than half their length before Winsorization. Therefore we have convincing evidence that the data were not normal to begin with.

COCHRAN What effect does the length of time before the response is known have on the general feasibility of the up-and-down technique? For instance, must the response be known in an hour, since one must know the answer from each step before starting the next step? I realize that one can, in some circumstances, start several sequences in series.

DIXON If one uses a nominal sample size, say 4, then the experiment will take about four times as long as it will if the animals are all tested at once. However, in many circumstances the experimenter cannot test all animals at once. The question is, how are tests to be done over time? If they are done with the up-and-down design, they will yield more information in the sense that design variables can be subsequently introduced into the problem and the observations are better placed for the desired estimation. Unless one knows which tests to make, can do them all at once, and has cheap test materials, one gains no particular advantage from the up-and-down method. In many of the problems I have worked with, the up-and-down method has not, in fact, prolonged the experiment. It has merely changed the order in which the tests were done.

CHAPTER TWELVE

Biomathematics*

MURRAY EDEN

1. Introduction

The principal concern of the applied mathematician is to take the observations and concepts developed from empirical knowledge and to recast them into the formal language of mathematics. If the translation into mathematical language is successful, one may be enabled to discover relations and consequences that could not easily have been expressed in the original language of experimental observation.

Is there any special mathematics for endocrinology or, more generally, for biology? Are there branches of mathematics (perhaps some of the more esoteric ones, such as topology or algebraic number theory) that are not particularly useful in physics or chemistry but that might find application in the life sciences? I think that the answer is a qualified "No." By and large, there is nothing particularly special about biology in this sense. The tools that a mathematician uses in physics or chemistry are the same as those he uses in biology. However, there is one striking difference, namely, the variability of the data with which he is confronted. It is appropriate that this conference is concerned mainly with statistics. In biology the chief problem in the interpretation of results is to give credence to the data. In general, instrumental error tends to be rather small relative to so-called biological variation. The only mathematical tools that are useful in giving this credence to biological data are those of statistics, such as experimental design, tests of significance and confidence-interval estimation. Although the mathematician and the statistician have similar interests, I distinguish between the two in that problems of quantitation tend to be the concern of the latter more than of the former.

Aside from statistics, what kinds of mathematics does one find in papers dealing with endocrinology? Precisely the same that one finds in papers dealing with problems in chemical kinetics and with problems involving flow and diffusion: for example, the treatment of tracer

* This work was supported principally by the National Institutes of Health Grants 5-P01-GM 14940-02 and 5-P01-FM 15006-02 and in part by the joint services of Electronics Program, Contract DA28-043-AMC-02536 (a).

measurements (so-called compartmental analysis and, to a certain extent, feedback analysis) involves the same mathematics. Parenthetically, feedback of a special kind has been known to the chemical world for at least a hundred years under the name of "reflux."

During the last ten years a number of engineers have become interested in the application of mathematical techniques to biological problems, including those with which endocrinology is concerned. Electrical, mechanical, and chemical engineering have a common denominator in that they deal with the relations between things, usually physical quantities that one can call inputs and outputs, such as flows of materials and currents. Moreover, engineering theory can concern itself with relations between abstract elements, especially the flow of information, and biological problems can often be cast in this format.

2. Linearity

Most practical situations that an electrical or mechanical engineer encounters exhibit the convenient property of linearity, at least within certain ranges for the variables of concern. The utility of linear-system models resides in the fact that a vast armamentarium of mathematical techniques has been developed for their solution and interpretation.

Let me attach two slightly different meanings to "linearity." Most problems, such as those of chemical kinetics, can be cast in terms of a differential equation. An equation is called linear if the sum of any two solutions or the product of any solution and some arbitrary constant is also a solution of the differential equation. Linearity also refers to a so-called linear system. One should distinguish between a linear system and a set of linear differential equations. They are closely related, but they are not the same.

A linear system may be conveniently described as follows. Consider a system in which one can label a given variable as input and another as output, and for which one can make the statement, "It is at rest." For instance, when all of the currents and voltages in an electrical system are turned off, if one waits long enough the system will come to rest. On the other hand, it is by no means necessarily true that a biological system "in equilibrium" is at rest. However, if it is at rest, and if it has what may be labeled input and output, one may regard the output as a function of the input. A linear system has the following convenient property. Let us imagine that two possible inputs to the system are denoted by x_1 and x_2. For the sake of concreteness we may consider an input to be the quantity of some chemical substance introduced into an organism and plotted as a function of time. Let us assume that the measured response, or output, corresponding to input x_1 is $T(x_1)$; this might be the concentration of some other chemical substance in the plasma of the organism, again considered as a function of time. Similarly, let us assume that the measured output corresponding to input x_2 is $T(x_2)$. What can we expect to find as the response to an input $Ax_1 + Bx_2$, where A and B are multiplicative constants? If the system is linear, we can predict that the measured response will be $AT(x_1) + BT(x_2)$. In fact, we can prescribe certain special input functions, measure the response to these particular inputs, and predict the response of the system to any input within the range of linearity.

In biology the argument is occasionally made that, since most biological systems are nonlinear, linear analysis has little to offer. It is true that most biological systems are nonlinear; so, too, are most inorganic systems. However, this does not vitiate the usefulness of linear-system analysis any more than the nonexistence of perfect gases vitiates the usefulness of the gas laws.

3. Utility of simple models

Insight is to be gained by using simple, approximate models before attempting to devise more precise and complicated ones. Let me give an instance from a small piece of research in which I once participated. It relates to a physiological process and has an adventitious connection with endocrinology. A well-known observation is that the difference between the partial pressures of CO_2 in the plasma and in the urine changes as a function of the buffer capacity of the urine. I will not go through the equations in any detail. An algebraic equation is derived, in which the rate of change of CO_2 concentration with time is related to the concentration of CO_2, H_2CO_3, and various anions, to pH, to various hydration and dissociation constants, and also to a catalytic coefficient (since the dehydration of carbonic acid is catalyzed by certain anions). The model of the system depends on little more than the notions of mass action, equilibrium, electroneutrality, and some other simple concepts of chemistry. The equation is

$$\frac{a_{\mathrm{H}}^2 + C_1 a_{\mathrm{H}} + C_2}{a_{\mathrm{H}}^3 + b_1 a_{\mathrm{H}}^2 + b_2 a_{\mathrm{H}} + b_3} \cdot \frac{da_{\mathrm{H}}}{dt} = -K_{\mathrm{D}} \tag{1}$$

The form of the equation is also simple, although from one point of view it is confusing. A number of terms must be summed, and one term involves a quadratic expression in the independent variable a_{H} (hydrogen ion activity) divided by a cubic expression.

When the indicated integration is performed, the resulting equation is

$$
\begin{aligned}
-K_D(t - t_0) = {} & (r_1 A + r_2 B + r_3 C) a_H \\
& + A(r_1^2 + C_1 r_2 + C_2) \ln(a_H - r_1) \\
& + B(r_2^2 + C_1 r_2 + C_2) \ln(a_H - r_2) \\
& + C(r_3^2 + C_1 r_3 + C_2) \ln(a_H - r_3) \\
& + \text{constant}
\end{aligned}
\tag{2}
$$

where r_1, r_2, and r_3 are the real roots of the cubic equation in the denominator of Equation 1. This equation is more unwieldy, although it is still a simple algebraic expression. From the mathematical point of view the problem is solved, in that the partial pressure of CO_2 has been related to experimental variables and relevant system constants in a closed, analytic form. The mathematician will say, "I have finished."

From the point of view of an investigator interested in verifying this equation in terms of some set of experiments this is, however, merely the beginning. For a numerical solution a tedious series of calculations is required, and it took myself and others an entire afternoon to compute two data points. I don't know how many of my readers know what the error rate is for human beings as computers. For the students and technicians who have worked with me an error rate of something on the order of 1% per atomic computation (1% per addition or multiplication or division) is not an unusually high figure. If a hundred arithmetic operations are required to compute one data point, the probability of getting one data point correct is rather small. I have had the traumatic experience of plotting a graph that theory indicated should be a straight line but that looked like a scatter diagram, simply because more than half of the computed points were in error. We therefore went with our basic equation to the National Bureau of Standards and arranged for an ENIAC computer to be programmed to yield numerical solutions.

By means of the equation we have derived we computed the values of pH as a function of time; they are depicted in Figure 1. Since an experimental test of the mathematical model was envisaged, changes in pH (which is relatively easy to monitor continuously) are shown rather than changes in the partial pressure of CO_2. Reasonable values were assigned to the constants required (some parameters, such as ionization constants, were obtained from the literature, and others were assigned values that, from an incomplete knowledge of the composition of the glomerular fluid, seemed plausible). It should be noted that for sufficiently high buffer strength a period of well over a minute is required before the CO_2 has equilibrated with the gas phase above it. In other words, the dissociation rate for carbonic acid is really quite slow, and in consequence we could demonstrate rather large differences in pH with time.

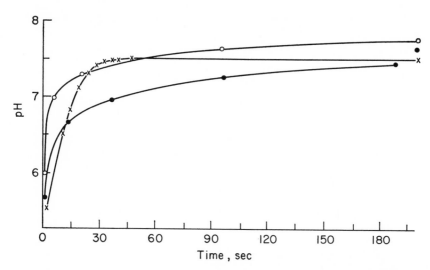

FIGURE 1 Plot of pH as a function of time, derived from a mathematical model. Buffer concentration, 1×10^{-1} M. Buffer pK: ($\times$) 1×10^{-5}; ($\bullet$) 1.66×10^{-7}; ($\bigcirc$) 1×10^{-8}. $K_{H_2CO_3}$ (the first ionization of H_2CO_3), K_D (the dehydration constant), and K_H (the hydration constant) are taken from Roughton (1935). From Kennedy et al. (1957).

For purposes of experimental verification we constructed a small model in which buffers at different pH's and with different amounts of carbon dioxide were bubbled with air, while we observed what happened to pH as a function of time. The fit of the mathematical model to the experimental observations of the physical model was quite good. A typical experimental run is shown in Figure 2.

An additional point is that it was unnecessary to solve the equation. Although it would not have given us a formal solution, the computer could certainly have performed the computations with the differential form rather than with the analytic solution. Since an analytic solution to the differential equation may simply not be found, it may be essential to employ the differential form in complicated systems.

However, there is another approach that may be tried. Rather than attempt to compute the numerical results for some complicated expression it is often instructive to simplify the model to such a point that its mathematical form can be solved readily. There are many instances in which an examination of the algebraic expression will provide one with greater insight than any particular set of numerical approximations to solutions. Many of the implications to be drawn concerning the relations between different parameters or between different variables are to be found, not by looking at graphs or columns of numbers but, rather, by looking at the algebraic expressions themselves. Of course, in making the

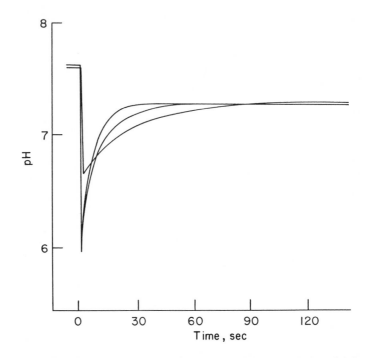

FIGURE 2   Plot of pH as a function of time, derived from a physical model. Buffer
pK, 6.78. Buffer concentration, μmol/lit: (upper curve) 0.005; (middle curve)
0.010; (lower curve) 0.35. From Kennedy et al. (1957).

simplification that permits a solution to be found it may be that one has
obtained simplicity but lost relevance. How simple can one make a
model and yet retain some hold on the real data? What I have been
talking about is the art, rather than the technique, of computation, and
consequently no prescribed answer can be given. It seems appropriate
to add that the art of mathematical use, like more conventional art forms,
requires a knowledge of the techniques as well as talent.

   As was mentioned earlier, statistics is clearly the most important tool
in much of the biology dealing with the problems of data evaluation. To
the engineers who have thought about biological problems perhaps the
most interesting aspect of data evaluation is that of modeling. Models
are created for a variety of purposes. They satisfy the æsthetic urge to
provide a rational explanation of the phenomena of nature. We like to
believe, after all, that biology is rational.

   Unfortunately, many of the phenomena that we should like to explain
are not very accessible to experimental measurement. Sometimes the
measurement is not justified, by reason of hazard to the organism being
observed. At other times techniques for obtaining the data with sufficient

accuracy, precision, or frequency are not available. The experimental biologist has learned to live with the notion of biological variability, but the cost is great. Consider, for example, the problem of studying pH or cation concentration changes in the circulation of a large mammal. Samples can be drawn and measurements made with a frequency not much greater than perhaps once every ten minutes; yet there is good reason to believe that the measured quantities can undergo substantial changes within seconds. In any study involving the injection of some chemical entity into the circulation and measurement of that entity the measurements should be made at very short intervals and preferably continuously. Despite this obvious need there are virtually no bioassays that yield continuous measurements. In the jargon of engineering, there is remarkably little information that can be obtained about a signal with considerable high-frequency content if the signal can be sampled only at relatively long time intervals.

4. Curve-fitting

In the face of biological variation curve-fitting is a valuable technique for reducing data to a compact form. However, it must be applied with a certain amount of caution. A conflict may very well develop between the characteristics of the proposed model and the desire to obtain a good fit to the data. When, for example, there is a tracer study of the distribution of some component in an organism, the usual practice is to fit the data to a sum of exponentials, on the assumption that this is the way certain first-order events manifest themselves and that these events can occur sequentially or in parallel or perhaps in other arrangements. A semilog plot of the tracer concentration as a function of time is often prepared and the question asked, "How many straight-line segments do I draw in order to fit this curve?" I believe that in many cases this is a fruitless exercise. Unless the data are remarkably precise and there is strong anatomical or physiological indication of a multiplicity of compartments, there is no particular reason to use the exponential form of the equation for fitting the data; one might choose from many other functions, perhaps for sounder reasons, and the search for a third compartment and then a fourth will add little to the analysis.

For those who like to play mathematical games I suggest the following exercise. Take a piece of graph paper, and with a spline or French curve draw a line that intersects the y axis at some positive value and that appears to be asymptotic to the x axis; in other words, draw a curve that "looks like" exponential decay, a curve without local extrema or points of inflection. Now try to fit this arbitrary curve by a sum of three exponentials and then by a sum of four exponentials. Plot the two estimates on the same piece of graph paper. It will be seen that only the unusual biological experiment will provide data that are sufficiently precise and reproducible to justify choosing the four-exponent over the three-exponent equation.

My feeling is that curve-fitting is a way of representing data in a form that can be entered in a notebook as an equation rather than as a column of numbers. Whether one happens to use a power series or a sum of exponentials or whatever makes little difference, unless there is a sound physiological or physicochemical reason for choosing one representation over another.

5. Pitfalls in model-building

In model-building we assume what we believe to be a plausible mechanism. In some sense this is the justification for such concepts as compartments, diffusion rates, and the like. To be sure, compartments and membranes exist in the objects under study. However, we have to be cautious in assuming that the mechanism underlying a model is correct simply because it is plausible.

An anecdote will illustrate the pitfalls of plausible argument. This concerns the statistics of birth rates. It seems reasonable to say at first sight that births conform to a binomial model, which assumes that they are independent events. One can make the simple computation that the probability of a live birth is estimated from the number of live births divided by the number of couples in a population. If the expected number of live births is given by np, where n is the number of couples, one would expect the standard deviation to be $\sqrt{np(1 - p)}$, or very nearly the square root of the number of live births. What does this mean? It means that in a country that has a million live births in a year one would expect the year-to-year fluctuations to be of the order of 1,000. We consulted the birth statistics, published by the World Health Organization, of the countries for which one could find reliable figures. The year-to-year variation proved to be from ten to forty times as great as the estimate based on the binomial trial model. It suggests that there are other factors that prevent the events from being truly independent. Although the model is unsuitable for this particular prediction, other deductions that it permits about birth processes may be correct.

Similar comments may be made regarding other issues in model-building that are relevant to endocrinology. Most chemical and physiological models assume continuity and homogeneity. It is my impression, however, that the architecture of the tissues that produce the variety of hormones is not homogeneous. Moreover, it seems reasonable to me that a cell that can manufacture a particular hormone is either "on" or "off."

This is very far from being a continuous process. It may be justifiable to argue that, since there is a large population of cells producing the enzyme, the concentration of some appropriate component in the system controlling the rate of production of the enzyme "averages out" over the population of cells. However, it is my impression that the process is fairly discontinuous, even when hormone production is observed at the drop level rather than the micro level. In other words, the stream rate is not a constant with time, even given that the other variables in the system are constant; there is fluctuation here too. Many models postulate the existence of compartments. By implication compartments are homogeneous in all the concentration variables, but there are practically no compartments in the body (and that includes the blood) in which one can expect the completeness of mixing that must be assumed in compartment analysis. Again, this is not to say that compartment analysis and the other assumptions made in tracer kinetics are unjustified. It depends upon the specific problem and upon the investigator's expertise. I will simply repeat what I said earlier: one should approach a model with a certain amount of care, for the assumptions may be unjustified.

6. Coda

If I appear to be discouraging the use of mathematics, that is not my intention. Every biologist should learn something of mathematics and its relevance to his field of interest. It is unrealistic and probably incorrect to advise biologists to develop a high level of mastery of mathematics, but in endocrinology and in other branches of biology that deal with control and execution of function it would be wise to cultivate a mathematical point of view. This implies a concern with precision of expression, with relations between variables rather than with causation, and with quantitation rather than description. The endocrinologist who has sufficient skill to set up a mathematical model can, in all likelihood, find the mathematical help needed to derive the consequences of the model.

DISCUSSION

GURPIDE I want to join the speaker in expressing pessimism concerning the validity of current methods of estimating the number of pools that exchange material with a circulating compound. This number is usually obtained by counting the exponential terms, the sum of which describes the disappearance from plasma of an intravenously injected tracer. However, even in irreducible systems (systems consisting of pools that exchange isotope with each other) the number of exponential terms may be much smaller than the number of pools in the system (Sharney, Wasserman, and Gewirtz, 1964). Furthermore, analysis of more than one specific-activity curve does not help to overcome the uncertainty about the number of pools in the system. On the other hand, since a large number of "fast mixing" pools certainly has to be considered with in vivo experiments, the drastic reduction in the number of exponential terms may be the result of a linear dependence in the specific activities of some pools (Hearon, 1963). In collaboration with Dr. Jonah Mann we have derived relationships, among the fractional rates of transfer between the pools, that are necessary and sufficient for a linear dependence among specific activities. There is a corresponding reduction in the number of exponential terms in all of the pools of a general, irreducible system.

Since representation of a compound in a tissue as a fast-mixing pool is unrealistic, smaller pools should be considered. They may represent a compound in individual cells or even in subcellular components, where fast mixing could be postulated. If one can invoke relationships among the rate constants of transfer between those small, fast-mixing pools and the circulation, one can predict curves of disappearance of the tracer from plasma that consist of a few exponential terms. By means of this approach more realistic models for interpreting the data may be postulated.

*SAVAGE The speaker is correct in emphasizing the importance of differential equations in the application of mathematics to biology, but major contributions can be made from other areas of mathematics, such as numerical analysis, combinatorics, topology, and algebra. The speaker mentioned the importance of statistics in the analysis of biological data, but one should not forget the use of probability theory throughout biology.

The speaker emphasized the need for mathematics in biology as soon as quantitative results are being considered. One of his remarks was to the effect that the most important contribution of mathematics to biology was in helping with the *exact* (closed) solution of systems of differential equations. In my opinion, a major contribution of mathematics in biology is in the qualitative description of phenomena, such as whether a system will reach an equilibrium point. Furthermore, for the systems of differential equations that are likely to arise in biological research I doubt whether exact solutions are available or desirable. The mathematical arsenal offers numerical analysis for one aspect of the problem. Other aspects involve topological and algebraic properties of the solutions.

* Comment submitted after termination of the Conference.

*EDEN Admittedly, differential equations are not the only tool of importance in endocrinological research. However, in my opinion analytic solutions have a great deal more to offer than numerical approximations. It has been my experience that such matters as the existence of solutions can be decided from the form of an equation, even though a numerical solution cannot be found analytically. Even so, I agree that numerical approximations can be useful and are sometimes the source of important insights.

* Comment submitted after termination of the Conference.

CHAPTER THIRTEEN

Interconversion and Production Rates of Steroids: An Example of Biomathematics

J. F. TAIT

The following describes briefly and in general terms a specific example of an application of mathematics in endocrinology. The field chosen is one in which such an approach may lead to predictions and therefore to new discoveries. This field comprises the measurement and consideration of the interconversion and production rates of steroids in vivo. The aim is a quantitative description of a total biological activity, such as androgenic or estrogenic activity, in terms of the secretions of known prehormones and hormones.

The study of steroids is characterized by somewhat unique problems, in that the active hormones, besides being secreted, may be formed peripherally from precursors (Baird et al., 1968). Fortunately, the rates of interconversions and metabolism of most steroids, being of intermediate speed, are favorable in analyses of the situations. Crucial in the analyses is the measurement of the specific activity of a steroid or one of its unique metabolites after injection of the labeled steroid and the calculation of a quantity, $R/\int_0^\infty \sigma \, dt$, where R is the amount of radioactivity injected, σ is the specific activity of the compound, and t is time. Various terms, such as secretion, blood production, and urinary production rate, have been assigned to this quantity, depending on the nature of the measurement and the viewpoint taken at the time. If the specific activity of a urinary metabolite is measured, and the urine is continuously collected, until no more radioactivity is excreted in the form of the metabolite, integration is automatically performed. Only one analysis of the urinary metabolite is then required. Moreover, if the radioactive steroid is infused continuously, until the specific activity of the free steroid in blood is constant, integration is, in effect, automatic. Again, only one measurement of the blood steroid is required. Both of these methods, which are simple to analyze, have been employed. Another approach involves the integration of the disappearance curve of specific activity of the steroid in blood after a single injection. However, since this entails a much more complicated analysis of the data, particularly in a calculation of errors, than does continuous infusion, the use of an infusion pump may be more convenient than the use of a computer.

In the first applications of this type of approach, made by Pearlman (1957) and others, $R/\int_0^\infty \sigma \, dt$ was assumed to be equal to the secretion rate of the steroid. In many situations this is quite valid. However, if the steroid is secreted into an anatomical compartment (such as the fetus) other than that into which the radioactive steroid is injected, or if it is synthesized from precursors peripherally, the simple expression will not hold. This was first explained by means of an anatomical model with two compartments (Laumas et al., 1961a,b).

In Figure 1 the quantities S^I and S^Q are secretion rates, and b', b, a, and e are rates of steroids transferred and irreversibly metabolized. In this simple model R/σ will not equal S^I, regardless of the steroid measured or the compartment from which the metabolite is derived, unless S^Q equals 0. Gurpide and Mann (1965) have applied a more general mathematical treatment both to chemical pools and to anatomical compartments; see Figure 2. Thereby they have obtained rigorous proof of many interesting theorems with even the most complicated model.

In all probability one of the most useful general concepts to emerge from the intuitive and formal considerations given by various groups of investigators is that of the blood production rate. When the specific activity of the free steroid in blood is measured, the simple expression $R/\int_0^\infty \sigma \, dt = S$ can be replaced with $R/\int_0^\infty \sigma \, dt = P_B$, where P_B is the blood production rate. This is the total rate of newly synthesized steroid entering the blood. The newly synthesized steroid may be secreted or

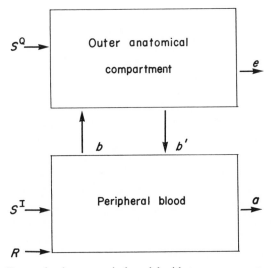

FIGURE 1   An anatomical model with two components.

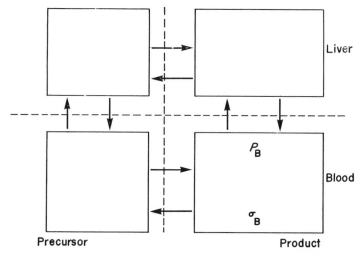

FIGURE 2   Simplest model with chemical pools and anatomical compartments.

may enter the blood after conversion from a precursor in any anatomical compartment. This is a general statement independent of the model, as shown formally by Gurpide and Mann and intuitively by Tait and Burstein (1964). In the model in Figure 1 we have $P_B = S^I + S^Q [b'/(b' + e)]$ or, if the outer compartment is the liver, $P_B = S^I + (1 - H)S^Q$, where H is the splanchnic extraction of the steroid.

In the case of a urinary metabolite $R/\int_0^\infty \sigma \, dt$ is a much more complicated matter to interpret in physiological terms. The metabolite may be formed from several anatomical compartments. Moreover, the secretion of the metabolite by an endocrine gland can seriously affect the value and interpretation of $R/\int_0^\infty \sigma \, dt$. It was this type of complication that enabled the group at Columbia University to discover the secretion of dehydroepiandrosterone sulfate by the normal adrenal gland. The investigators at first measured the specific activity of this substance as an index of the secretion of free dehydroepiandrosterone, but they later concluded, from a mathematical analysis of the data and a careful quantitative investigation of other possibilities, that it must be secreted (Vande Wiele et al., 1963). This must, I think, be classified as a significant discovery in endocrinology that resulted chiefly from mathematical analysis.

As previously mentioned, the blood production rate of a steroid may be interpreted in terms of the secretion of a steroid plus its peripheral synthesis from other precursors:

$$S^T = \frac{P_B^T - [\rho]_{BB}^{AT} P_B^A}{1 - [\rho]_{BB}^{AT}[\rho]_{BB}^{TA}}$$

$$P_B^T - S^T - [\rho]_{BB}^{AT} P_B^A = \; > 0$$

where T and A are product and precursor, and $[\rho]_{BB}^{AT}$ is the proportion of precursor converted to product. When there are n precursors, $n + 1$ simultaneous equations can be solved. Using this approach, which again owes much to the theoretical treatments of Gurpide and Mann, Horton and I (1966) found that in the female the androgenic activity (assuming testosterone to be the active androgen) is actually about one half due to conversions from the secreted prehormone, androstenedione. With this approach there may be a "remainder," after contributions from known hormones and prehormones are subtracted from the blood production rate. It is then that interesting predictions of unknown secretions can be made from the analysis. In certain situations involving estrogens this seems to be the case, according to recent work (Baird et al., 1968).

It has also been found useful to compare $R/\int_0^\infty \sigma \, dt$ for a steroid in blood and for its metabolite in urine. The most important sites of conversions and other interesting information may thereby be revealed. Injection of the radioactive steroid into sites other than blood is now being employed as an approach with the same aim.

However, all theoretical treatments at present assume a nonisotopic steady state, and this is not true of most hormones. The validity of conclusions drawn from measurements of steroids from the same compartment at a particular time is probably not affected thereby. However, the same cannot be said of comparisons of urinary and blood production rates and certain other considerations. Theoretical and experimental work with the nonsteady state must therefore be continued in such investigations. Of course, in investigations concerning control mechanisms a nonsteady state is of fundamental importance.

Finally, if the appropriate experimental situation were available, most of the theoretical concepts and expressions derived from the in vivo situation could be applied to in vitro biosynthetic processes. The S^I value would be for a product not formed from known precursors. Correct quantitative analysis of such processes has, in my opinion, been much neglected in endocrinology. There is now hope that this can be accomplished in the near future by the use of superfusion, in which the radioactive precursors are continuously infused into an incubating tissue in vitro (Tait et al., 1967).

DISCUSSION

ALBERT   Would the speaker elaborate on his studies concerning the metabolism of estrogen?

TAIT   The investigation is in the preliminary stage. However, it is beginning to appear that the estrone in male plasma cannot be accounted for in terms of the known hormones and precursors. But here again, of course, we have the problem of possible nonsteady-state complications.

GURPIDE   Are you implying the possible conversion of androstenedione to estrone or of testosterone to estradiol?

TAIT   No, I am saying that even if we allow for conversion from all the known precursors, including androgens, we cannot account for the blood production rate of estrone in the male.

EMMENS   Is this also true of testosterone in the female?

TAIT   No. On the whole we can account for the blood production rate of testosterone in the female. We would say that 50% came from androstenedione, probably mostly secreted by the adrenal gland, about 15% from dehydroepiandrosterone, and the remainder from secreted testosterone.

CHAPTER FOURTEEN

Pituitary-Adrenal Feedback: An Example of Biomathematics[*]

SALLY B. FAND AND RICHARD P. SPENCER

1. Introduction

Mathematical models of biologic systems serve two functions. First, they can be employed in an effort to match known data. Second, they can suggest previously unexpected relationships or point to unexplored areas.

Although the first of these functions has been examined with regard to the contribution of circulating peripheral target-gland hormones to feedback control of pituitary tropic hormones (Yates and Urquhart, 1962; Ungar, 1964; Yates and Brennan, 1967), the second has been relatively neglected. We have therefore constructed simple models of the pituitary-adrenal relationship and have illustrated them by means of solutions obtained on an analogue computer. That is, the computer was programmed to demonstrate the pituitary and adrenal changes as a function of time, and the rate constants were varied until the computer output agreed with known data.

2. Basic models

For the initial model we shall consider only the quantity of hormone in the blood stream and shall neglect stores in the pituitary and peripheral organs. At the core of the model are the following equations, where P is the appropriate pituitary hormone in the blood, in our example assumed to be adrenocorticotropic hormone (ACTH), and A is adrenal hormone in the blood:

$$dA/dt = mP - \lambda A \tag{1}$$

$$dP/dt = -rA \tag{2}$$

Here m, λ, and r are rate constants; that is, they have the units of reciprocal time, such as 1/hour. The equations state that the rate of

[*] Supported by USPHS Grants CA-06519, AM-07430 and AM-09429, and by the James Picker Foundation.

change of adrenal hormone is equal to a pituitary entry term minus an expression for utilization (which is described as a destructive process proportional to the blood level of the adrenal hormone). The rate of change of the pituitary hormone is set equal to a negative adrenal feedback term.

In the case of hypophysectomy ($P = 0$), Equation 2 disappears ($dP/dt = 0$), and Equation 1 reduces to

$$dA/dt = -\lambda A \tag{3}$$

This is the conventional first-order decay equation. From literature data (Nugent et al., 1961; Yates and Urquhart, 1962) we note that the adrenal cortical hormones in most species have a half-time in the blood of about 30 minutes, or 1/48 day. Therefore, λ has the value of about 33/day, or $\lambda = 0.693/T_{1/2} = 0.693/(1/48)$.

After adrenalectomy ($A = 0$), Equation 1 disappears, and Equation 2 simplifies to

$$dP/dt = 0 \tag{4}$$

In other words, in the absence of the adrenals the pituitary output of the appropriate tropic hormone (ACTH) would be some constant value: d (constant)/$dt = 0$.

Equations 1 and 2 and their simplifications can be solved by the analogue computer. A suitable computer diagram is shown in Figure 1. Included are amplifiers from which dP/dt and dA/dt can be obtained; the reason for needing such outputs will be discussed later.

We neglect for the moment the utilization of the adrenal hormone by setting $\lambda = 0$. Then Equation 1 reduces to

$$dA/dt = mP \tag{5}$$

Numerical values for an initial analogue-computer trial of this simplified model were obtained from Galicich et al. (1963) and from Ungar and Halberg (1963). Blood corticosterone in mice varies between 10 and 40 µg per 100 ml with a mean of 25 µg. To show the cycling, we expressed the values in terms of

$$\frac{\text{observed value} - \text{mean value}}{\text{mean value}} \times 100$$

Hence, the mean becomes 0 in the new variable, 40 becomes $(40 - 25)/25 \times 100 = 60$, and 10 becomes $(10 - 25)/25 \times 100 = -60$. A similar system was used for expressing pituitary ACTH levels in the blood (reported in the literature as percent variation from the mean).

The constraints were as follows. The system had to cycle with a period of 1 day, the pituitary output peak had to precede the adrenal, and

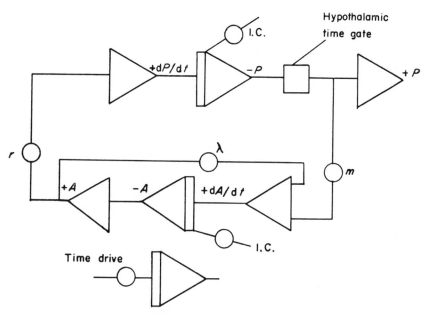

FIGURE 1 Analogue computer flow chart for solution to differential Equations 1 and 2. I.C. signifies "initial conditions." Conventional symbols are employed to identify the component functional modules: circles represent potentiometers (multipliers), triangles represent inverting or summing amplifiers, and triangles with lines through them represent integrating amplifiers. The apices of the triangles point in the direction of flow.

the amplitude of the peak had to agree with the values obtained from the literature cited above. An analogue-computer solution meeting these conditions is shown in Figure 2; it exhibits a typical sine wave with a period of 1 day. The pituitary output peak precedes the adrenal by some 6 hours, which is in approximate agreeement with the available data. Adrenal output reaches a minimum at 0600 h whereas, according to the data of Ungar and Halberg (1963) on the mouse, it reaches a minimum at 0400 h.

To change the time relationships between the pituitary and adrenal outputs simple time-delay circuits can be used (Carlson and Hannauer, 1964). Brodish (1964) has reported that hypothalamic lesions delay, but do not prevent, the stress-induced release of ACTH. Hence, a hypothalamic input probably should be placed after the pituitary output amplifier marked $-P$, where it could act as a delay circuit. Available data indicate that negative feedback control of ACTH release is limited to the region of the median eminence, stalk, and anterior pituitary (Kendall et al., 1964) and are consistent with our model. Subsequent approaches of greater sophistication will necessarily include an evaluation

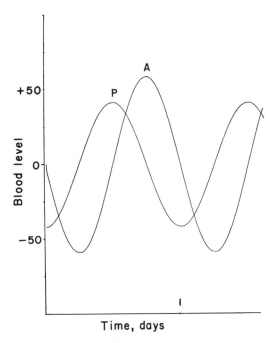

FIGURE 2   Percent departure of blood corticosterone levels, A, and of blood ACTH levels, P, from their respective means over a 24-hour period, determined from the analogue computer solution of Equations 1 and 2. The solution was obtained by letting 1 second of computer time equal 7,862 seconds of real time (a scaling factor of 1.27×10^{-4}). The value of m was 1.02×10^{-4}, and that of r was 0.51×10^{-4}. The initial condition of the adrenal integrator was set at zero.

of variable peripheral utilization. Yates (1967) has pointed out that the attainment of a new steady-state level of the peripheral hormones is more quickly achieved (when feedback is present) if the liver has some inherent regulating function.

3. Energy loss due to damping

The basic model can be made to cycle, but it is unrealistic since it neglects destruction of adrenal hormone. As soon as a value of λ other than zero is employed, the solutions of the equations exhibit damping, as shown in Figure 3. When in reality λ is 33/day, damping would quickly occur if it were not for the continual input of energy (presumably due to both pituitary and adrenal glands). There are a number of ways to measure the damping of such systems. The logarithmic decrement L is defined (Kotter, 1960) as

$$L = \ln (A_n/A_{n+1}) \tag{6}$$

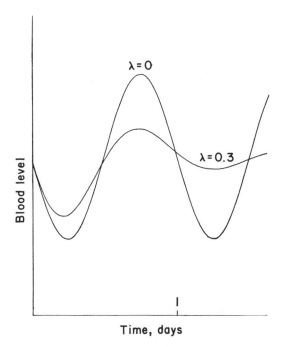

Time, days

FIGURE 3 Percent departure of blood corticosterone level from its mean over a 24-hour period as determined by analogue computer solution of differential Equations 1 and 2 when the peripheral utilization of adrenal cortical hormone is and is not neglected: that is, $\lambda = 0$ and $\lambda = 0.3$ (times the scaling factor), respectively.

where A_n and A_{n+1} are the values of two successive maximal quantities. In a system without damping L is zero. For the example in Figure 3 with $\lambda = 0.3$ the logarithmic decrement L is approximately 1.6.

4. Additional considerations

In the initial model the pituitary and adrenal glands were depicted as responding to the circulating level of hormone. It is possible that the response depends partially upon the rate of change of circulating hormone rather than solely upon its absolute level. Equations 1 and 2 then become

$$dA/dt = mP - \lambda A + s\, dP/dt \tag{7}$$

$$dP/dt = -rA - q\, dA/dt \tag{8}$$

where s and q are new rate constants.

The complete system has interesting problems of stability, which will not be pursued here. The point of importance that emerges is that the

system, which damps as long as λ, the decay constant for blood corticoids, is nonzero, shows less damping when the adrenal gland is set to
respond not only to the level of pituitary hormone but to its rate of
change as well. That is, the additional term in Equation 7 has an appreci-
able impact upon the theoretical results.

As yet no data are available that enable us to decide whether the rate
of change of pituitary hormone level has any biological importance.
Clinical investigations (Nugent et al., 1961) seem to suggest that intermittent ACTH therapy (which would cause the term $s\,dP/dt$ to vary
abruptly from zero to some maximum) is less likely to result in a steroid
withdrawal syndrome (diminished adrenal responsivity) after therapy
has been stopped. Intermittent corticoid therapy may be thought of as
indirectly inducing changes in pituitary outputs of endogenous ACTH.

5. Data on levels of tropic hormones

In a more rigorous analysis of the system under discussion
there are at least four compartments: pituitary gland, adrenal gland,
blood level of pituitary hormone, and blood level of adrenal hormone.
Further, each compartment has a quantity of hormone that depends on
the product of the concentration and the volume of the compartment.
The rate constants for release of the hormones might be under metabolic
control. At present the data are insufficient to allow us to determine
whether the feedback responses are dependent on the total amount of
hormone in the organs or on the concentrations (amount per unit weight
or per unit water content), but it appears that synthesis and release
typically move together, in the same direction. The data in Table 1
suggest, at least with respect to growth hormone and ACTH, that
pituitary stores alone are insufficient to yield any biologically important
hypertropic hormone states; an increase in production is required.

6. Further approaches

Further approaches to quantitation of the pituitary-adrenal
relationship might include the following:

1. There may be a pituitary system for comparing the blood level of
adrenal hormone, A_B, with some intrapituitary component, A_P. That is,
the relationship might be, in place of Equation 2,

$$dP/dt = -r(A_P - A_B) \qquad (9)$$

The "variable set point" discussed with regard to pituitary models
(Yates and Urquhart, 1962) may be thought of as a variation in the A_P
term.

TABLE 1   Daily Production of Two Tropic Hormones: Relation to Pituitary Hormone Content

	Growth hormone	ACTH
Amount in 1 cm³ of blood plasma	10 mμg (Utiger et al., 1962)	2×10^{-14} mol (Wajchenberg et al., 1964; Yalow et al., 1964)
Amount in extracellular fluid	140 μg (Parker et al., 1962)	2.9×10^{-10} mol
Half-life	27 min (Parker et al., 1962; Glick et al., 1964)	15 min (Yalow et al., 1964)
Fractional turnover rate	2.6%/min	4.6%/min
Turnover per minute	3.64 μg	1.3×10^{-11} mol
Turnover per hour	0.218 mg	7.8×10^{-10} mol
Turnover per day (daily production)	5.2 mg	1.87×10^{-8} mol
Amount in anterior pituitary	10 mg	1×10^{-7} mol
Ratio of anterior pituitary hormone content to average daily production	1.92	5.35

2. The exact relationship between adrenal and pituitary cannot be truly linear. That is, it is likely that the adrenal gland can respond only to some maximal value when pituitary hormone is given. Equation 1 might take the form

$$dA/dt = \frac{fP}{k + P} - \lambda A \qquad (10)$$

When very small amounts of pituitary hormone are given ($P \ll k$), this reduces to

$$dA/dt = \frac{f}{k} P - \lambda A \qquad (11)$$

When large quantities of pituitary hormone are administered ($P \gg k$), this becomes

$$dA/dt = f - \lambda A \qquad (12)$$

That is, the adrenal output reaches some maximal value given by f.

3. The descriptions of ACTH-secreting pituitary tumors (Salassa et al., 1959) in patients adrenalectomized for Cushing's disease raise the question of why tumor formation with excess ACTH production is almost never seen in Addison's disease or after bilateral adrenalectomy for other causes. The models suggest two possible explanations: (a) Equation 4, describing the pituitary output of ACTH in the absence of the adrenals, indicates that the output would reach but not exceed a constant value; (b) an input of energy is required for the production of physiological levels of ACTH. The energy considerations would themselves militate against unchecked compensatory ACTH production in the absence of yet another abnormality serving to drive pituitary ACTH production and release. The model is thus consistent with the interpretations drawn by Drucker et al. (1965) in their study of abnormal pituitary-adrenal relationships in patients with Cushing's disease.

DISCUSSION

FORTIER   We too have been interested in models of the pituitary adrenocortical feedback control system but have used a somewhat different approach from that presented by the speaker (Normand et al., 1966). Before developing a model a biologist must ask what objectives it will serve: will it provide answers to otherwise insoluble problems, and will it have predictive value? These objectives are best achieved by means of an analytical approach and with appropriate experimental data rather than fragmentary observations from the literature. As a preliminary to the study of a whole system under increasingly complex conditions, a systematic analysis is made of the time–response characteristics of isolated components. Control engineers make use of this approach in electromechanical systems. The underlying principle is to determine the transfer function of a system element through rupture of the loop, stimulation of the element from an initial resting state, and quantitative study of the dynamics of stimulus and response. Increasingly comprehensive mathematical formulation is achieved by simulating at each step, on an analogue computer, the behavior of a given subsystem. By so-called computer synthesis the interconnections between subsystems are then varied, until the behavior of the system is successfully imitated. For example, a mathematical model of the adrenal cortex can be derived from the assessment of the corticoidogenic response of the gland to graded doses of ACTH in the hypophysectomized rat. A similar approach may be applied to determination of the transfer function of the pituitary gland; that is, ACTH secretion (output) is related to graded doses of the corticotropin releasing factor (input) after appropriate blockade of the endogenous secretion of the latter. To develop a model of the whole hypothalamopituitary-adrenocortical system, one must accommodate the characteristics of the individual system elements constituting the response pattern of the intact animal to environmental stimuli of graded intensity. This is an arduous task. It implies deriving the mathematical model from the results of experiments and then performing new experiments to test its predictions. Since the speaker's elegant approach is at the other end of the spectrum, may I ask what are her particular objectives?

FAND   Let me cite one prediction from this very simple model. Equation 4 states that after adrenalectomy the ACTH output from the pituitary stabilizes at a constant level. This prediction provides a rationale for the clinical observation that the incidence of pituitary tumors secondary to removal of target gland is much lower than one might expect if there were no upper bound to maximal trophic hormone output. Our model permits a rigorous analysis of simple relations between endocrine glands and may thus have an advantage over more complex models.

BIRMINGHAM   Can the speaker's model explain the fact that, when one cannulates an adrenal vein, one cannot block the pituitary ACTH output? When one cannulates the adrenal, one places such a stress upon the organism that no amount of steroid-evoked feedback can lessen the output of ACTH.

FAND   Are you saying that ACTH output is not a constant but keeps rising?

BIRMINGHAM   ACTH secretion is no longer affected by steroid secretion.

FAND   Are you saying that the output of ACTH does not peak but increases continually under the experimental conditions you describe?

BIRMINGHAM   If one places stress upon the rat by an adrenal vein cannulation, one just fires off the pituitary and cannot block the release of ACTH.

BARTOSIK   That's not the same as saying it reaches a maximum. What Dr. Fand is saying is that eventually ACTH secretion reaches a maximum, which it cannot exceed, not that it cannot continue to rise to reach that maximum.

BIRMINGHAM   So her model fits.

ROMANOFF   In the case of adrenalectomy the speaker's model has $dP/dt = 0$, which indicates either maximal or *minimal* output of ACTH.

FAND   Dr. Romanoff is right. Our Equation 3 simply states that the output of ACTH equals a constant. The empirical facts tell us that the constant is a maximum.

FORTIER   Some of the speaker's assumptions seem questionable. For instance, the postulated inversely proportional relationship of circulating ACTH to blood corticosteroid concentration disregards the fact that the actual variable is the free (unbound to proteins), not the total, steroid concentration. We have, for example, observed a concurrent increase of ACTH and corticosterone secretion as a result of thyroxine administration to rats and the inverse situation as a result of thyroidectomy (Labrie et al., 1965). Equally questionable is the assumption that the clearance rates of ACTH and of corticosteroids are unaltered by different experimental situations. Many observations in the literature contradict this postulate. Finally, I question the validity of assessing the dynamic performance of a system from data obtained under "steady state" conditions.

FAND   So far as Dr. Fortier's first two points are concerned, they are certainly well taken. However, the model could be altered to make provision for them. All one would need to do would be to modify the utilization term. I agree that more data would be useful.

PEARLMAN   I believe that this meeting is intended to encourage persons like myself, who until recently had no great need for analogue computers to solve problems in endocrinology, and who may feel overwhelmed at the sight of a set of differential equations. In my experience the simplest analogue computer that I could set up was a hydrodynamic system. Only the simplest laboratory equipment was needed: erlenmeyer flasks, water, dye, a colorimeter, and pumps such as are used in column chromatography. I found this a wonderful way to begin. One can then readily move on to the electrical analogue computer. With the hydro-dynamic analogue computer one can study both nonsteady and steady states. I am under the impression that the electrical analogue computer can handle only steady-state systems, but I may be mistaken.

ROMANOFF There are many electrical devices that will do whatever your hydrodynamic model will do, but one visualizes the system more clearly with the hydrodynamic model than with any of the electrical devices. For instance, for modeling purposes one can learn from one of the problems in the transmission of electrical power, which is "surging." If you know something about synchronous motors, then you are familiar with the problem of "tramping," which is the alternate speeding up and slowing down of a motor. Surging and tramping have their analogues in biological phenomena and illustrate nonsteady electrical states.

Although nonsteady states are analyzed by Dr. Fand's model, it implies a sine wave. Many biological phenomena are not described by a sine wave formulation. Something starting off as a sine wave will often be converted into a nonsine wave, which is something Dr. Pearlman has been discussing. How does your model cope with this?

FAND Our model does not. Models can be made with the use of other differential equations and without our restrictions. But a different model probably would be required.

CHAPTER FIFTEEN

An Introduction to Computers

EDWARD M. KAPLAN AND JOHN P. GILBERT

1. Introduction

Some endocrinologists have been using digital computers for years to analyze their data. However, most are just embarking upon the application of such equipment to their data-processing and reduction problems. The only way in which the latter group — and, in fact, many of those who have already used computers — can effectively apply these devices is to understand the basic philosophy underlying their operation. It is the purpose of this chapter, therefore, to provide insight into the workings of these machines. Instead of preparing a treatise, couched in the mysteries of technical jargon, we have attempted to describe in simple terms the basic logic inherent in most digital computers. At the end of this chapter are descriptions of some applications of digital computers, included neither to impress nor to awe but, rather, to show the broad utility of general-purpose computers and, perhaps, to stimulate thought toward the applications of these machines to endocrinology.

There are two basic types of computer: digital and analogue. The digital computer works with coded information, and the analogue computer has electric circuits to simulate actual mathematical relationships. In the analogue computer it is the actual voltage or current that represents the quantities being dealt with. Various changes are made in those quantities by means of specific circuits. The way in which these circuits are arranged determines what the computer is programmed to perform. For this reason analogue computers tend to be utilized for specialized applications. We shall herein concern ourselves almost entirely with the digital computer.

People who are unfamiliar with computers tend to think of them as devoted to doing arithmetic day and night. Although most of what the computer does is essentially arithmetic, the information that is coded in a digital computer can and often does represent many kinds of information. An example is the use of the computer to sharpen the photographs of the moon taken by satellites. Other examples are the uses of computers to play chess and to prove mathematical theorems.

2. How a computer works

There are many levels of explanation and description at which we could describe the workings of a computer. If we were considering how a cat walks, we could describe the way it places its feet, or we could discuss the actual mechanism of its nervous system, the neurons and axons of the nerves. Here we shall be dealing with the gross anatomy of the computer and not with the physical processes that go on within it.

Before considering how present-day computers work we shall consider the computers of the early nineteen-fifties. These stand in the same relationship to modern computers as the Model T stands to the present-day automobile: most of the same parts are there, but in a much simpler form. The computer we have in mind consists of an arithmetic, or logical, unit, a program-control unit, a memory, and a method of entering data and programs into memory and of getting the results of computation out of memory. The arithmetic unit together with the program-control unit is usually referred to as a central processing unit. It contains registers and special wiring that allows it to add, subtract, multiply, and divide numbers as well as make logical comparisons as, for example, to test whether one number is greater than another. Generally speaking, it is the central processing unit that is actually doing what one usually thinks of as computing. The memory serves to store, not only the data on which the computer is to operate, but also the programs that specify these operations. The memory is organized much like an old country post office, with the difference that the letter boxes in the computer can hold only one number at a time. We must avoid confusing the number of the mailbox and the number that is in it. When Mrs. Jones looks in her mailbox, the fact that hers is Box #3 does not affect the letters she finds. What is important is the fact that she and the postmaster agree that it is her box, and any of the available boxes would have served as well.

To illustrate these concepts, we assume that we have a simple computer with fifty random-access memory locations, each of which can hold a four-digit number. We assume that, in addition, it has an accumulator, or working register, and a program register and that it operates sequentially. The instructions for this computer will consist of two parts. The first tells what operation is to be performed, and the second indicates the memory location involved in the operation. In order to write a program for adding two numbers and storing the answer in memory, we will need four operation codes, denoted by 00, 01, 02, and 03. The meaning of these codes will be:

00 Stop.
01 Clear the accumulator, and load it with the contents of the number contained in the indicated memory location.

02 Add the contents of the indicated memory location to the number already in the accumulator.

03 Store a copy of the number in the accumulator in the indicated memory location.

To write our program, we must specify in which locations of the computer's memory each instruction is to be found besides what the instruction is:

Location	Contents
01	0120
02	0230
03	0340
04	0000

The first two digits of each of the numbers in the content column are the operation code; the second two, the memory location involved. Thus, the first instruction directs the computer to clear the accumulator and load the contents of memory location 20 into the accumulator. The second instruction directs it to add to the number in the accumulator the contents of memory location 30. The third instruction directs it to store the contents of the accumulator, which are now the sum of the first two numbers, in location 40. We did not add the numbers 20 and 30; we added the numbers in those locations and stored the sum in location 40. The last instruction informs the computer that the operation is complete. If location 20 had contained the number 4 and location 30 had contained the number 12, then after this program was finished, these two locations would contain the original numbers, while location 40 would contain the sum of these two numbers, or 16. The instructions for this program have been coded as numbers and, like the data, they were stored in the memory. There, as shown in the table, they were stored in locations 01, 02, 03, and 04.

Instead of stopping at the fourth instruction, location 04, we could change our program, making it slightly longer, as follows:

Location	Contents	Location	Contents	Location	Contents
01	0120	05	0212	09	0213
02	0230	06	0301	10	0303
03	0340	07	0213	11	0401
04	0101	08	0302	12	0001
				13	0110

Locations 12 and 13 are used merely to store constants employed by the program.

The first three instructions are as before. Instructions 04, 05, and 06 have the effect of adding the contents of location 12 to the first instruction. Since location 12 contains the number 0001, this will change instruction 01 to read "0121." The next two instructions have the effect of adding 0110 to the number left in the accumulator. Since this is 0121, the result will be 0231. This number is now stored in location 02. The next two instructions have the same effect by adding 0110 to the number now in the accumulator; they produce the number 0341, which is then stored in location 03. At this point we introduce a new operation, which we have coded 04. Its interpretation is that the program is to get its next command from that location mentioned in the address part of the instruction; that is, the computer is now to go back to location 01 and start over. However, at this point it finds a new instruction in location 01. The instructions in 01, 02, and 03 now have the effect of adding the number in 21 to the number in 31 and storing it in location 41. Instructions 04 through 10 again add the number 1 to instructions 01, 02, and 03, modifying them to say, "To the number in 22 add the number in 32, and store in 42." Instruction 11 again causes the computer to start over at location 01. The computer will go on and on, until it comes to an instruction that no longer makes sense. A real computer can count how many times it makes such a loop and can be programmed to repeat this ten times and then to stop or begin another part of the program. The second program illustrates one of the most important properties of the digital computer: its ability to modify its own program. If we had had to write the analogue of steps 1, 2, and 3 twenty times to add twenty pairs of numbers, we would not have taken much less time than we would have in doing it by hand. What gives the computer tremendous power is the fact that we can write a loop, such as the one illustrated, that will generate the program necessary to add twenty pairs or, indeed, seven hundred pairs of numbers. As regards the manner of their storage in memory, there is no difference between numbers used as data and numbers used as instructions, and the distinguishing factor is the central processing unit register in which the number is placed. Thus, if numbers are put into the accumulator, they are treated as data. If they are put into the program register, they are treated as operations and addresses or, in other words, as instructions. We have ignored how those numbers are entered into the computer and how the computer is started. The essential point is that the computer, once given a location from which to start, puts that instruction in its program register, performs that instruction, and goes on to the next sequential location in memory to obtain its next instruction. It then performs that instruction and goes to the next sequential location in memory to get its third instruction. Thus, it will go from instruction 01, 02, 03, 04, etc., unless it comes to a special instruction, such as the one we have coded as 04, which is called a *jump*, or a *branching instruction*. This tells it the new place to start, and it then proceeds from there sequentially. Thus, the computer has two types of operation that are performed in sequence: it obtains and interprets an instruction, and it performs whatever that instruction directs. Note that each new instruction must be obtained from the memory and stored in the program register. Note also that the interpretation of each instruction usually requires that the computer obtain a number from memory or store a number in memory. Thus, at most instructions the computer has to gain access to memory twice. The speed of the computer therefore depends mainly upon the time required to insert a number from memory into the central processing unit. This quantity is called the *memory access time*. In present-day computers access times are of the order of one microsecond.

It is clear from the example given that even a computer expert could not cope with all of these numbers for long. Soon people began to use the computer to help write its own programs. The first step in this process was to substitute mnemonics for the operation codes. For example, instead of saying "01," the programmer would write "CLA" for "clear, and load the accumulator"; instead of "02," he would write "ADD" for "add"; instead of the operation code "03," he would write "STO" for "store." The program is thereby made much easier to understand. Thus, our first program would have been written

CLA 20, ADD 30, STO 40 and STP 00

Before such a program can actually be run on the computer, it must be translated into its original form. However, it is not hard to program a computer to make this translation. To run a program written in mnemonics requires two steps: a special program is first run to translate the mnemonics into the original number format, and the output from this translation is then run as a program.

At this point the machine is doing two jobs: first, it is translating and, second, it is computing. The extent to which the machine can ease the task of the programmer depends upon the capabilities of the computer itself; hence, a small computer is seldom as easy to program as a large one, because it is less able to help write its own programs.

3. Second-generation computers

The invention of ferrite core memories with their faster *cycle times* (the time it takes to transfer a number from memory to the central processor) led to the development of the "second generation" computers. Though much more expensive than their predecessors, they could do more, both per unit time and per dollar. Because of their higher cost it became imperative to devise more efficient ways of operating them. The two principal problems were to reduce the time spent transferring data and programs into and out of the computer and to reduce the time required to switch from one user to the next.

The importance of the first of these problems is illustrated by the fact that it could easily take five minutes to read in data cards for a problem requiring less than one minute of actual computing. In order to avoid this waste of computer time, most second-generation computer installations utilize a second, less expensive, computer that reads the program and data cards and rewrites them onto magnetic tape. The input tape is read into the main computer at a much faster rate. Data can be read from magnetic tape at approximately thirty times the rate it can be read from cards. The main computer writes its output onto another magnetic tape, which the secondary computer reads and prints on a line printer. Using this arrangement, the programmer's communication with the computer is almost entirely via the magnetic-tape intermediary.

To appreciate the need for an efficient way to switch the computer from one user to the next, we must realize that, in addition to longer jobs, a university computing center may have from one hundred to three hundred jobs in a day, each of which takes less than one minute to run. Clearly, it is no longer possible to ask the user to come into the computer room, mount his tapes, and operate the machine, as was done with the first-generation computers. The solution to this problem has been to put the user programs and their data onto an input tape one after the other; a "super" program reads in the first program, determines its needs, and starts it running. When this program has finished, control returns to the superprogram, which proceeds to the next user program as well as makes a note of how much to charge the first user. Such a super program is called an "operating system," and the art of writing these superprograms is called "systems programming." These programs must be able to provide the correct compiler to translate the original program into machine language; they must also be able to incorporate into the user program the various subprograms supplied to the user program by the system. Examples of such subprograms are those which read the data from magnetic tape and execute various mathematical functions (e.g., square root, logarithm). In addition, they must be able (a) to stop the user program when it commits an unpardonable blunder, such as trying to divide by zero, (b) to print a relevant, if irreverent, error message, and (c) to find and start the next program on the input tape. Since many programs are run for the purpose of checking for errors, or "debugging," it is quite common for programs to stop short of completion. This is one of the reasons for there being so many one-minute jobs.

In summary, most second-generation computers are operated by first writing the input decks of ten to twenty jobs onto magnetic tape by using a secondary computer. The input tape is then entered into the main computer under the control of an operating system. The results are written on an output tape by the main computer and are finally printed by the secondary computer. This mode of operation is called *batch-processing*.

Another important development spurred on by the capacity of these computers was the devising of a variety of sophisticated programming languages. Thus, instead of dealing merely with the simple operation by operation directions of our examples, programs were written in terms that could involve fairly extensive calculations for each command written in the program. Languages were developed for many special purposes. Some of these languages are FORTRAN, LISP, SLIP, IPLV, ALGOL, SNOBOL, and COBOL.

It must be kept clearly in mind that a computer language consists of two separate parts. One comprises the grammatical rules, which the programmer must follow if he is to write a correct program in the language. A correct program in the language constitutes as clear a set of directions to another person who knows the language as it does to the computer. For example, if you wished a laboratory assistant to perform a rather complicated analysis on a desk calculator, you might write the instructions in, say, FORTRAN. These would provide explicit directions for the calculations without necessitating the involvement of a computer. The other part of a computer language constitutes the interpreting, or "compiling," program in the computer. This translates the directions given in, say, FORTRAN into a machine-language program. One must make a distinction between the program as written in FORTRAN and the result of the translation by the computer. Thus, two different computers may both be able to interpret FORTRAN. However, the resultant "object," or machine-language, programs may be quite different in the two systems. An important aspect of these computers is the set of "languages" (i.e., language-translating programs) that they possess and the system or supervisory programs that they utilize in their operation. It is these facilities, as a whole, which are referred to as *software*, in contrast to *hardware*, which is the actual computer. Without programs, of course, the computer is powerless.

4. Third-generation computers

The third-generation computers have now arrived. They have had a little trouble getting started. However, we can discuss some of the problems that these computers present and some of the solutions proposed to solve them. The cycle time of these computers is so short that even the fastest input and output devices are excessively slow in comparison to the time that it takes the computer to do its calculating. This means that if the computers were run as second-generation batch processors were run, too much of their capability would be standing idle during the time that it takes to get data into and out of the computer. In order to utilize this extra capability, several proposals have been made. One of these is called *multiprogramming*.

In multiprogramming several programs are in the computer simultaneously. The hope is that while one program is waiting for input or output, another program can be using the central processor. In order to accommodate several programs in the computer simultaneously, the core memory is divided into five or six parts, and a different program is stored in each. They all take turns using the same central processor. Since these computers have separate facilities for getting data in and out that do not need to use the central processing unit, the programs waiting for input or output do not use the central processor but leave it free for computation. To the user the multiprogramming computer looks very much like the second-generation batch processor, since he is not aware that his program is sharing the computer with other programs. He simply submits his job to the computing center and gets it back after a certain length of time. The simultaneous presence of four programs in the computer requires that its memory be four times the size of that required for a single program, and this presents somewhat of a problem. One method of reducing the amount of memory needed is to divide the memory requirements of a program into units, called *pages*. With such a division the entire program and its data need not be "in core" at any particular time. All that need be in core are the pages that are being referenced and the particular part of the program that is being run. When the program comes to a reference that is not in core, it waits while the computer obtains a new page and puts it in core. While the first program is waiting, another program will be using the central processing unit. Provided that at least one program is always ready to use the central processing unit, this system will use the computer efficiently.

A different but closely related solution to the problem is called *time-sharing*. In this system many users interact with the computer during the same period of time. Each utilizes a small fraction of the computer's total capability. Thus, if there are ten users, each gets essentially a tenth of the computer's time. The computer gives each a small turn, one after the other. If the program of a particular user is not ready to employ the central processing unit because it is waiting for input or output purposes, its turn is skipped, and the next user gets his turn. With this scheme, if ten users are sharing a fast computer, it looks to each as though he had a somewhat slower computer all to himself. One of the advantages of this system is that it gives the user the capability of close interaction with the computer. This resembles the interaction he enjoyed with the small first-generation computers and forfeited with the second-generation machines, which required batch-processing. The user has almost immediate interaction with the computer, which he did not in the batch-processing system, which necessitated his waiting until all the other programs in the batch had been run and the output separated and put in bins, before he could resubmit his job with the required corrections. In addition to the on-line interaction which the time-sharing of a large computer offers the user, it provides the facility for higher-level languages. I shall take the liberty of discussing the time-sharing system at Harvard, not because of any chauvinistic feeling, but because it is the system that I know most intimately.

Structurally, the time-sharing system consists of a central processing unit, a core storage unit, a rapid-access drum memory, a large disk-file memory, and provisions for connecting as many as thirty-two teletype-writers simultaneously to the computer. In addition, the computer is designed to respond to a priority system of *interrupts*. If program A is running and an interrupt comes in, A is saved and program B, which copes with that particular interrupt, is started. If at this point a higher-priority interrupt comes in, B is saved and the second interrupt is taken care of. B is then restarted, and when B has finished with its work, the original program A is resumed. When, for example, someone types a letter on a teletype, this causes an interrupt which initiates the program that takes care of teletype input. Because in the time scale of the computer this is rather a leisurely process, such a teletype interruption has a very low priority. Let us look at this computer in action.

At any given time a running program will be in core storage and will be using the central processing unit. In addition, other programs, or at least pages of other programs, will also be resident in core storage. Some programs will be waiting for input from their respective teletypes and will therefore not be in line to use the central processing unit. Other programs must wait until data that they have sent to the teletypes have been typed before continuing with their problems, and will likewise not be waiting for the central processing unit. In addition, programs that need to have additional pages brought to the core storage unit from the rapid-access memory will be waiting. All programs that are involved with connected teletypes are stored either in core storage or on the rapid-access memory. One of the tricks utilized to get programs in and out of core storage more rapidly is to keep track of whether a page has been changed or not. When a page is taken from the rapid-access memory and put into core, its image is also left on the rapid-access memory. If that page is not changed by the computer, it does not need to be recopied onto the rapid-access memory. Such savings help to make the system more efficient. Ideally, the user is unaware of this. The only hint he has that other people are using the computer is that the teletype may be sluggish. This is because it takes the computer a little longer to service the interrupts from his particular teletype messages.

As the result of these developments we shall soon have a continuum ranging from small computers, somewhat limited in their programming languages and capabilities, to the "computer utility" looming over the horizon from MIT. Some of the more vexing problems of the time-sharing and the computer utility type of installation involve the communication links. The teletypewriters that we have connected to the Harvard system use part of the regular telephone voice network. However, when one is working on an involved problem, a typical computing call may last as long as two or three hours. This is much longer than the average voice call, which lasts approximately three minutes. Thus, a teletypewriter call can tie up the telephone switching network for as long as forty or fifty voice calls. We should also like to have terminals that utilize a higher data rate than these teletypes. Thus, we should like to provide television screens under the control of the computer. Such units are in operation; however, because of this high-frequency link they are usually limited to being close to the computer. If the telephone companies should get to the point where they have picture phones, these might make a very useful input-output device for people using the computer from remote locations. At present almost all the terminals on the market are expensive and not very satisfactory.

Another class of problem involved with these third-generation computers is the amount of time spent in bookkeeping. The computer must keep track of the location of everyone's program, whose turn is next, which program gets the input from each input device and, most important of all, who gets charged how much for what. To illustrate this last point, the Harvard system currently charges users for three separate items: the amount of permanent memory used to store programs and data, the number of hours they have been connected to the computer, and the number of minutes of actual central-processor time used. If the computer spends as much time performing overhead functions as it would have wasted in doing input-output in the batch-processing mode, nothing has been gained by upgrading to multiprogramming. Thus, the true speed and cost of these computers depends as critically upon the efficiency with which their operating systems perform the necessary bookkeeping tasks as upon the rapidity with which the hardware performs its functions.

5. On-line computer systems

Let us consider for a moment the "processor-controller" class of computer or, to use a term more in vogue, the *on-line real-time* computer system. Unlike the large batch-processing or time-sharing computer systems, which are essentially "stand alone" devices, this is somewhat smaller and more specialized. Although basically a general-purpose digital computer, the on-line system has certain characteristics and performs certain functions not generally required or found in the larger computer systems. An on-line computer is an integral part of a larger system in which computation per se is not the principal objective. Rather, the computation, speed, and decision-making logic inherent in a digital computer are permitted to interact with one another and are utilized to control a particular process or experiment. The computer, being the central portion of the entire operation, accepts as input various signals representing the operational status of the instrumentation being used. These signals are interpreted and condensed by the computer, and the results of the decision-making logic are then made available either to the equipment actually involved in the process or to the operator or experimenter, so that he may exert manual control. The progress of the experiment is thereby automatically controlled by what may be considered positive or negative feedback action. The real-time aspects of such a system are incorporated in the responses of the computer with respect to the operational characteristics of its external environment; all processing and logic is performed in a time frame that is minimally equivalent and maximally shorter than the basic time frame or major cycle time of the experiment. Thus, we are now considering the computer as a piece of equipment incorporated into a larger processing system rather than as *the* system without any additional equipment.

Characteristically, on-line computers do not have the capacity, i.e., storage capability, of the stand-alone systems. This is principally because they are designed to handle manageable amounts of continually changing data *as they are being generated* rather than to manipulate vast quantities of information, gathered over several weeks or months, at what amounts to a single entry. That is, the quantity of data may be the same for either system, but the rate of data entry in an on-line system is limited by the rate at which an instrument can produce it; in a batch system all the data have been generated, and the more the computer can accept at any given time, the more efficient the processing of the data becomes.

Since computation is not in most cases the overriding consideration in an on-line system, this capability is usually compromised to some degree in favor of more powerful and flexible logical and decision-making capabilities. In fact, there are on-line applications controlled by computers that cannot multiply or divide unless such operations are simulated by programmed algorithms, which are generally quite slow. Since control and data management are the main functions of this class of computer, the characteristics of the machines reflect these needs. In addition, they are generally dedicated merely to a single application and user and, hence, for economic reasons are smaller and more basic machines. However, if desired, supplementary units can be acquired for these computers so that, like their big brothers in data-processing centers, they can be made as computationally powerful (and expensive).

Perhaps the biggest difference between on-line computers and the other classes of machine is in their input-output structure, that is, in the manner in which they communicate with the external environment. Typically, on-line computers derive their basic data directly from an analogue signal without any intermediate storage device such as magnetic tape or cards. A digital computer operates on discrete pieces of information, whereas the analogue signal is a continuous-voltage waveform representation of a physical phenomenon. Therefore, an "interface," also called an *analogue-to-digital converter*, is required for entering the data into the computer. This device takes the analogue signal, which is a voltage or time plot, and selects points, or voltages, at specified times for conversion. These voltage values are the digital representation of the analogue signal. The number of values selected per unit time, the conversion or digitizing rate, is a function of the frequency. On-line computer systems are being used to control chemical-processing plants, to run experiments in x-ray crystallography, and to monitor critical heart patients.

6. Summary

In this paper we have presented an admittedly oversimplified account of how computers are programmed and how technical developments and economic considerations have influenced the manner in which they are used. The advent of time-sharing installations with remote terminals and interactive programming languages now makes programming much easier to learn than heretofore. Indeed, these developments have taken programming out of the hands of experts and "bright" graduate students and have rendered the computer almost as simple to use as the desk calculator. Since it is impossible to appreciate the strengths and weaknesses of computing devices without direct trial, we hope that the ease with which programming can now be accomplished will encourage endocrinologists who are unfamiliar with computers to acquire first-hand experience. The only danger in this is that a number of you may decide that programming is more fun than endocrinology.

Bibliographical notes

For further reading see Bartee (1966), Bernstein (1963), Gilbert (1967), McCracken (1961), and Piel (1966).

Addendum

At the time of this writing most of the computations for the statistical analyses with which this book is concerned, such as analysis of variance, analysis of covariance, estimation of potency from quantitative and quantal assays, are available in program libraries and are accessible to most computer installations.

CHAPTER SIXTEEN

Supplementary Discussion

EDITORS' NOTE: The purpose of this session was to enable the Workshop participants to raise questions that had not been covered in the formal program. We have retained such discussion as we feel to be of general interest to the readers of this volume.

Statistical significance more likely with increasing number of observations

BORTH   I should like to bring up the problem of statistical significance at a selected level as a function of the number of observations. With few observations no effect will ever be "significant," whereas with many a small effect will be "significant." I find it disturbing that increasing the number of observations sufficiently will make anything become "significant." This has, parenthetically, a relevance to bioassay in the testing for parallelism: with a sufficient number of animals parallelism will vanish from most bioassays.

MUSSETT   You simply do not do an analysis of variance.

FORTIER   The issue raised by Dr. Borth is disturbing to many biologists. They seek to ascertain the validity of their findings. However, perhaps because of too elementary a training, they tend to place undue reliance on statistical tests of significance.

ARMITAGE   I think the answer is to put much less emphasis on significance tests and much more on estimation (for example, the determination of confidence intervals).

BORTH   Even if one has discovered a statistically insignificant effect, one should not forget to examine it for relevance to the particular research situation.

ARMITAGE   In the case of the problem with parallelism one can express limits for the difference between the slopes. We do not know how important differences of various magnitudes may be. One of the points that emerged from the discussion following Professor Cornfield's talk is that, although one may get away with slight differences, there may be real differences that one has not detected but that may be important. We do not know very much about the consequences of differences in slope from assay to assay.

MCHUGH Perhaps it is more relevant to ask when one should use significance tests.

FINNEY One must recognize that sometimes significance tests are almost totally irrelevant: for example, when one is seeking to maximize the measure of a gain from some policy. When forced to take an immediate decision, one does not care in the least about significance. A different situation is that in which the aim is to choose the best of a group of materials according to some criterion. One selects the material that has the highest mean, regardless of whether it is significantly different from the second best or whether it differs by a minute fraction of the standard error.

EMMENS We encounter this problem continually in studies of mammalian spermatozoa, in which the number of replicates available from the ejaculate is unlimited: one can subdivide the total sperm collection into fractions each of which contains hundreds of thousands of cells. The accuracy of determinations of response to changes in osmotic pressure, salt and sugar content, and so forth is very high, and one can pick up 1 or 2% differences which, I am sure, have no profound physiological meaning. But one is continually embarrassed in the formal analysis of variance by high-order interactions that turn out to be significant. These can be obliterated only by pooling the high-order interactions with error, so that the small differences between ejaculates no longer interfere. What it amounts to is that differences of the order of 5 or 10% between the ejaculates do not, physiologically speaking, matter at all. The effects of interest are of the order of 50 to 100%.

COCHRAN It is my feeling that significance tests have, on the whole, done more good than harm to the scientist. A good feature is that they serve to temper the incautious investigator. By the use of some reasonably objective tests he must first show that there is a significant difference before he can start writing papers that influence the direction of research, perhaps in unfruitful ways.

If one does not obtain a significant difference, it is worth while to determine whether the experiment was so small that only a very big difference would have shown up. Occasionally one may overlook a promising lead by finding something apparently nonsignificant and concluding that the true difference was either zero or unimportant, whereas the fact may simply be that the experiment was too small to measure the true difference at all precisely.

Sequential statistical analysis: addition of observations until significance is achieved

BORTH   A procedure that, I think, arises frequently is the following. An investigator compares two drugs with a group of, say, twenty patients. He examines the data and calculates his t test, χ^2 test, or whatever, and finds the result to be "not significant." However, what difference he finds is in what might be called the right direction. He proceeds to collect another ten or twenty cases so that his test will become "significant." I am informed that it is not appropriate to increase the number of observations until the test becomes significant, but I do not understand why.

ARMITAGE   The point is that if one performs repeated tests of significance with accumulating data, examining, for example, every twenty or forty cases, one is making more than one test, and the chance of finding a significant difference increases with the number of tests. If one continued the testing indefinitely, one would eventually obtain significant results at even the one-in-a-million level.

BORTH   Isn't this simply the phenomenon of increasing the number of observations?

ARMITAGE   No, because in every test that one performs one takes account of the number of observations that have been used so far, usually in determining the standard error. Yet, if one employs many significance tests, one runs quite a high risk of finding at some time or another a difference that is significant at whatever level one likes, even if the tests are not all independent, and even if they are made on different accumulations of the same body of data. To work in this way is perfectly reasonable. However, one should take some sort of precaution, perhaps by doing tests at the 1% level rather than the 5%. Actually, there are more precise ways of doing sequential procedures. These are designed to achieve a significance level defined in advance (Armitage, 1960). If one does not wish to be quite so precise at the outset, the rough rule of continuing until one achieves a significance level more stringent than that ultimately selected will probably be adequate.

FINNEY   Let me state the case rather firmly and rigidly. If one has two drugs that literally do not differ in the slightest degree, and if one continues to test them on patients, performing a test of significance after every twentieth patient, eventually one will obtain a result that is apparently statistically significant. The proof of this statement is difficult, but it is a logical consequence of mathematical argument.

A standard dose–response curve based on cumulative experience versus one based on a concomitant standard

BROWN   I should like to bring up the question of using laboratory values from previous tests. Is it a common procedure to use standard curves from previous experience rather than the standard curve estimated from the data of the day?

EMMENS   Many laboratories, particularly commercial ones, accumulate data and have a standard dose–response line. They view the week's testing in the light of the experience of years. It is not so commonly done in research, because one is always suspicious that changes may be occurring.

BROWN   Is it not done quite often in clinical laboratories where routine assays are done as well?

ALBERT   I am rather biphasic about this. For research purposes a standard is always run concomitantly with the unknown. For routine diagnostic assays I use a composite standard dose–response curve. This curve has been built up over many years and is tested periodically. Because of the numbers and replications that this curve embodies it provides more satisfactory results than could be obtained with a single assay of standard against unknown.

EMMENS   Do you find that you can depend on the constancy of both position and slope of the standard dose–response curve? In my experience the slopes remain fairly constant but the positions vary.

ALBERT   After a while the extent of the variation is defined.

BROWN   When, in these routine diagnostic assays, you locate the intercept and use the composite slope, do you still check the slope of the day? If it appears to be in line with past experience, do you then use the composite slope?

ALBERT   Yes, and then we incorporate the slope obtained that week or that month in the composite.

FINNEY   In circumstances like that would there be an advantage in not taking a simple, unweighted mean but in giving, say, three times as much weight to the most recent assay and twice as much to the next most recent? Thereby one would place rather more emphasis on one's most recent experience.

ALBERT   Such a procedure probably would be advantageous. That is what we should do if we found that the most recent assays were the most precise.

BROWN   Do you observe any systematic variations?

ALBERT   No, none.

EMMENS   Seasonal variation in the response has occasionally been described.

ALBERT   In most animal houses today there is no such thing as season. Rats in a well-run colony are bred according to schedule, and the environment is constant with respect to temperature, humidity, heat, light, food, water, and even personnel. One year there seemed to be some mysterious effect whereby the rats knew that it was spring: our rat production went up two or three times. Since I hadn't noticed any kind of seasonal effect on the reproductive quality of the rat, I began looking into this. I found that there had been a change in keepers and that one of them was slipping on the job. A new man was brought in, and when more attention was paid to weeding out the littermates and so forth, the effect disappeared.

EMMENS   When I worked for the Medical Research Council thirty years ago, my colony of ovariectomized mice showed a great deal of seasonal change. It was undoubtedly related to the fact that daylight and temperature varied and, probably, other things as well. Now my mice are kept at a constant temperature and have twelve hours of daily lighting, etc., and we don't see any fluctuations.

The pooling of interactions with error in an analysis of variance

BIRMINGHAM   When is one allowed to pool insignificant interactions in the error term in an analysis of variance?

FINNEY   It is never legitimate to do so, but it is sometimes desirable — which is true of a lot of things in life.

BIRMINGHAM   That is fine, because I thought that it was necessary.

FINNEY   I don't think one can defend the point that it is necessary. Sometimes it is, or seems to be, for gaining degrees of freedom. Personally, I would not pool unless I were very short of degrees of freedom, with, say, fewer than ten or fifteen for error. Pooling inevitably introduces some confusion and risk of misunderstanding, and one has to judge whether the advantages more than compensate.

BROWN   I certainly agree that in most experiments one does not need additional degrees of freedom for error. Once there are twenty or so in the error term, pooling will not change a statistic or F ratio much, unless the estimates one is pooling are discrepant — in which case one would really have cause for concern.

FINNEY   There are a few instances in which out of sheer laziness one might pool, for example, with a highly complicated design in which the isolation of high-order interactions is intractable unless one has access to a computer program. Then, from general experience, I would pool if the effort of doing anything else were not worth while.

Confidence limits on a ratio of relative potencies

ALBERT   I should like to consider the determination of 95% confidence limits on a ratio of follicle-stimulating hormone to luteinizing hormone. Suppose that a 24-hour sample of urine of a menopausal patient on day 1 of a series is analyzed for both FSH and LH. The FSH content, determined by a parallel-line bioassay, is, say, 101 IU per 24 hours, with a 95% confidence interval of 79 to 132. The LH content, determined by an independent parallel-line bioassay, is, say, 48 IU per 24 hours, with a 95% confidence interval of 27 to 83. The ratio of FSH to LH is, therefore, $101/48 = 2.10$. What are 95% confidence limits on this ratio?

BROWN   An approximate short-cut solution is that $79/83 = 0.95$ and $132/27 = 4.89$ are 90% confidence limits. In general, if 95% confidence intervals are N_L to N_U for the numerator of a ratio of random variables and D_L to D_U for the denominator, then N_L/D_U to N_U/D_L is a $(95\%)^2 = 90.25\%$ confidence interval on that ratio. To obtain a 95% confidence interval one would need $\sqrt{95\%} = 97.5\%$ confidence intervals on the numerator and denominator of each.

ARMITAGE   A more appropriate method which, incidentally, yields narrower limits, is to take the logarithm of the ratio, so that one obtains the difference between the logarithms of the two estimated potencies; that is,

$$\log_{10}(R_{FSH}/R_{LH}) = \log_{10} R_{FSH} - \log_{10} R_{LH}$$
$$= \log_{10} 101 - \log_{10} 48 = 0.323$$

Since each of the two assays is of the parallel-line type, each potency estimate has the following form (see Equation 3 of Chapter 4):

$$\log_{10} R = (\bar{x}_S - \bar{x}_U) - (\bar{y}_S - \bar{y}_U)/b \tag{1}$$

If the calculations for the potency estimates can be retrieved, then an approximate variance for $\log_{10} R$ (Finney, 1964, p. 115, eq. 4.14) is

$$\frac{s^2}{b^2}\left[\frac{1}{N_S} + \frac{1}{N_U} + \left(\frac{\bar{y}_S - \bar{y}_U}{b}\right)^2 \frac{1}{\sum(x_S - \bar{x}_S)^2 + \sum(x_U - \bar{x}_U)^2}\right] \tag{2}$$

ALBERT   For the data cited the respective variances were calculated as

$$\text{var}(\log_{10} R_{\text{FSH}}) = 0.002459 \quad \text{and} \quad \text{var}(\log_{10} R_{\text{LH}}) = 0.011884$$

ARMITAGE   Since the two assays involved were independently conducted, it follows that the standard error (SE) of the difference of the logarithms of the estimated potencies is

$$\begin{aligned} \text{SE}(\log_{10} R_{\text{FSH}} &- \log_{10} R_{\text{LH}}) \\ &= \sqrt{\text{var}(\log_{10} R_{\text{FSH}}) + \text{var}(\log_{10} R_{\text{LH}})} \\ &= \sqrt{0.002459 + 0.011884} = 0.120 \end{aligned} \qquad (3)$$

Consequently, 95% confidence limits on $\log_{10} R_{\text{FSH}} - \log_{10} R_{\text{LH}}$ are obtained by adding and subtracting two standard errors. This gives

$$0.323 \pm 2(0.120) = 0.083, 0.563$$

Finally, a 95% confidence interval on the ratio of relative potencies is obtained by taking the antilogs of these:

$$\text{antilog}_{10} \, 0.083 = 1.21 \quad \text{to} \quad \text{antilog}_{10} \, 0.563 = 3.66$$

This method is valid provided that the expression for $\text{var}(\log_{10} R)$ is a satisfactory approximation. According to the guideline set forth by Finney (1964, p. 29), the approximation is satisfactory when the g, the index of significance of the regression, calculated for each of the assays does not exceed 0.2.

If the calculations for each of the relative potencies cannot be retrieved, then one can roughly estimate $\text{var}(\log_{10} R)$ from the confidence limits. The logarithms of the 95% confidence limits on R span roughly four standard errors. Hence the variance is approximated by squaring one quarter of the difference of the logs of the 95% confidence limits. For example, the given 95% confidence limits on FSH potency are 79 to 132. Then,

$$\text{var}(\log_{10} R_{\text{FSH}}) \approx [(\log_{10} 132 - \log_{10} 79)/4]^2 = 0.0031$$

Correspondingly, for LH, whose given 95% confidence limits are 27 to 83,

$$\text{var}(\log_{10} R_{\text{LH}}) \approx [(\log_{10} 83 - \log_{10} 27)/4]^2 = 0.0149$$

Both variances are larger than the more precise estimates retrieved from the original calculations. Hence, the resulting confidence limits are somewhat wider (1.14 to 3.90).

ALBERT   How many degrees of freedom is one allowed when making these determinations?

ARMITAGE   One need not worry about the degrees of freedom, since they are not relevant in this situation. These are approximate results, and errors are regarded as normally distributed on the scale of log potency.

ALBERT   Would it be wrong statistically to consider weighting the numerator and denominator? The FSH value in the numerator is perhaps three to five times as good as the LH value in the denominator. Although the error is actually the sum of the two, would it not be possible somehow to weight the variances?

EMMENS   In the analysis that Dr. Armitage suggested such weighting is implicit, in that the denominator has wider limits. Even if the FSH assay were absolutely accurate, the error in LH alone would determine the limits on their ratio.

FINNEY   The precision of the ratio of two variates will always be worse than the worst of the two. I don't think one can hope for anything that can be called an exact solution to this problem.

ALBERT   If one now determines the FSH/LH ratio for the menopausal patient on another day, how can one tell whether the two ratios differ? Suppose that the FSH/LH ratio on this other day, say the sixth day of a series, is $241/45 = 5.36$. Further, on this subsequent day

$$\mathrm{var}\,(\log_{10} R_{\mathrm{FSH}}) = 0.001576 \quad \text{and} \quad \mathrm{var}\,(\log_{10} R_{\mathrm{LH}}) = 0.011904$$

ARMITAGE   Provided that the four assays involved are independently conducted, one can continue with the process of taking logarithms of the ratios. For the first day one has the ratio and the variance of its logarithm. For the subsequent day one has another ratio and can determine the variance of its logarithm. One can add these two variances together to obtain the variance of the difference between the logarithms of ratios.

For example, with the results of the sixth day one has

$$\log_{10}\,(R_{\mathrm{FSH}}/R_{\mathrm{LH}}) = \log_{10} 5.36 = 0.729$$
$$\mathrm{var}\,(\log_{10} R_{\mathrm{FSH}} - \log_{10} R_{\mathrm{LH}}) = 0.001576 + 0.011904$$
$$= 0.013480$$

The difference between the log ratios for the two days is

$$0.323 - 0.729 = -0.406$$

with standard error

$$\sqrt{0.013480 + 0.014343} = \sqrt{0.027823} = 0.167$$

The ratio of the difference to its standard error is

$$-0.406/0.167 = -2.43$$

From a table of the normal distribution (or t tables with infinite degrees of freedom) one can conclude that the ratio on the sixth day is significantly higher than that on the first ($P < 0.05$).

*ALBERT If two multiple assays, one for FSH and one for LH, were conducted and the number of unknowns corresponded to the number of days on which extracts were obtained, how would the procedure be modified?

*COLTON If the FSH and LH potencies for the first and sixth days were determined by testing the extracts in multiple assays, and if the values for the sixth day are denoted by a prime, then the difference in log ratios for the two days is

$$(\log_{10} R_{\text{FSH}} - \log_{10} R_{\text{LH}}) - (\log_{10} R'_{\text{FSH}} - \log_{10} R'_{\text{LH}}) \qquad (4)$$

Rearranging terms gives

$$(\log_{10} R_{\text{FSH}} - \log_{10} R'_{\text{FSH}}) - (\log_{10} R_{\text{LH}} - \log_{10} R'_{\text{LH}}) \qquad (5)$$

Since R_{FSH} and R'_{FSH} are from a multiple assay having common slope and residual variance, it follows that

$$\log_{10} R_{\text{FSH}} - \log_{10} R'_{\text{FSH}} = (\bar{x}_{\text{U}'} - \bar{x}_{\text{U}}) - (\bar{y}_{\text{U}'} - \bar{y}_{\text{U}})/b \qquad (6)$$

If there were only three preparations in the multiple assay (one standard and two unknowns for both days), the approximate variance of Equation 6, analogous to Expression 2 for a single assay, would be

$$\frac{s^2}{b^2} \left[\frac{1}{N_{\text{U}}} + \frac{1}{N_{\text{U}'}} + \left(\frac{\bar{y}_{\text{U}} - \bar{y}_{\text{U}'}}{b} \right)^2 \right.$$

$$\left. \times \frac{1}{\sum (x_{\text{S}} - \bar{x}_{\text{S}})^2 + \sum (x_{\text{U}} - \bar{x}_{\text{U}})^2 + \sum (x_{\text{U}'} - \bar{x}_{\text{U}'})^2} \right] \qquad (7)$$

By performing this calculation separately for the FSH and LH assays and adding the resulting variances one obtains the variance of the required difference. By taking the square root to find the standard error one can then proceed either to calculate confidence limits on the ratio of the FSH/LH ratios or to compare the two FSH/LH ratios with a test of significance.

*ALBERT Multiple assays for FSH and LH with the data previously described give the following results:

* Remarks added after termination of the Conference.

	Multiple FSH assay	Multiple LH assay
R (day 1)	101	48
R' (day 6)	241	45
$\log_{10} R$	2.004	1.681
$\log_{10} R'$	2.382	1.653
$\log_{10} R - \log_{10} R'$	-0.378	0.028
s^2	625.81	40.10
b (pooled slope)	315.08	32.47
N_{U}	4	4
$N_{\mathrm{U'}}$	8	4
$\bar{y}_{\mathrm{U}} - \bar{y}_{\mathrm{U'}}$	22.7	0.85
$\sum (x_{\mathrm{S}} - \bar{x}_{\mathrm{S}})^2$	0.1812	1.4499
$\sum (x_{\mathrm{U}} - \bar{x}_{\mathrm{U}})^2$	0	0
$\sum (x_{\mathrm{U'}} - \bar{x}_{\mathrm{U'}})^2$	0.1812	0

*COLTON The estimate which, of course, is the same as that derived when single assays are assumed, becomes

$$(\log_{10} R_{\mathrm{FSH}} - \log_{10} R'_{\mathrm{FSH}}) - (\log_{10} R_{\mathrm{LH}} - \log_{10} R'_{\mathrm{LH}})$$
$$= -0.378 - 0.028 = -0.406$$

For the variance of $\log_{10} R_{\mathrm{FSH}} - \log_{10} R'_{\mathrm{FSH}}$ one obtains, by using Expression 7,

$$\frac{625.81}{(315.08)^2} \left[\frac{1}{4} + \frac{1}{8} + \left(\frac{22.7}{315.08} \right)^2 \frac{1}{0.1812 + 0 + 0.1812} \right]$$
$$= 0.002454$$

and for the variance of $\log_{10} R_{\mathrm{LH}} - \log_{10} R'_{\mathrm{LH}}$ one obtains

$$\frac{40.10}{(32.47)^2} \left[\frac{1}{4} + \frac{1}{4} + \left(\frac{0.85}{32.47} \right)^2 \frac{1}{1.4499 + 0 + 0} \right] = 0.019035$$

The variance of the estimate is

$$0.002454 + 0.019035 = 0.021489$$

and the standard error is

$$\sqrt{0.021489} = 0.147$$

This is in good agreement with the standard error of 0.167 calculated previously by assuming that all assays were independent.

These results do not show the multiple-assay technique to its best advantage. With these data there were indications of strong heterogeneity of variance. Under more favorable circumstances the multiple-assay approach is preferable, since it conserves experimental effort and could be expected to yield a smaller standard error (see Finney, 1964, p. 305, for a discussion of the statistical advantages).

* Remarks added after termination of the Conference.

I
Theoretical Aspects

CHAPTER SEVENTEEN

Introduction

Chemists and immunologists have traditionally been concerned with the quantitative aspects of the reactions of substrates with specific reactor substances. Commonly the substrates are immunogenic materials, antigens, and the specific reactors are their homologous antibodies. Within the past decade endocrinologists have become keenly aware of the contributions that quantitative immunological methods can offer to their discipline. Hormones, especially polypeptide hormones, are present in plasma at concentrations as low as 10^{-12} to 10^{-10} M. Since the hormonal polypeptides often do not contain elements that would allow their detection by specific chemical means and are present in a milieu in which the total protein concentration is as great as 10^{-4} to 10^{-3} M, highly specific and delicate methods are required for measuring these hormones in plasma. An awareness that immunological methods have both great specificity and great delicacy has prompted their widespread and successful empirical use by many endocrinologists. Since these techniques are based on firm mathematical formulations, and since many of the participants in this Workshop Conference have interests both in mathematics and the quantitative aspects of endocrinology, the Organizing Committee considered it worth while to raise for discussion here certain theoretical aspects of these methods.

The following two chapters are concerned with the mathematical formulations that underlie the competitive inhibition of binding of labeled hormones to their specific reactor substances. This technique, referred to as *radioimmunoassay*, is discussed by Drs. Yalow and Berson with particular reference to polypeptide hormones and their homologous antibodies. Drs. Ekins, Newman, and O'Riordan prefer the term *saturation assay* and include in their discussion reference to substances that are not usually considered immunogenic (steroid hormones, thyroxine, and vitamin B_{12}). The points considered by both groups relate principally to the sensitivity and precision of these methods.

CHAPTER EIGHTEEN

Radioimmunoassays

ROSALYN S. YALOW AND
SOLOMON A. BERSON

Hormonal potency must, by definition, be expressed in terms of some effect upon a biological system. Therefore, if feasible, it would be advantageous to utilize bioassay procedures for the measurement of plasma hormones. Some in vivo assays for plasma insulin in specially prepared small animals have been described. However, at best their sensitivity barely suffices for a measurement of the elevated levels of insulin found in unextracted plasma after glucose administration (for review, see Yalow and Berson, 1960a). In vitro bioassays for insulin with adequate sensitivity have usually lacked specificity (for review, see Berson and Yalow, 1966). The bioassay for melanocyte-stimulating hormone, described by Shizume et al. (1954), possesses exquisite sensitivity but requires preliminary extraction of urine and plasma for satisfactory specificity. Plasma adrenocorticotropic hormone (ACTH) has been measured by a specific bioassay developed by Lipscomb and Nelson (1960) and has been used by them and by Liddle et al. (1962) to gain valuable information concerning the regulation of ACTH secretion. However, dynamic studies of normal subjects have not been extensively pursued with this technique, which requires relatively large volumes of plasma. For most of the other peptide hormones bioassay methods have provided neither adequate specificity nor the sensitivity required by the low concentrations present in plasma. Although several immunological assay techniques have been developed to overcome these difficulties, radioimmunoassay, which possesses distinct advantages in terms of sensitivity, specificity, precision, and simplicity, has been the most widely used.

Radioimmunoassay had its origin more than a decade ago, when antibodies capable of binding ^{131}I-labeled insulin were demonstrated in human subjects treated with a mixture of commercial beef and pork insulin. Using the techniques of paper electrophoresis and chromato-electrophoresis, Berson et al. (1956) showed that the percentage of insulin bound to antibody decreased as the insulin concentration in the incubation mixtures was increased and that unlabeled insulin could displace labeled insulin from the insulin–antibody complexes.

The principle of competitive inhibition derived from these observations is summarized in the following reaction:

$$\left(\begin{array}{c}\text{free}\\\text{hormone}\end{array}\right)_{-^{131}\text{I}} + \left(\begin{array}{c}\text{hormone}\\\text{antibody}\end{array}\right) \rightleftharpoons \left(\begin{array}{c}\text{antibody-bound}\\\text{hormone}\end{array}\right)_{-^{131}\text{I}}$$

(F) (B)

+

unlabeled hormone
(in known standards
or in body fluids)

⇅

antibody-bound
unlabeled hormone

As a result of the competitive inhibition the ratio of the concentrations of antibody-bound (B) to free (F), or unbound, labeled hormone, denoted by B/F, diminishes as the concentration of unlabeled hormone increases. The concentration in an unknown sample can be obtained by comparing the inhibition observed with that produced by standard solutions containing known amounts of hormone; see Figure 1.

The sensitivity (about 250 to 500 μU/ml) available with the human antiserum to the mixture of beef and pork insulins (Figure 2) that was used in the original study was comparable to that obtained by in vivo bioassay but was far from adequate for measuring endogenous insulin in plasma. However, an immunoassay was developed on these principles (Berson and Yalow, 1957), and by selection of more suitable human antisera the sensitivity was improved sufficiently to measure the rate of disappearance from plasma of a small, intravenous dose of insulin in the rabbit (Berson, 1957; Berson and Yalow, 1958). When it was found that human insulin reacted more strongly with some guinea pig antisera to beef insulin than with human antisera (Berson and Yalow, 1959a), an immunoassay for endogenous human insulin in unextracted plasma became feasible (Yalow and Berson, 1959 and 1960b); see Figure 2. Within the next two years a further improvement in the assay (Figure 2) followed the observation that guinea pigs immunized with pork insulin provided still more sensitive antisera for the immunoassay of human insulin (Yalow and Berson, 1961a), probably because of the virtual identity of pork and human insulins, which differ only in the C-terminal amino acid of the B chain (Nicol and Smith, 1960).

The sensitivity and simplicity of radioimmunoassays led to a burgeoning of interest in the application of this technique to the measurement of other circulating peptide hormones. We have been primarily concerned with the assay of insulin, growth hormone, adrenocorticotropic hormone, and parathyroid hormone. Others have successfully applied the method to the assay of glucagon, luteinizing hormone, follicle-stimulating

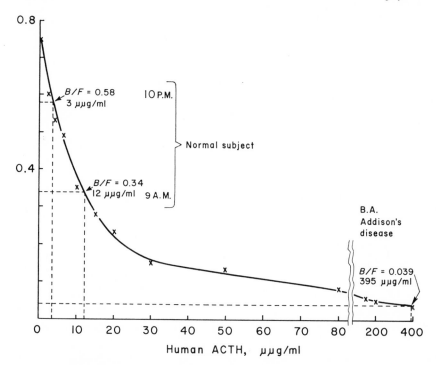

FIGURE 1 Standard curve for ACTH assay. The ratio of antibody-bound to free ACTH–^{131}I is plotted as a function of unlabeled, standard ACTH in incubation mixtures. For determination of ACTH concentrations in unknown samples the abscissa corresponding to the ratio B/F (bound to free) in the unknown is found by reference to the standard curve. All plasma samples were assayed at a dilution of 1:5. From Berson and Yalow (1969).

hormone, thyroid-stimulating hormone, placental lactogen, vasopressin, angiotensin, and other peptide hormones.

The principles of radioimmunoassay have been extended to non-immune systems and to the measurement of substances other than hormones. The generalization of the assay method — the competitive inhibition of the binding of a labeled substrate to any specific reactor, which may or may not be an antibody — is described in the following set of competing reactions:

$$\text{S*} + \text{specific reactor} \rightleftharpoons \overline{\text{S*–R}} \dashrightarrow \text{products*}$$

$$\begin{array}{cccc} \text{(F)} & \text{(R)} & \text{(B)} & \text{(P*)} \\ & + & & \\ & \text{S} & & \\ & \text{\Updownarrow} & & \\ & \overline{\text{S–R}} & & \\ & \downarrow & & \\ & \text{P} & & \end{array}$$

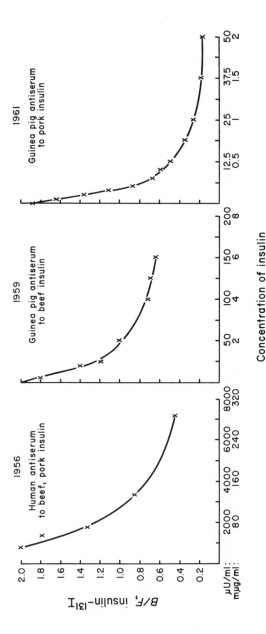

FIGURE 2 Typical standard curves for the radioimmunoassay of insulin in the years shown. For the curve on the left beef insulin was used as standard (from Berson et al., 1956, Fig. 9b). For the other two curves human insulin was used as standard (from Yalow and Berson, 1959 and 1961b).

where S is any substance to be measured, R is a specific reactor for that substance, P is the products that may result from the interaction when R and S are enzyme and substrate, respectively, and F and B are as defined above. The asterisk indicates labeling.

In this more general form the principle has been applied to the assay of plasma vitamin B_{12} by using intrinsic factor as the specific reactor (Rothenberg, 1961; Barakat and Ekins, 1961), of folic acid by using folic acid reductase as the specific reactor (Rothenberg, 1965), and of thyroid hormone (Murphy and Pattee, 1964) and steroid hormones (Murphy et al., 1963) by using specific binding proteins from plasma.

The mathematical formulations that provide the basis of immunoassay will be the principal concern of this chapter, and only such description of experimental techniques as is necessary for a fuller understanding of the theory will be interposed.

Information gleaned from our studies of the kinetics of the reaction between insulin and insulin-binding antibody serves as a foundation for the mathematical analysis basic to radioimmunoassay (Berson and Yalow, 1959b). In these studies we assumed that the law of mass action is applicable to the reaction between insulin and antibody and considered the possible consequences of three models of this reaction, which are as follows.

A. Univalent insulin as antigen (Ag) reacting with a single order of antibody combining sites (Ab):

$$[Ag] + [Ab] \underset{k'}{\overset{k}{\rightleftharpoons}} [\overline{AgAb}] \tag{1}$$

B. Univalent insulin (Ag) reacting with two or more different orders of antibody combining sites (Ab_a, Ab_b, etc.):

$$[Ag] + [Ab_a] \underset{k'_a}{\overset{k_a}{\rightleftharpoons}} [\overline{AgAb_a}] \tag{2a}$$

$$[Ag] + [Ab_b] \underset{k'_b}{\overset{k_b}{\rightleftharpoons}} [\overline{AgAb_b}] \tag{2b}$$

C. Divalent insulin reacting with a single order of antibody combining sites:

$$[Ag] + [Ab] \underset{k'}{\overset{k}{\rightleftharpoons}} [\overline{AgAb_1}] \tag{3a}$$

$$[AgAb_1] + [Ab] \underset{k'_c}{\overset{k_c}{\rightleftharpoons}} [\overline{AgAb_2}] \tag{3b}$$

The brackets indicate molar concentrations of reactants, and the unprimed and primed k's indicate the forward and reverse velocity constants, respectively, for the various reactions.

Models of multivalent insulin reacting with multiple orders of antibody combining sites may be formulated as extensions of the simpler models.

These equations can be solved for the ratio B/F as a function of B. From a comparison of experimental data with the theoretical models it was found that the reaction of insulin with human antisera was best described by model B, that of univalent insulin reacting with at least two orders of antibody combining sites. The equilibrium constants for the reactions ranged from 10^7 to 2×10^{10} lit/mol. From these studies we concluded that there was little likelihood of finding human antisera suitable for immunoassay.

To appreciate the reasoning behind this conclusion, consider the case of the reaction of univalent antigen with a single order of antibody combining sites. From Equation 1 we obtain the equilibrium constant K:

$$K = \frac{k}{k'} = \frac{[\overline{AgAb}]}{[Ag][Ab]}$$

Now let $[Ab°]$ be the molar concentration of antibody combining sites such that $[Ab°] = [Ab] + [\overline{AgAb}]$. Then, substituting $F = [Ag]$ and $B = [\overline{AgAb}]$, we obtain

$$B/F = K([Ab°] - B) \qquad (4)$$

If the concentration of antibody is in marked excess over the concentration of hormone being determined, even the complete binding of all the unlabeled hormone would not significantly diminish the antibody available for the binding of labeled hormone, and the competitive inhibition would hardly be detectable. It is therefore necessary to dilute the antiserum sufficiently to lower the antibody concentration to the same order as the lowest hormone concentration to be measured. From Equation 4 it is evident that $B/F \le K[Ab°]$. This condition sets a practical limit to the dilution possible for any designated B/F value. Suppose that we desire a B/F ratio of 1.0; then the antibody concentration cannot be lowered beyond the value determined by $[Ab°] \ge K^{-1}$.

Since the molar concentrations of many peptide hormones in the nonstimulated state range from 10^{-12} to 10^{-10} M (Table 1), the antibody concentration $[Ab°]$ should be in this range to yield a B/F ratio of 1.0. Antisera suitable for the immunoassay of peptide hormones in plasma must therefore have equilibrium constants of approximately 10^{12} to 10^{10}, respectively. The highest equilibrium constants are required for detecting the hormones in lowest concentration in the plasma. In only an occasional human anti-insulin serum is K equal to or greater than 10^{10} for the reaction with beef insulin, and the equilibrium constant is even smaller for the reaction with human insulin (Berson and Yalow, 1959c).

Table 1   Concentrations of Some Hormones in Human Plasma

Hormone	Molar concn. $M \times 10^{-12}$
Insulin	100
Glucagon	100
Growth hormone	60
Parathyroid hormone	30
Adrenocorticotropic hormone	1 (P.M.) to 10 (A.M.)

Fortunately, guinea pig antisera for many peptide hormones often exhibit equilibrium constants several orders of magnitude higher. These considerations serve as a theoretical guide in immunoassay.

The ultimate requirement for successful radioimmunoassay is, of course, a suitable antiserum. As we have seen, the criterion of suitability is not titer or antibody concentration but, rather, a property related to the energy of interaction between antibodies and hormonal antigen. The parameter of energy that determines the potential sensitivity of the antiserum is the equilibrium constant characterizing the reaction between the hormone and that class of antibodies for which the product of the equilibrium constant K and the antibody concentration [Ab°] predominates in the antiserum.

In considering the sensitivity of an immunoassay we are not concerned directly with B/F as a function of B but, rather, we are concerned with the extent to which B/F or b, the fraction bound, varies with a change in the total hormone concentration, [H]; evidently, $b = B/[H]$. For consideration of precision we are concerned with how B/F or b varies with the fractional change in hormone concentration (Yalow and Berson, 1968a).

These relationships are complicated. However, by substituting $[H] - B = F$ in Equation 4 we can solve for B in terms of [H] in order to evaluate B/F as a function of [H]. This gives

$$B/F = K[\text{Ab}°] - \tfrac{1}{2}(\varphi - \sqrt{\varphi^2 - 2\lambda[H]}) \qquad (5)$$

where the new symbols are $\varphi = K[\text{Ab}°] + K[H] + 1$ and $\lambda = 2K^2[\text{Ab}°]$. Expanding $\sqrt{\varphi^2 - 2\lambda[H]}$ according to the binomial theorem, we obtain a convergent series,

$$\frac{B}{F} = K[\text{Ab}°] - \frac{1}{2}\left[\frac{\lambda[H]}{\varphi} + \frac{1}{2}\left(\frac{\lambda^2[H]^2}{\varphi^3}\right) + \cdots + \right] \qquad (6)$$

Since it will be shown that sensitivity is optimal at $[H] \ll [\text{Ab}°]$ and $K[\text{Ab}°] < 1$, we can neglect the higher-order terms beyond the first term in the parentheses. Differentiating this equation with respect to [H] and simplifying, we obtain

$$\frac{d(B/F)}{d[H]} = -\frac{(B/F)^2}{[Ab^\circ](K[Ab^\circ] + 1)} \tag{7}$$

This equation determines sensitivity, since $d(B/F)/d[H]$ is, by definition, the slope of the dose–response curve, B/F versus [H]. This slope increases as $[Ab^\circ]$ decreases. From Equation 4 it is evident that $B/F \leq K[Ab^\circ]$ and that $[Ab^\circ] \to (B/F)/K$ as $B \to 0$ or, that is, as $[H] \to 0$. If now we substitute the minimal value of $[Ab^\circ]$, we obtain the *maximal* sensitivity at any given B/F:

$$\frac{d(B/F)}{d[H]} = -\frac{B/F}{B/F + 1} K \tag{8}$$

It follows that this degree of sensitivity will be obtained when the concentration of labeled hormone is sufficiently low for B to be much less than $[Ab^\circ]$. At higher concentrations, such that this condition is not fulfilled, B/F is less than $K[Ab^\circ]$, and the sensitivity is less than that given by Equation 8.

Although under these conditions $d(B/F)/d[H]$ increases with B/F to a maximal absolute value of K, when B/F is very high even large changes in B/F may not be measurable with precision. For example, even a fall in ratio from 1,000:1 to 100:1 means that b has decreased only from 0.999 to 0.990. It is therefore desirable to find the B/F value at which the absolute value of $db/d[H]$ becomes maximal. It has been shown (Yalow and Berson, 1968a) that this is attained at $b = \frac{1}{3}$, which occurs at $B/F = 0.5$, and that under these conditions

$$\frac{db}{d[H]} = -\frac{4}{27} K \tag{9}$$

This is the equation for maximal change in b with [H]. Thus, maximal sensitivity is dependent on K and is obtained as [H] approaches 0, when, that is, only a negligible fraction of the antibody combining sites is occupied.

Precision is defined in terms of the extent of change in B/F or b with fractional change in hormone concentration:

$$\frac{d(B/F)}{d[H]/[H]} \quad \text{or} \quad \frac{db}{d[H]/[H]}$$

From Equation 7 it can be shown (Yalow and Berson, 1968a) that

$$\frac{d(B/F)}{d[H]/[H]} \approx -B/F\left(1 - \frac{B/F}{K[Ab^\circ]}\right) \tag{10}$$

Unlike maximal sensitivity, maximal precision is obtained, not at trace concentrations of hormones, but at concentrations that result in virtual saturation of the antibody combining sites, that is, at $B/F \ll K[\text{Ab}^\circ]$. Under such conditions $B \approx [\text{Ab}^\circ]$ obtains.

Since by definition b equals $B/[\text{H}]$, then under the conditions described

$$b \approx \frac{[\text{Ab}^\circ]}{[\text{H}]}$$

which, when logarithms are taken, becomes

$$\ln b \approx \ln [\text{Ab}^\circ] - \ln [\text{H}] \tag{11}$$

Differentiating this equation with respect to [H] yields

$$\frac{1}{b} \cdot \frac{db}{d[\text{H}]} = -\frac{1}{[\text{H}]}$$

and rearranging yields

$$\frac{db}{d[\text{H}]/[\text{H}]} = -b \tag{12}$$

Unlike sensitivity, the maximal precision is independent of K. A plot of $\ln b$ versus $\ln [\text{H}]$ is a straight line (in the region of $K[\text{Ab}^\circ] \gg B/F$) and has the same slope for all antisera, regardless of K.

Under conditions of $B/F \ll [K\text{Ab}^\circ]$ precision is maximal when b approaches 1 (that is, when B/F approaches ∞) but decreases only 2-fold when b is 0.5 (that is, when B/F is 1). Generally, a convenient operating range for obtaining good precision is one in which b is between 0.4 and 0.75 (when B/F is between 0.67 and 2.0).

Antisera are generally heterogeneous with respect to the affinities and concentrations of various orders of antibodies. Therefore, the use of a too highly concentrated antiserum can result in diminished precision if antibodies of low affinity but high concentration begin to bind a significant fraction of labeled hormone at high hormone concentration. A diminution of precision at higher hormone concentrations, due to the influence of a second antibody combining site of lower energy, is shown in Table 2. The table was constructed by assuming values of F and using the formulas shown at the top of the table for evaluating B_1, B_2, H, and b. It can be seen that the decrements in fraction bound are similar over a 6-fold change in hormone concentration with antiserum diluted 1:1,000 and over a 2.5-fold change with antiserum diluted 1:10,000. Precision is poorer in the former situation, in that a greater change in [H] is required to produce the same change in b. This effect is attributable to the influence of the second antibody combining site in the more concentrated antiserum.

TABLE 2   Values of Bound Fraction Corresponding to Different Hormone Concentrations with Antiserum Containing Two Orders of Antibody Combining Sites at Dilutions of $1:1,000$ and $1:10,000$*

Undiluted antiserum: $K_1 = 10^{12}$, $[\text{Ab}_1^\circ] = 10^{-7}$; $K_2 = 10^9$, $[\text{Ab}_2^\circ] = 10^{-6}$

$B_1/F = K_1([\text{Ab}_1^\circ]/n - B_1)$, $B_2/F = K_2([\text{Ab}_2^\circ]/n - B_2)$, where $n =$ dilution factor

$B_1 + B_2 + F = H$, $b = B/H$

$n = 1,000$		$n = 10,000$	
$H,$ $M \times 10^{-10}$	b	$H,$ $M \times 10^{-11}$	b
2.34	0.705	1.08	0.72
2.90	0.655	1.24	0.67
4.65	0.572	1.38	0.64
6.3	0.525	1.64	0.57
9.33	0.465	2.02	0.50
13.45	0.405	2.59	0.42

* See text for definition of symbols.

Although the mathematical considerations just described depend on identical behavior of labeled and unlabeled hormone, the validity of the radioimmunoassay method requires only that the hormone to be measured and the standard hormone behave identically in the immune system.

The sensitivity of the assay is evaluated experimentally from the initial slope of a plot of either b or B/F versus $[H]$; see Figure 3. Experience has shown that antisera from different animals of the same species, immunized on the same schedule, may vary greatly in their sensitivity for the detection of hormone. Antisera are tested at an appropriate dilution to give $B/F \approx 1$ with the minimal practical concentration of labeled insulin. Standard curves are obtained at this dilution, and the antiserum with the sharpest initial slope is selected. Because antisera generally are used in very high dilution, each milliliter of antiserum usually suffices for a hundred thousand to several million determinations.

To achieve maximal sensitivity it is necessary, as is already deduced from theoretical considerations, to keep the concentration of labeled hormone to a minimum. Thus, the combining sites of the highly sensitive antibody are not saturated by the labeled hormone alone. Experimentally it is observed that an increase in the size of the tracer gradually obliterates the region of sharpest slope from the dose–response curve; see Figure 4. Where possible, it is desirable to reduce the concentration of labeled hormone enough for the maximal slope to be reached. Further reduction of tracer will then result in no further improvement. For a

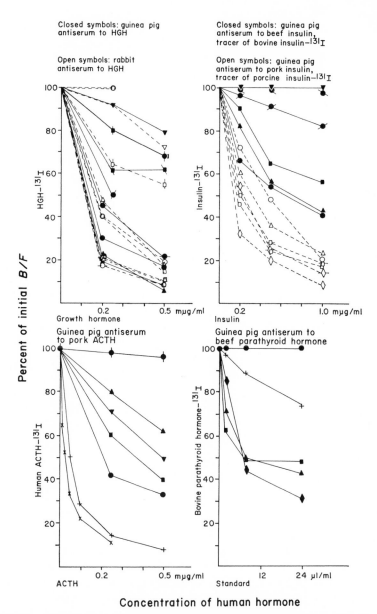

FIGURE 3   Comparison of various antisera for sensitivity in measurement of human peptide hormones. Each curve represents a different antiserum. The antiserum giving the steepest slope will provide the most sensitive assay. The standards used were as follows: human growth hormone (Wilhelmi, Raben), human insulin (Novo, Mirsky), and human ACTH (Li). Since a suitably bioassayed and standardized preparation of human parathyroid hormone is not available, plasma from a hyperparathyroid patient was used as standard by diluting the standard plasma in hypoparathyroid plasma. The labeled preparations of human growth hormone and ACTH were the same as the standards. However, the insulin–^{131}I was prepared from crystalline porcine insulin (Novo or Mirsky). Bovine parathyroid hormone–^{131}I was prepared from highly purified hormone supplied by Dr. G. Aurbach and Dr. J. T. Potts, Jr., or by Dr. H. Rasmussen, Dr. C. Arnaud, and Mr. C. Hawker. From Berson and Yalow (1968).

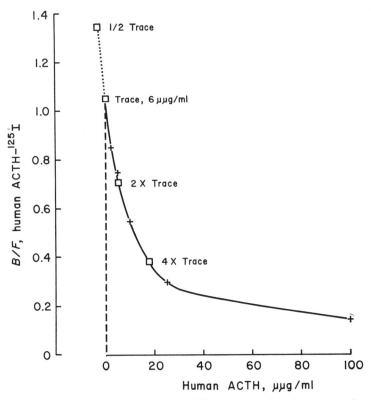

FIGURE 4   Ratio B/F of human ACTH–^{125}I as a function of concentration of unlabeled human ACTH ($\times$) and human ACTH–^{125}I. All mixtures for the standard curve contained the same concentration of "trace ACTH–^{125}I," estimated to be 6 μμg/ml, and varying concentrations of unlabeled ACTH. Other mixtures were prepared without added unlabeled ACTH but with 0.5 to 4 times the concentration of trace ACTH–^{125}I ($\square$). Labeled and unlabeled ACTH fall along the same curve in this assay. From Yalow and Berson (1968b).

given counting rate it is evident that reduction of the chemical concentration of labeled hormone can be effected principally by increasing the volume of incubate assayed, the efficiency for detection of the labeled hormone, and the specific activity of the labeled hormone. We have considered these problems in detail elsewhere (Yalow and Berson, 1968a); here we note only that isotopes with long half-lives, such as ^{14}C and ^{3}H, cannot produce labeled proteins of sufficiently high specific activity to be used in the assay of peptide hormones in plasma, even were it possible to substitute many radioactive atoms; labeling of the ortho positions of the tyrosyl residues with either ^{131}I, whose half-life is 8 days, or ^{125}I, whose half-life is 57 days, has proved the most satisfactory.

In developing each new assay it is necessary to ensure its validity by demonstrating that endogenous plasma hormone and standard hormone react with the antibodies identically and that conditions are maintained such that other substances in the plasma do not affect the determination. A necessary, though not sufficient, condition for identical reactivities of standard and unknown is that the concentration of the unknown hormone fall linearly with the dilution factor; that is, the concentration calculated for undiluted plasma must be the same, regardless of the dilution used for assay; see Figure 5. A failure of the plasma's concentration to fall linearly with dilution may be due either to a lack of identity between the standard and the endogenous hormone or to nonspecific chemical

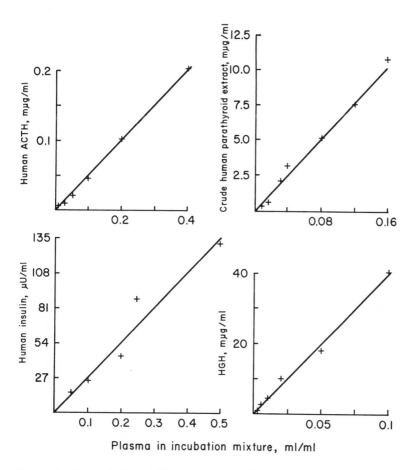

FIGURE 5   Effect of plasma dilution on measured endogenous hormone concentration. Hormone concentrations in individual, diluted plasmas determined by reference to standard curves. From Berson and Yalow (1968).

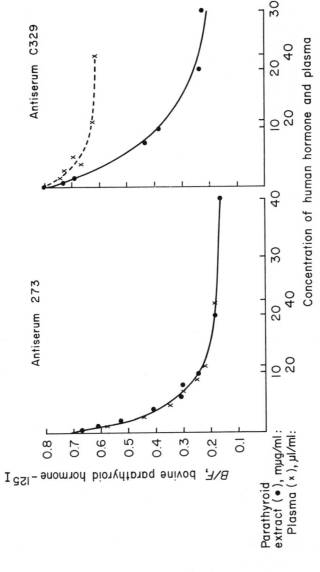

FIGURE 6 Competitive inhibition of binding of beef parathyroid hormone—^{125}I to antibody by extracts of human parathyroid adenomata and by human plasma. The abscissa scale for the human plasma was chosen to match the standard curve of human parathyroid hormone extract for antiserum 273 at a single point, and over the range of concentrations measured the curves were superimposable. The same abscissa scales were then used for antiserum C329, but the plasma and extract curves were not superimposable. From Yalow and Berson (1968b).

effects that interfere with the immune reaction. In certain cases a super-imposition of the dilution curves of standard and endogenous hormones over a 50-fold range has been possible with one or more antisera, while another antiserum may recognize the hormones as distinctly different; see Figure 6. On the basis of these discrepancies we have presented evidence for the immunochemical heterogeneity of plasma thyroid hormone. Comparing the dilution curves with several standards, several plasmas, and several antisera greatly diminishes the probability that immunologic distinctions between standard and plasma hormone will remain unrecognized.

The question may well be asked, whether it is desirable to assay unknown samples in duplicate or greater replicate. To answer this question properly requires an appreciation of physiologic changes in plasma hormone levels. A release of the majority of the peptide hormones can be acutely stimulated by an appropriate physiologic factor. Such stimulation can effect a 5-fold to 50-fold increase in the plasma concentration of the hormone, sometimes in a matter of minutes; see Table 3. After a suppression of hormonal secretion the disappearance of peptide hormones from the plasma is quite rapid, the half-times ranging from 15 minutes to less than an hour; see Figure 7. Although we generally include 400 to 800 samples in a single assay, we prefer to perform assays on multiple specimens taken at appropriate times during stimulation or suppression studies, rather than to assay replicates of a single specimen.

TABLE 3   Plasma Concentrations of Adrenocorticotropic Hormone, Measured by Duplicate Determinations at Beginning and End of Same Assay, Compared with Serial Changes Occurring in Response to Insulin-Induced Hypoglycemia and to Electric Shock Therapy

| Duplicate determinations in same assay | | Stimulus | | | |
| | | Insulin-induced hypoglycemia | | Electric shock | |
Beginning	End	Time, min	Concn., $\mu\mu$g/ml	Time, min	Concn., $\mu\mu$g/ml
70	55	−5	55	0	25
40	35	0	55	5	280
20	40	5	55	15	230
110	120	30	55	30	165
80	55	50	80	60	115
15	20	60	370	90	30
10	15	90	370	120	<5
<10	<10				
30	30				
60	80				

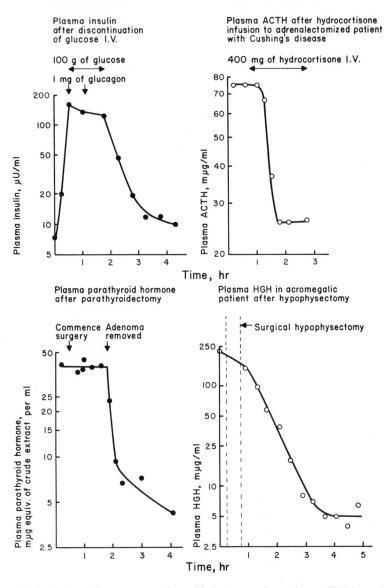

FIGURE 7   Rate of disappearance of peptide hormones from plasma. Highly purified human hormone preparations were utilized as standards for insulin, ACTH,
and growth hormone. Standard for parathyroid hormone was obtained by extraction from human parathyroid adenomata. We are indebted to Drs. G. Aurbach and
J. T. Potts, Jr., for the extraction. From Berson and Yalow (1968).

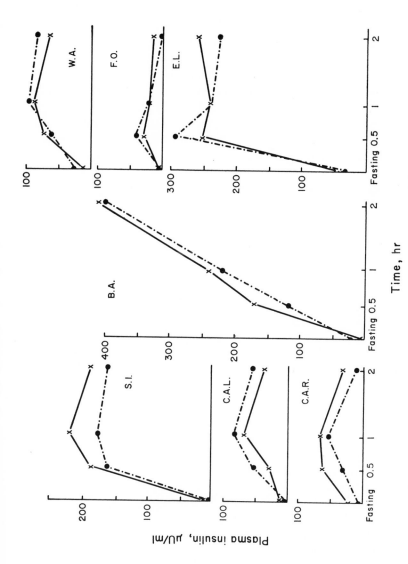

FIGURE 8 Reproducibility of plasma insulin determinations made with the same plasma samples with different lots of insulin–131I and performed one or more months apart. Plasmas were stored frozen between determinations. From Yalow and Berson (1960b).

This is because the differences between duplicate determinations of the same plasma samples are usually quite small compared to the acute changes that can be produced by appropriate stimulation or suppression (Table 3). However, to establish reproducibility it is necessary to evaluate replicate determinations in separate assays of the same plasma samples, which in the interim have been stored in the frozen state; see Figure 8.

It should be noted that immunoassay, unlike the traditional bioassay, is dependent on specific chemical reactions that obey the law of mass action and are not subject to errors introduced by the biological variability of test systems. Random errors due to pipetting, counting, etc. can be reduced to less than 1% or 2% without much difficulty. Nonrandom errors resulting from lack of specificity and difficulties arising from inadequate sensitivity should be minimized by improved experimental design rather than by statistical manipulation.

CHAPTER NINETEEN

Saturation Assays

R. P. EKINS, G. B. NEWMAN, AND
J. L. H. O'RIORDAN

One of the most exciting advances in endocrinology during the past decade has been the development of radioimmunoassay in the laboratory of Berson and Yalow. It must be emphasized, however, that much of the theory underlying radioimmunoassay is applicable to other assay systems which have an equally long history and which, no doubt, will ultimately attain to an equally important position in endocrinology. We refer, of course, to methods that have been developed for the assay of the thyroid and steroid hormones, of certain vitamins, and of other important compounds which, though nonantigenic, nevertheless interact specifically with saturable reagents, such as specific serum or tissue binding proteins and specific enzymes. Such substances thus can be assayed by the same fundamental approach as that applied to the protein hormones by the methods of Berson and Yalow. Indeed, our interest in this form of assay began, not with the advent of radioimmunoassay, but with the development of a technique for the estimation of serum thyroxine. Though little recognized at the time, this method (Ekins, 1960) represented the first practical application of the principle of competitive binding to the measurement of any human serum hormone. In view of the broad implications of the use of specific saturable reactants, whether antibody or naturally occurring binding protein (such as thyroxine-binding globulin and vitamin-B_{12}–binding protein) or specific enzymes, Ekins suggested the term *saturation analysis* for this group of techniques (Barakat and Ekins, 1961; Ekins, 1962).

In this chapter we wish to consider some theoretical aspects of these systems and to examine their specificity, sensitivity, and precision. We must first define the parameters that determine the shape of the standard "response" curve and, in particular, analyze three special situations, those in which (a) the specific reactant is composed of a single species of reacting or binding sites (that is, all of the reactive or binding sites on the reagent are identical in reaction energy vis-à-vis the compound under assay), (b) the specific reactant comprises a multiplicity of such species, and (c) there exist chemical or immunological differences between the standard used and the endogenous hormone present in the "unknown" samples.

1. Assay of univalent hormone with specific reactant carrying a single order of reacting site

The simplest system is a mixture of binding protein (Q) carrying a single order of binding site and a univalent hormone (P) labeled with a chemically and structurally identical radioactive hormone, the reaction between P and Q being governed by the law of mass action.[1]

From this premise may be derived equations relating the experimental variables, which are the total concentrations of P and Q in the system (denoted herein by p and q), and the experimental observation. As much for historical reasons as because to do so introduces significant advantages, we usually take the latter as the ratio of the free radioactive moieties to the bound. This practice differs from that initiated by Yalow and Berson, who have customarily expressed results in terms of the ratio of bound to free, but there is no fundamental mathematical difference between the two. However, many workers now measure the radioactivity in the free or the bound moiety alone. Such a procedure carries different statistical implications and yields an analysis differing in some details and in certain of its conclusions from that presented here. Nevertheless, we do not propose to explore the differences in this chapter, since the basic approaches, the topic with which we are especially concerned, are similar.

The fundamental equations relating the variables p and q and the distribution of radioactive hormone are

$$R_{f/b}^2 + R_{f/b}\left(1 - \frac{p}{q} - \frac{1}{Kq}\right) - \frac{1}{Kq} = 0 \tag{1}$$

$$R_{b/f}^2 + R_{b/f}(1 + Kp - Kq) - Kq = 0 \tag{2}$$

where $R_{f/b}$ and $R_{b/f}$ are the ratios of free to bound and bound to free radioactive moieties, respectively, and K is the equilibrium constant governing the reaction (for their derivation see Ekins et al., 1968).

---

[1] For brevity the compound to be measured is subsequently referred to as a "hormone," although the principle of the method clearly is applicable to many compounds, both organic and inorganic, and even to certain elements. For the same reason the reaction is referred to as a "binding" reaction, and the specific reactant employed is referred to as a "binding protein." The term "order of binding site" is employed herein, after Berson and Yalow (1959b), rather than the term "species," to avoid confusion in the use of the latter. In the context of this analysis, independent binding sites whose behavior can be described by the same equilibrium constant are regarded as belonging to the same order, whether or not they exist on the same molecule.

Equation 2, upon substitution of [H] for p and [Ab°] for q and solving for $R_{b/f}$, is equivalent to Equation 5 of Yalow and Berson (this volume).

Alternative forms of these equations, the significance of which will become more evident when we consider multiordered reactions, are

$$\frac{1}{R_{f/b}} = \frac{q}{\dfrac{p}{1 + 1/R_{f/b}} + \dfrac{1}{K}} \tag{3}$$

$$R_{b/f} = \frac{q}{\dfrac{p}{1 + R_{b/f}} + \dfrac{1}{K}} \tag{4}$$

When q is regarded as constant, Equations 1 and 2 define hyperbolæ. In each case one asymptote is the horizontal (that is, the p) axis. When p is plotted against $R_{f/b}$, the slope of the second asymptote is given by $1/q$, and the intercept on the vertical (that is, the ratio) axis is given by $1/Kq - 1$; conversely, the slope of the second asymptote of the $R_{b/f}$ curve is equal to $-K$, and the intercept on the vertical axis is equal to $Kq - 1$. The form of the curves is shown in Figure 1.

It follows that when $R_{f/b}$ is plotted against p, the curve in the positive quadrant (Figure 1) approaches a straight line, the slope of which is given by the reciprocal of the concentration of binding protein or antibody in the system. Thus, assuming the binding constant K governing the reaction to remain constant, the lower the concentration of binding protein employed, the steeper the resulting response curve, although its intercept on the vertical axis will concurrently tend to higher values of $R_{f/b}$ (Figure 2). It likewise follows that the hormone response curve, expressed as a function of $R_{b/f}$, increases both in steepness and in intercept value on the vertical axis with an increase in the magnitude of K, assuming q to be kept constant (Figure 2).

Despite the simplifications involved, the analysis based on a single order of binding site yields a qualitative picture in close agreement with experimental observation. Thus, Figure 3 shows a series of standard curves (obtained in the assay of vitamin B_{12} by Ekins and Sgherzi, 1964) in which the ratio $R_{f/b}$ is plotted against the concentration of vitamin B_{12} in the system. A reduction in the concentration of binding serum employed increases the slope of the curves and displaces the intercepts toward higher values of $R_{f/b}$. However, in many assays the picture is somewhat more complex; in particular, the binding reagent may comprise many orders of binding site, each characterized by its own equilibrium constant.

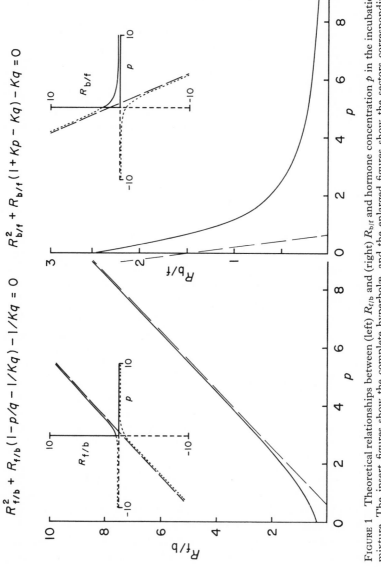

FIGURE 1   Theoretical relationships between (left) $R_{f/b}$ and (right) $R_{b/f}$ and hormone concentration p in the incubation mixture. The insert figures show the complete hyperbola, and the enlarged figures show the sectors corresponding to positive values of R and p. To compute these curves values of 1.0 and 2.5 have been assigned to q and K, respectively. The dimensions of p and q are mass per volume; of K, volume per mass.

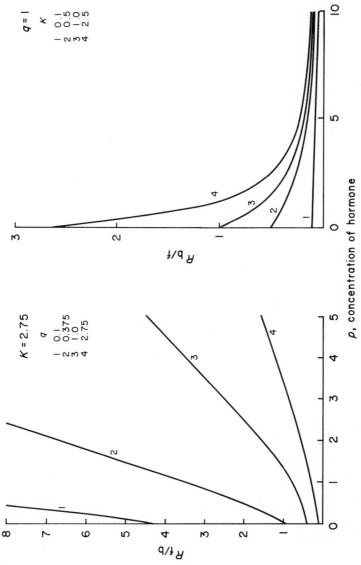

FIGURE 2 Effects on response curves $R_{f/b}$ and $R_{b/f}$ of change in (left) binding site concentration q with K constant and (right) K with binding site concentration constant, respectively.

2. Assay of univalent hormone with binding protein mixture carrying multiple orders of binding site

A binding protein mixture carrying multiple orders of binding site may be represented by the equation

$$P + Q_i \rightleftharpoons PQ_i$$

where Q_i is the binding site of the ith species, i being 1, 2, 3, ..., n.

From this may be derived (see Ekins et al., 1968) the general equation, which may be compared with Equation 3:

$$\frac{1}{R_{f/b}} = \sum_{i=1}^{n} \frac{q_i}{\dfrac{p}{1 + 1/R_{f/b}} + \dfrac{1}{K_i}} \tag{5}$$

Substituting different values for the various parameters, it is a simple matter to predict the form of response curve that can be observed in

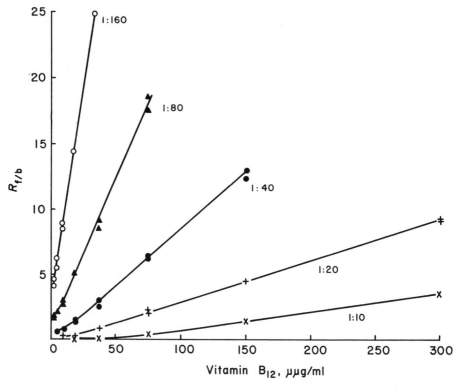

FIGURE 3   Calibration curves obtained in an assay of vitamin B_{12} by the method of Ekins and Sgherzi (1964), showing the dependence of slope on the concentration of binding protein employed in the system.

assays with multiple binding sites. The curves range from configurations essentially indistinguishable from those seen in assays with single binding sites, to various sigmoid forms and, ultimately, to curves that display a progressive reduction in slope for any increase in hormone concentration. Such curves are frequently encountered in practice and are exemplified by the results of assays for insulin and thyroxine, as shown in Figures 4 and 5.

Other factors may, of course, contribute to a deformation of the standard response curve from the simple hyperbolic shape defined by Equation 1. They include impurity in the tracer hormone, inefficiency of the technique used to sequester free from bound moieties, and such nonspecific effects as the binding of tracer material to glassware. Faced

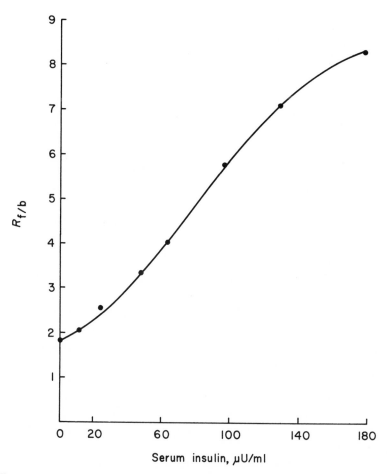

FIGURE 4 Sigmoid calibration curve observed in a radioimmunoassay of insulin.

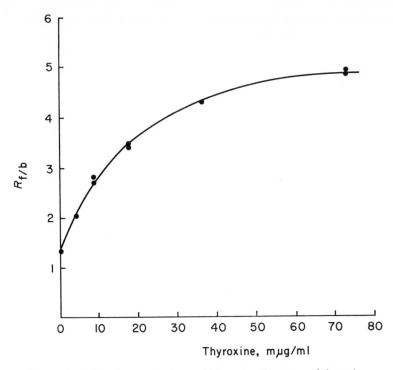

FIGURE 5   Calibration curve observed in a saturation assay of thyroxine.

with the consequent complexity in the shapes of response curves, the statistician has a very difficult task in attempting to devise transformations that will convert experimental data to a form to which he can apply standard statistical techniques.

3. Effect of differences between equilibrium constants of reactions of specific reactant and tracer, reactant and standard hormone, and reactant and unknown hormone

In the preceding sections the assumption has been made that the chemical and physical structure and, hence, the binding characteristics of the labeled hormone are identical with those of the non-radioactive hormone in the system. Except for tracer impurities, this assumption is likely to be valid for such compounds as thyroxine, vitamin B_{12}, and cortisol, in which the substitution of a radioactive nuclide will have no effect on the configuration of the molecule. On the other hand, in the case of the protein hormones (which are usually tagged with radioiodine) the tracer material will necessarily differ from the nonradioactive molecules in consequence of the conversion of constituent tyrosine residues into mono- and diiodotyrosine derivatives. Under such circumstances it cannot be assumed that the binding characteristics exhibited by the tracer remain unaffected. In addition, there may be species differences between the labeled and the unlabeled hormones in the system.

A mathematical consideration of this situation is particularly relevant to an understanding of the consequences of a difference between the hormone used as a reference preparation for the construction of the standard response curve and the endogenous hormone present in unknown samples. In these circumstances tracer hormone introduced into the incubation mixtures must necessarily differ from at least one of the unlabeled hormones with which it is mixed. Clearly, such a possibility might arise as a consequence of chemical alterations undergone by the standard hormone in the course of extraction from the parent gland or might, as in the case of the tracer, reflect a species difference between the two hormones.

The theoretical implications of these possibilities may be revealed by consideration of the simple case in which only one binding site, displaying equilibrium constants of K^* and K_h in its reactions with tracer hormone and unlabeled hormone, respectively, is involved in the reaction. If we denote the initial concentration of tracer hormone by p^* and that of competing unlabeled hormone by h, we can derive (see the Appendix) the following equation defining the response curve:

$$R_{f/b}^2 + R_{f/b}\left(1 - \frac{p^*}{q} - \frac{1}{K^*q}\right) - \frac{1}{K^*q}$$
$$- \frac{(h/q)(R_{f/b} + 1)R_{f/b}}{(K^*/K_h)R_{f/b} + 1} = 0 \quad (6)$$

A corresponding equation in terms of $R_{b/f}$ may also, of course, be derived.

This equation may now be applied to the situation in which the standard hormone (S), the "unknown" hormone (U), and the tracer hormone (P*) react with the same binding site but with different binding constants, given by K_S, K_U, and K^*, respectively. At very low values of $R_{f/b}$ (that is, $R_{f/b} \ll K_h/K^*$) or, conversely, at high values of $R_{b/f}$ the shape of the response curve is relatively independent of the value of K_h. This conclusion implies that for values of R in this range the response curves yielded by the two hormones S and U will be closely similar.

For high values of $R_{f/b}$, on the other hand, the position of the response curve with respect to the p ordinate is strongly dependent on K_h; nevertheless, the curve yielded by hormone U may be made to superimpose that yielded by hormone S by multiplying concentrations of U by the factor K_S/K_U.

It follows from these deductions that two response curves yielded by hormones differing in reaction energy with respect to a single binding site cannot be exactly superimposed (if R ranges from very low to very high values) by multiplying one of the curves by an appropriate normalizing factor. However, if assay conditions are so selected that values of R fall within a restricted range, it may be possible almost to superimpose two such curves by this means.

These conclusions clearly have relevance to the question of assay specificity, since a commonly employed criterion of the identity of an endogenous hormone with a standard one is that the dilution curves yielded by the "unknown" and standard are exactly superimposable. An alternative expression of this criterion is that the two dilution curves are parallel when dilutions of each preparation are plotted on a logarithmic scale.

Our analysis suggests that, although in certain circumstances this criterion may distinguish between hormones differing in reaction energy, the assay conditions selected may nevertheless be such that differences in the dilution curves would be extremely difficult to detect.

That these predictions have experimental validity is illustrated in Figures 6, 7, and 8. Figure 6 shows results obtained when the response curves of both vitamin B_{12} and corrin, a corrinoid compound containing no cobalt, were determined from an assay system relying on serum B_{12}-binding protein as the specific reactant and labeled B_{12} as the tracer. Plotted on a logarithmic scale, the two curves become parallel at the higher values of $R_{f/b}$, in agreement with the theoretical prediction that in this range they would differ by a constant factor. However, we see that multiplication of the hormone concentration values on the corrin curve by this factor yields a normalized corrin curve that is not exactly superimposable on the B_{12} curve.

This constitutes strong evidence that the corrinoid material reacts with serum B_{12}-binding protein but with an equilibrium constant markedly different from that governing the reaction with B_{12} itself; moreover, the results imply that the effect cannot be ascribed to B_{12} contamination of the competing corrinoid preparation.

By contrast, theoretical response curves plotted in terms of the parameter $R_{b/f}$ for two hormones differing in reaction energy by a factor of 10 are illustrated in Figure 7. It will be noted that in this example a value $R_{0,b/f}$ (the observed ratio corresponding to zero hormone) of unity has been chosen and that with an increase in hormone concentration all values of $R_{b/f}$ fall below unity (in practice, assay conditions yielding curves with these general characteristics are often selected). It is evident from this illustration that experimental work of great precision would be required to distinguish between the two dilution curves — assuming,

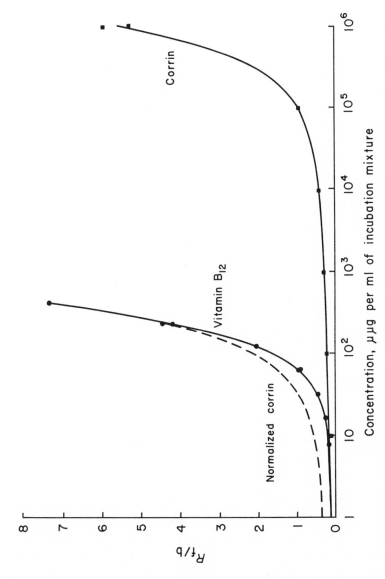

FIGURE 6 Experimental response curves yielded by corrin and vitamin B_{12} in competition with radioactive B_{12} for sites on serum B_{12}-binding protein.

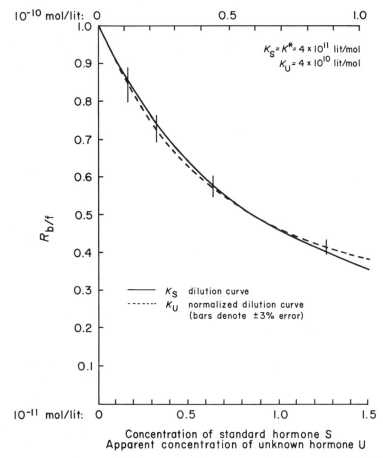

FIGURE 7 Superimposed dilution curves for two cross-reacting hormones differing in equilibrium constants by a factor of 10. In this example the superimposition is achieved by dividing the concentrations of the hormone of lower K by the factor 7. All points on the displaced curve fall within 3% of the standard dilution curve.

of course, that the absolute concentrations of hormone in one set of dilutions are unknown.

On the upper scale of this figure are shown the true concentrations of the hormone designated U. It is clear that an assay point yielded by hormone U could, if referred to the standard curve constructed by the use of hormone S, result in an error in the estimate of U by a factor between 6 and 10 (the factor used to normalize the U curve in this figure is 7). Thus, since a difference of this magnitude in the binding constants manifested by standard and unknown hormones might easily escape

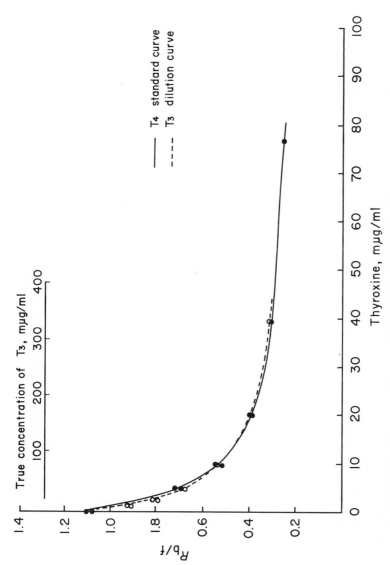

FIGURE 8 Experimental response curves yielded by thyroxine (T_4) and triiodothyronine (T_3) in a saturation assay system relying on the reaction between ^{125}I-labeled thyroxine as tracer and serum thyroxine-binding protein. Although T_3 is bound less avidly than T_4, the response curve yielded by the former may be super-imposed on the T_4 curve by contraction of the T_3 concentration scale by a factor of approximately 8.

detection, unsuspected errors in estimates of concentrations of U of the same order as this difference could readily be concealed within the assay data.

This theoretical prediction carries with it somewhat disturbing implications and obviously requires experimental verification. Fortunately, the saturation assay of thyroxine provides a relatively simple system with which the theory may be tested. In particular, this assay may be used to study the response curves yielded by two hormones reacting with identical binding sites but with different energies of reaction. The results of such an experimental enquiry are illustrated in Figure 8. Dilution curves yielded respectively by triiodothyronine and thyroxine, both reacting with serum thyroxine-binding globulin in the presence of radioactive thyroxine, have been superimposed by suitable adjustment of the concentration scales. The clear indication is that it is impossible, on the basis of dilution data alone, to be certain whether a thyroid hormone extracted from serum and subjected to the thyroxine assay procedure is thyroxine or triiodothyronine or a mixture of both. Neither is it possible, without additional chemical evidence concerning the identity of the thyroid hormone circulating in the blood, to regard the measured hormone concentration as possessing any absolute significance.

The position is more complicated when more than one order of reacting site on the binding protein or antibody is implicated. In such case certain of the sites involved in the reaction with one hormone may not be involved in the reaction with the other. Thus, an antiserum raised against a particular protein hormone may comprise a range of different binding sites directed against dissimilar antigenic groupings on the hormone molecule. A second, cross-reacting, hormone might be expected to present some but not all of the antigenic groupings characterizing the first and thus to react only with certain of the binding sites on the antibody molecule. This would clearly increase the possibility and magnitude of differences arising in both the slopes and shapes of the dilution curves yielded by the two cross-reacting hormones and thus give some theoretical justification for the use of dilution-curve criteria in testing for assay specificity.

Nevertheless, it is possible for substantial differences in the binding energies displayed by standard and unknown hormones with respect to a single site to exist without an observable divergence of their respective dilution curves, leading to gross inaccuracies in estimates of endogenous hormone concentration. Indeed, the belief that saturation assays in general and radioimmunoassays in particular yield results for serum hormone concentration that bear any resemblance to the true values rests on assumptions concerning the identity of the reactivities of endogenous and standard hormones, for which there is rarely substantial direct experimental evidence.

4. Assay sensitivity and precision: definitions

We now wish to turn to the subject of assay sensitivity and precision and, in particular, to show how the equations defining the standard response curve may be used to optimize these quantities. Before doing so it is necessary that we define exactly what we mean by sensitivity and precision, since our definitions and the conclusions that can be drawn therefrom differ fundamentally from those of Berson and Yalow (Berson and Yalow, 1964; Yalow and Berson, 1968a).

Our definition of sensitivity, the minimal detectable concentration of hormone, is best understood by reference to Figure 9. It is designated Δp and is equal to the standard error in the determination of R_0 divided by the slope of the response curve at R_0, where R_0 is the free-to-bound (or bound-to-free) ratio yielded by an incubation mixture containing only tracer hormone. It thus corresponds (to a close approximation) to

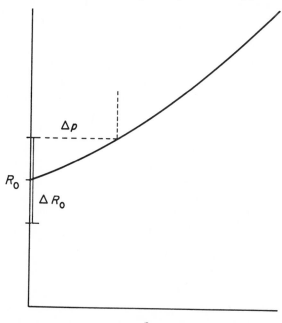

p

FIGURE 9   Diagram illustrating the definition of assay sensitivity as that concentration Δp of unlabeled hormone which in the presence of tracer hormone changes the isotope distribution ratio R_0 by an amount equal to ΔR_0, the standard error of R_0. The value of Δp is approximately equal to ΔR_0 divided by the slope of the response curve at R_0 and is equal to $\Delta p = \Delta R_0 \times \mathrm{d}p/\mathrm{d}R_0$.

the standard error of the estimate of unlabeled hormone concentration when the latter is equal to zero. It can therefore be said to represent the minimal detectable concentration of hormone, although the confidence level in this assertion is low. In normal practice Δp would be multiplied by some factor, to yield an appropriate level of confidence; however, this adjustment does not affect the main conclusions stemming from the following analysis and has therefore not been taken into account. The essential difference between this definition of sensitivity and that of Yalow and Berson is that the former takes into consideration the errors in the determination of distribution ratios and does not ascribe high sensitivity to an assay simply on the grounds that it yields a response curve with a steep slope.

The definition of sensitivity can be extended to encompass the definition of precision shown in Figure 10. Our definition of precision, the error in assessment of the hormone concentration, is analogous to the so-called index of precision, λ, familiar to all workers in bioassay. For the measurement of a concentration h of unlabeled hormone we denote precision by Δh and define it as the standard error in the determination of the ratio R_h divided by the slope of the response curve at

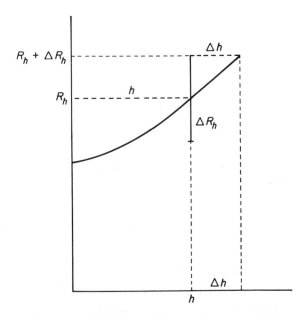

FIGURE 10   Diagram illustrating the definition of assay precision in the measurement of the hormone concentration h as that increment Δh in hormone concentration corresponding to an increment in the isotope distribution ratio ΔR_h, the standard error of R_h. The value of Δh is approximately equal to ΔR_h divided by the slope of the response curve at R_h.

R_h. The ratio R_h represents the distribution ratio yielded by an incubation mixture containing tracer hormone together with unlabeled hormone at a concentration of h. It should be noted that sensitivity and precision are equivalent when the hormone concentration h is put equal to zero.

It will be intuitively apparent that assay conditions (that is, concentrations of specific reactant and of tracer hormone) can be so selected as to maximize the precision of measurement of *any* chosen hormone concentration and, in particular, to maximize the sensitivity of the assay.

In this chapter we wish to dwell almost entirely on the maximization of assay sensitivity. Not only does this present the simpler mathematical problem, but also saturation assays are commonly employed to measure exceedingly low hormone concentrations. Hence, the optimization of assay sensitivity constitutes the more important requirement.

5. Assay sensitivity

Assuming that the only error in the determination of R stems from the counting errors implicit in any measurement of radioactivity, it is a simple matter to calculate the error in R_0 if such parameters as the amount and specific activity of tracer employed in the incubation mixture are known. The expression for fractional standard error or coefficient of variation $\Delta R_0/R_0$ of a single measurement of R_0 under such circumstances is given by

$$\frac{\Delta R_0}{R_0} = \sqrt{\frac{R_0 + 1}{R_0 p^* S T V}}\,(1 + \sqrt{R_0}) \tag{7}$$

where p^* is the concentration of tracer hormone in the system, S is the specific activity of the tracer (in counts per minute, per unit weight), T is the total time devoted to counting each pair of samples (that is, each free and bound pair), and V is the volume of incubation mixture that is subjected to separation and to radioactive measurements (in milliliters).

In these expressions R_0 is taken to represent the free-to-bound ratio. For the derivation of Equation 7 see the Appendix.

The slope of the response curve at any point may also be readily derived and expressed in terms of the concentrations of reactive sites and hormone present and of the equilibrium constant of the reaction. The slope at R_0 is obtained by the differentiation of Equation 1, with K and q as constants,

$$\frac{dR}{R\,dp} = \frac{1}{qR_0 + 1/KR_0} \tag{8}$$

for any value of R.

An estimate of Δp, the minimal detectable hormone in the system, is obtained by dividing Equation 7 by Equation 8, which gives

$$\Delta p = \frac{1 + \sqrt{R_0}}{\sqrt{SVT}} \left(qR_0 + \frac{1}{KR_0} \right) \sqrt{\frac{R_0 + 1}{p^* R_0}} \tag{9}$$

In this expression there exist as independent variables the concentration of binding sites, q, and the concentration of tracer hormone, p^*. By a judicious selection of these two concentrations it is possible to minimize Δp and hence to maximize the sensitivity of the system. Mathematically, this constitutes a simple procedure, the details of which are given by Ekins et al. (1968).

The optimal values are $q = 3/K$ and $p^* = 4/K$, and the value of R_0 obtained by using these concentrations of reactant and tracer is unity. Under these circumstances the minimal detectable concentration of unlabeled hormone is given by

$$\Delta p_{\min} = \frac{4\sqrt{2}}{\sqrt{KSVT}} \tag{10}$$

This approach enables us, in principle, to select optimal concentrations of reagents and to predict the maximal sensitivity attainable in the system. However, the predictions based on this simple treatment are of no great practical value. They rest on the supposition that the only errors implicit in the measurement of isotope distribution ratios are those associated with counting, and they neglect the experimental errors associated with, for example, the separation of free and bound moieties. Nevertheless, it is possible to take the latter into account and, by making certain simple assumptions, to arrive at predictions of much greater value regarding the composition of assay mixtures.

We have approached this extension of the analysis by assuming that the *minimal* experimental (relative) error in the determination of R_0 occurs when R_0 is equal to unity; it is given by ε.[2] If we introduce the latter term into our original expression for the standard error in R_0 (defined in Equation 7), it becomes possible to derive more complex relationships which define optimal concentrations of Q and P. Thus, the optimal concentration of binding sites is given by

$$\varepsilon^2 STV(q - 1/K)^2 + 2(q - 1/K) - 4/K = 0 \tag{11}$$

This expression defines the curve relating the parameter $\varepsilon\sqrt{STV/K}$ to the optimal concentration of binding sites; see Figure 11. The optimal

---

[2] Other assumptions regarding the variation of ε with R_0 may be made and introduced into the analysis. In this presentation we have postulated that ε is a minimum when R_0 is unity, since this relationship can be demonstrated experimentally in many assays, though it is unlikely to apply to all.

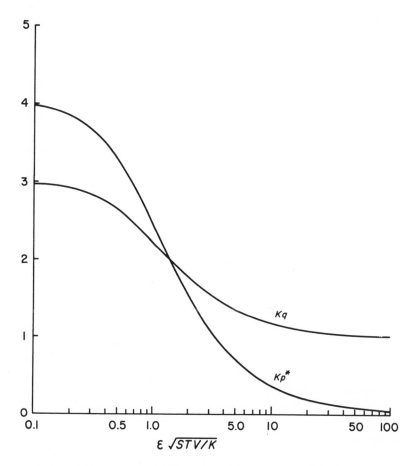

FIGURE 11 Curves relating optimal concentrations of binding site, q, and of tracer, p^* (multiplied in each case by the equilibrium constant), to the product $\varepsilon \sqrt{STV/K}$. The product Kq is asymptotic to the values 3 and 1; the product Kp, to the values 4 and 0.

concentration of tracer hormone has been similarly computed and also plotted in the figure.

It will be seen from these plots that, as the experimental errors (that is, pipetting and other manipulation errors) decrease toward zero, Kq tends to 3 and Kp^* to 4, the values obtained earlier in this analysis, regardless of the values of S, T, V, and K. It will also be noted that, when ε equals zero, the optimal amounts of tracer and binding protein are independent of the specific activity of the tracer used; however, if experimental errors are finite, an increase in the specific activity of the tracer implies the use of less tracer. Nevertheless, for all values of ε

greater than zero there clearly exists an optimal value of the concentration of tracer that should be introduced into the incubation mixtures. The use of either more tracer or less than is optimal will result in a loss of sensitivity.

At this juncture it is necessary to emphasize that these conclusions, regarding the composition of assay mixtures yielding maximal sensitivity, differ in essence from those drawn by Berson and Yalow (1964) and by Yalow and Berson (1968a). In particular, those workers have frequently stated that it is essential to employ the smallest tracer concentration permitting reasonable counting accuracy.

We are in fundamental disagreement with this contention although, given normal experimental errors, the optimal concentrations of tracer suggested by our analysis will, in practice, frequently fall within limits commensurate with Yalow and Berson's somewhat imprecise recommendations. It is notable, however, that in discussing sensitivity Yalow and Berson neglect errors in the determination of isotope distribution ratios and consider only the slope of the response curve. This difference in approach undoubtedly accounts for the contrasting conclusions that we have respectively drawn.

It is possible, by using optimal concentrations of tracer and of binding sites, based on estimates of the values of ε, S, T, V, and K, to calculate the maximal assay sensitivity obtainable under any given conditions and with any given reagents. This has enabled us to derive useful insights into the variation of sensitivity with changes in various of these assay parameters. Some of these insights are illustrated in Figures 12 and 13.

Figure 12 shows curves relating sensitivity to the magnitude of the equilibrium constant governing the reaction for different values of the experimental error. In this illustration the value of the product SVT has been taken as 1,000 ml/$\mu\mu$g, which corresponds very roughly to the value that it will assume for a tracer of high specific activity, taking usual incubation volumes and times of counting of samples. It is clear from this figure that no antibody of equilibrium constant less than 10^9 lit/mol would normally be usable in sensitive assays of such hormones as insulin or parathormone. Moreover, assuming reasonable experimental errors, only a value greater than 10^{11} lit/mol would be acceptable for assays of these hormones in plasma at the incubation-mixture dilutions necessary to obviate incubation damage to the tracer hormone.

Figure 13 exemplifies the relation between minimal detectable hormone concentrations and the product STV (in this case the calculations have been applied specifically to the assay of insulin). This plot is of particular interest since, if we consider that T and V are held constant, the abscissa corresponds to the specific activity of the labeled hormone used in the assay. Thus, by taking, for illustration, the product TV to be

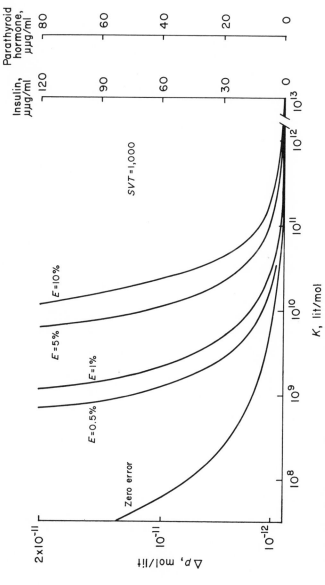

FIGURE 12   Sensitivity Δp as a function of K for different values of the relative error ε in the measurement of the value R_0 due to pipetting and other causes not connected with statistical errors of counting.

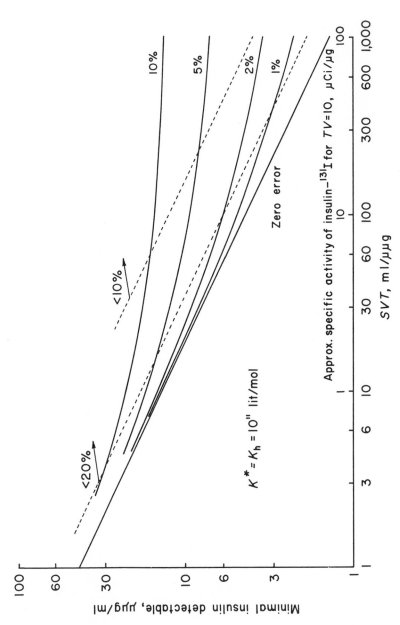

FIGURE 13 The relation between assay sensitivity (represented here by minimal detectable insulin concentration) and the product SVT for different values of the experimental error ε. If the terms T and V are given values of 10 min and 1 ml, respectively, the abscissa represents the specific activity of the ^{131}I-labeled insulin employed as the tracer. The values of tracer specific activity are based on a counter efficiency such that one microcurie per microgram is identically equal to one count per minute, per micromicrogram. In areas to the right of the broken lines the increases in sensitivity for a doubling of tracer specific activity are less than 20 and 10%, respectively.

equal to 10 ml·min we are able to demonstrate the variation in sensitivity with specific activity of the tracer insulin employed expressed in microcuries per microgram.

The curves in this diagram are plotted for different values of the experimental error and reveal that for all finite values of ε an increase in tracer specific activity becomes increasingly unrewarding in terms of assay sensitivity as higher values are approached. Thus, the broken lines in this figure delineate areas such that at all points above and to the right of these lines the increase in sensitivity consequent upon a doubling of tracer specific activity will be less than 20 and 10%, respectively. Moreover, it can be shown that the curves are asymptotic to the value $2\varepsilon/K$; this implies that even with a tracer of infinite specific activity a sensitivity better than this value could not be obtained.

These findings are particularly relevant to the problems associated with the synthesis of hormones of high specific activity. Not only do such

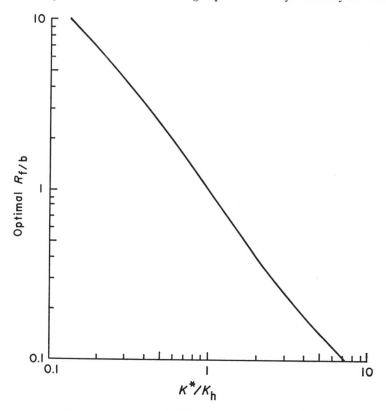

FIGURE 14   The relation between K^*/K_h and $R_{0,f/b}$ for concentrations of reagents yielding maximal assay sensitivity (errors of counting only). Binding constants: tracer, K^*, and unlabelled compound, K_h.

syntheses occasionally present substantial logistical problems, but the stability and reactivity of the resulting tracer hormone may be critically impaired. However, the computation of theoretical sensitivities, exemplified by Figure 13, can give a precise indication of the advantage in terms of sensitivity to be gained by increased tracer specific activity.

6. Effect on sensitivity of difference between equilibrium constants of tracer and unlabeled hormone

A further factor that affects assay sensitivity is the difference between the equilibrium constant of the tracer employed and that of the inactive hormone under study. The difference occurs, for example, when labeled bovine insulin is used in a radioimmunoassay for human insulin, and it is not uncommon for a competing labeled steroid to be different from the steroid being measured.

This problem may be dealt with essentially in the manner outlined

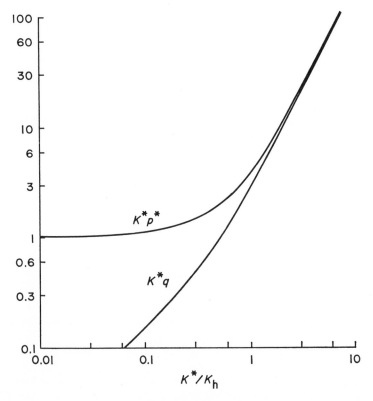

FIGURE 15   Concentrations of binding sites and tracer hormone for maximal sensitivity, as a function of K^*/K_h (errors of counting only).

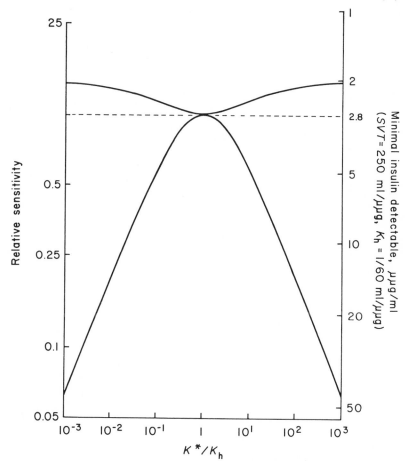

FIGURE 16   Assay sensitivity as a function of K^*/K_h with K_h constant. The upper curve shows the variation when R_0 is adjusted to its optimum value; the lower, the variation when R_0 is restricted to unity. Both curves are based on the premise that only counting errors contribute to the error in R_0 ($\varepsilon = 0$).

above; however, its solution is more complex and cannot be attained without making certain simplifying assumptions.

Again, the analysis is probably best exemplified by considering first a situation in which the only errors arising in the determination of distribution ratios are those of counting. The analysis based on this premise (for details see Ekins et al., 1968) yields a value for the optimal concentration of binding protein that is given by

$$q = \frac{1}{K^* R_{0,f/b}}\left(2 + \frac{1}{R_{0,f/b}}\right) \tag{12}$$

where $R_{0,f/b}$ is given by the equation

$$K^* R_{0,f/b}(R_{0,f/b}^{3/2} + 2R_{0,f/b}^{1/2} + 1) - K_h(R_{0,f/b}^{3/2} + 2R_{0,f/b} + 1) = 0$$

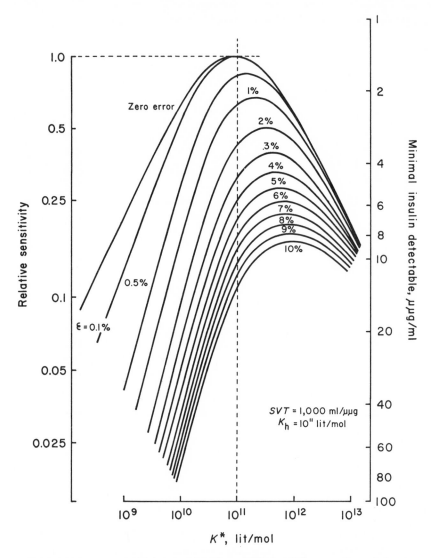

FIGURE 17   Assay sensitivity as a function of K^* for different values of the experimental error ε. Optimal concentrations of reagents consistent with the restriction $R_0 = 1$ have been assumed throughout the computation.

and K^* is the equilibrium constant of the tracer hormone and K_h the equilibrium constant of the unlabeled hormone. Figure 14 is a plot of the relationship between K^*/K_h and $R_{0,f/b}$ as defined by this equation. Corresponding curves relating K^*p^* and K^*q derived from Equation 12 are shown in Figure 15. These equations and the curves they define indicate that, when binding constants of tracer and inactive hormones differ, the maximal assay sensitivity is no longer achieved when $R_{0, f/b}$ equals unity.

It is also possible to calculate the sensitivity that will be achieved under optimal assay conditions when K^* differs from K_h. The results of a computation based on change in the equilibrium constant K^* of the tracer while K_h is kept constant are plotted in Figure 16, the minimal detectable concentration of hormone being here expressed as a fraction of the value derived when K^* equals K_h.

It will be observed that theoretical sensitivity *increases*, as K^* departs from K_h, in the directions both of increasing and of decreasing K^*. However, this finding is not applicable to experimental situations, since experimental errors, inevitably introduced into the assay procedure, tend to increase as the distribution ratio R_0 departs from unity. Thus, the increase in assay sensitivity which, the simple theory suggests, would be obtained by using a tracer with an equilibrium constant different from that of the unlabeled hormone, might be lost through the increased error implicit in the measurement of the indicated optimal ratio.

A solution of this dilemma cannot be achieved without a precise knowledge of the variation in the experimental error with change in R_0. However, since many experimenters set up assays such that R_0 is close to unity, it is relevant to consider the effect on the optimal assay sensitivity of a change in the tracer equilibrium constant when R_0 is restricted to this value. The results of such an enquiry are summarized in Figures 16 and 17. It is clear from these figures that even when the experimental error is zero, the sensitivity will fall dramatically as K^*/K_h departs from unity, in consequence of the restriction placed on R_0. The curves obtained for finite values of ε are, however, particularly interesting. They indicate that maximal sensitivity is achieved when the equilibrium constant of the tracer hormone is somewhat higher than that of the unlabeled hormone, the extent of the advantage depending upon the magnitude of the experimental errors involved. Conversely, it is clear that a fall in sensitivity will inevitably result from the use of a tracer with a lower equilibrium constant than that of the unlabeled material.

To conclude this discussion of assay sensitivity, it is perhaps relevant to illustrate the foregoing analysis as applied to various saturation assays carried out in our own laboratory. One of the most sensitive[3]

[3] In computing "experimental" sensitivities we have used the formula

$$\text{sensitivity} = \frac{\text{mean difference between duplicate estimates of } R_0}{1.1 \times \text{slope of response curve at } R_0}$$

which estimates sensitivity as defined in the theoretical analysis (Pearson and Hartley, 1954).

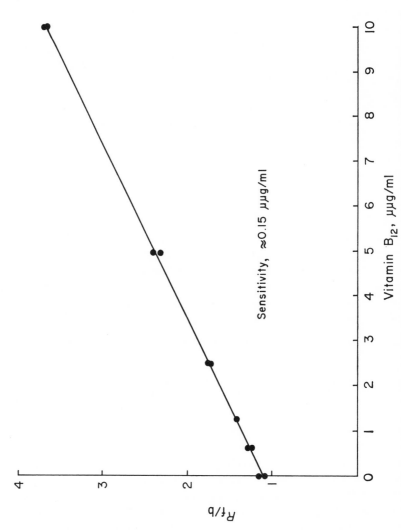

FIGURE 18   Saturation assay of vitamin B_{12} by the method of Ekins and Sgherzi (1964) with optimal concentrations of labeled vitamin B_{12} and binding serum for maximal sensitivity.

assays, though not for a hormone, is that for vitamin B_{12} (Ekins and Sgherzi, 1964). The standard response curve obtained under maximal sensitivity conditions is shown in Figure 18; the sensitivity of the method is of the order of 0.15 μμg per milliliter of incubation mixture. Sensitivities recorded in our laboratory for insulin, testosterone, and thyroxine, assayed by procedures as yet unpublished in detail, are respectively of the order of 1, 150, and 200 μμg per milliliter of incubation mixture. In each case these sensitivities achieved experimentally have been found with assay mixtures prepared as required by the theoretical analysis discussed in this chapter and have accorded closely with the values theoretically predicted.

7. Assay precision

As emphasized earlier, the terms "sensitivity" and "precision" are related in the sense that the expressions "high sensitivity" and "high precision for hormone levels at or close to zero" are tautological. In principle, the equations derived above may be generalized so as to apply to *any* unlabeled-hormone concentration selected. However, since we have not fully completed this extension of the analysis, it would be premature to present our final conclusions.

Where experimental errors contribute to the total error in the measurement of distribution ratios, it would appear that the selection of optimal assay conditions requires a foreknowledge of the variation in the experimental error for different values of the radioisotope distribution ratio and that relatively sophisticated computer optimizing techniques will be necessary to deal with this information. However, the simple case in which only counting errors are significant can be resolved without resort to computer methods.

The results of this analysis, which has yet to be published in detail, are depicted in Figures 19 and 20. Figure 19 shows the relationship between h, the concentration of unlabeled hormone to be measured, and q and p^*, the optimal concentrations of binding sites and tracer hormone required to maximize the precision of measurement of h. In Figure 20 is plotted the relationship between the product Kh and R_h, the free-to-bound ratio that will be observed in the incubation mixture containing both tracer hormone and unlabeled hormone at concentration h. The variations of Δh (the standard error in the determination of h) and $\Delta h/h$ with h also are plotted as functions of Kh.

From the resulting curves it is clear that, ideally, the composition of each set of assay incubation mixtures (standards and unknown) should be so selected as to match exactly the hormone concentration to be

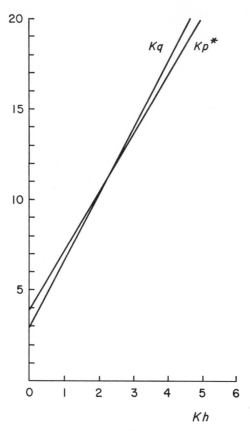

FIGURE 19   Optimal concentrations of tracer and binding site required for maximizing the precision of measurement of the hormone concentration h.

measured. It is also clear from Figure 20 that maximal assay precision must depend, as does assay sensitivity, on the equilibrium constant of the reaction. This finding contrasts with that of Yalow and Berson, who claim to show that maximal assay precision is independent of the equilibrium constant. They also maintain that near-optimal precision is likely to be attained by using antiserum concentrations ten or twenty times greater than those yielding optimal sensitivity (Yalow and Berson, 1968a).

Their conclusions appear to us curious, particularly in the light of our belief that sensitivity constitutes merely a special case of assay precision, as applies in the limiting circumstance of zero unlabeled-hormone concentration. Neither can we reconcile Yalow and Berson's contention with our conclusion that the composition of assay mixtures of optimal precision will depend on the exact concentration of hormone to be

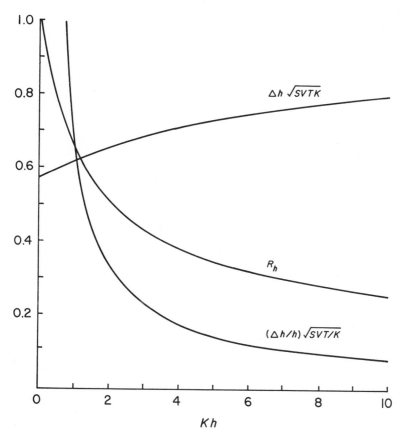

FIGURE 20 The precision of measurement of the hormone concentration h as a function of Kh. For a given value of the latter one may read off the values of R_h, $\Delta h \sqrt{SVTK}$, and $(\Delta h/h)\sqrt{SVT/K}$. Subsequently, assuming that the values of S, V, T, and K are known, the precision of measurement of h (under optimal conditions) can be calculated, expressed either as Δh or as the coefficient of variation, $\Delta h/h$. Assuming SVT and K to be constant, the curves labeled $\Delta h \sqrt{SVTK}$ and $(\Delta h/h)\sqrt{SVT/K}$ represent, in form, the variation of Δh and $\Delta h/h$ with h.

measured, a finding which accords with intuitive expectation. Thus, it might be anticipated that the composition of an assay mixture designed for the precise measurement of high hormone concentrations would differ markedly from that of a mixture intended to measure hormone concentrations close to zero.

In this connection it will be noted that in the plots shown in Figures 19 and 20 the optimal concentrations of binding sites and tracer and the resulting value of R_h converge on the values corresponding to high sensitivity as h tends to zero.

Undoubtedly the reason for this divergence of views on the composition of assay mixtures stems from the difference in the respective definitions of sensitivity and precision. It is our opinion that statements concerning sensitivity and precision are meaningless if based solely upon consideration of the slopes of assay response curves, without reference to the accuracy with which the points along such curves are determined.

APPENDIX

Derivation of Equation 6

Let the labeled hormone be designated P* and the competing unlabeled hormone H. The two reactions may be represented by $P^* + Q \rightleftharpoons P^*Q$ and $H + Q \rightleftharpoons HQ$, governed by equilibrium constants K^* and K_h, respectively, such that

$$K^* = \frac{[P^*Q]}{[P^*][Q]} \tag{A1}$$

$$K_h = \frac{[HQ]}{[H][Q]} \tag{A2}$$

Then, if $R_{f/b} = [P^*]/[P^*Q]$, an equation defining the response curve can be derived as follows:

$$[Q] = q - [P^*Q] - [HQ] \tag{A3}$$

$$[P^*] = p^* - [P^*Q] \tag{A4}$$

$$[P^*Q] = \frac{p^*}{R_{f/b} + 1} \tag{A5}$$

If these values are substituted in the expression

$$K^*[P^*][Q] = [P^*Q] \tag{A6}$$

the equation takes the form

$$K^*\left(p^* - \frac{p^*}{R_{f/b} + 1}\right)\left(q - \frac{p^*}{R_{f/b} + 1} - [HQ]\right) = \frac{p^*}{R_{f/b} + 1} \tag{A7}$$

Rearranging gives

$$R_{f/b}^2 + R_{f/b}\left(1 - \frac{p}{q} - \frac{1}{K^*q}\right) - \frac{1}{K^*q}$$
$$- \frac{[HQ]}{q}(R_{f/b} + 1)(R_{f/b}) = 0 \tag{A8}$$

An expression for [HQ] can be derived from the fact that

$$[H] = h - [HQ] \tag{A9}$$

and, from a combination of Equations A1 and A2,

$$[H] = \frac{[HQ]R_{f/b}}{K_h/K^*} \tag{A10}$$

From Equations A9 and A10 it follows that

$$[HQ] = \frac{h}{R_{f/b}K^*/K_h + 1} \tag{A11}$$

Combining Equations A8 and A11 gives

$$R_{f/b}^2 + R_{f/b}\left(1 - \frac{p^*}{q} - \frac{1}{K^*q}\right) - \frac{1}{K^*q} - \frac{(h/q)(R_{f/b} + 1)R_{f/b}}{(K^*/K_h)R_{f/b} + 1} = 0$$

Derivation of Equation 7

If the activity in the bound fraction at $R_{0,f/b}$,

$$b_0 = \frac{p^*SV}{R_{0,f/b} + 1}$$

is equal to k and that in the free fraction,

$$f_0 = \frac{p^*SVR_{0,f/b}}{R_{0,f/b} + 1}$$

is equal to $kR_{0,f/b}$ and if this pair of fractions is counted for a total counting time T in such a way as to minimize the relative error in the free-to-bound ratio,[4] the standard error $\Delta R_{0,f/b}$ of a single measurement of $R_{0,f/b}$ under these circumstances is

$$\frac{\Delta R_{0,f/b}}{R_{0,f/b}} = (1 + \sqrt{R_{0,f/b}})\sqrt{\frac{R_{0,f/b} + 1}{p^*SVTR_{0,f/b}}}$$

The standard error of b_0 in time t_b is $\sqrt{b_0/t_b}$, and the fractional standard error of b_0 is

$$\frac{\sqrt{b_0/t_b}}{b_0} = \sqrt{\frac{1}{b_0 t_b}} = e_1$$

---

[4] The optimal division of total sample counting time T is given by

$$t_f/t_b = \sqrt{b_0/f_0} = \sqrt{1/R_{0,f/b}}$$

where t_f and t_b are the times for counting free and bound fractions, and f_0 and b_0 are the corresponding counting rates (see also Ekins et al., 1968). Then $t_b = \sqrt{R_{0,f/b}}\, t_f$ and $T = t_b + t_f = \sqrt{R_{0,f/b}}\, t_f + t_f = t_f(1 + \sqrt{R_{0,f/b}})$.

The fractional standard error of f_0 in time t_f is

$$\sqrt{\frac{1}{f_0 t_f}} = e_2$$

and the fractional standard error of the ratio is

$$\sqrt{e_1^2 + e_2^2} = \sqrt{\frac{1}{b_0 t_b} + \frac{1}{f_0 t_f}} = \sqrt{\frac{1}{k t_b} + \frac{1}{k R_{0,f/b} t_f}}$$

Thus, the minimal fractional error in R_0 is

$$\frac{\Delta R_0}{R_0} = \sqrt{\frac{1}{k\sqrt{R_{0,f/b}} t_f} + \frac{1}{k R_{0,f/b} t_f}} = \sqrt{\frac{1}{k T R_{0,f/b}}} (1 + \sqrt{R_{0,f/b}})$$

which, upon substitution for k, becomes

$$\sqrt{\frac{R_0 + 1}{p^* S V T R_{0,f/b}}} (1 + \sqrt{R_{0,f/b}})$$

CHAPTER TWENTY

Discussion

MCHUGH   Could the speakers please state what methods they use in the fitting of the standard calibration curves? In the sensitivity and the precision studies was Dr. Ekins concerned only with the simpler situation or with the multiplicity-of-binding-sites case also?

O'RIORDAN   My calibration curves were freehand drawings.

MCHUGH   And, in practice, is this also the way you estimate potency?

O'RIORDAN   Yes.

YALOW   For standard curves we make a plot of B/F as a function of hormone concentration and make a freehand drawing of the best fit. We generally use a twelve-point standard curve for each assay. However, if there were concern about best fit, a twenty-point or thirty-point standard curve would not be onerous, since we generally assay five hundred or more samples in a single run.

EKINS   In the greater part of the precision studies we have been dealing with the single-binding-site situation, which is particularly amenable to relatively simple algebraic treatment. However, in the case of multiple binding sites a good approximation for determining optimal sensitivity conditions is embodied in the concept of an effective equilibrium constant and an effective, or equivalent, binding site concentration. The equivalent single equilibrium constant is given by

$$\overline{K} = \sum K_i^2 q_i / \sum K_i q_i$$

and the equivalent single-binding-site concentration by

$$\bar{q} = (\sum K_i q_i)^2 / \sum K_i^2 q_i$$

These expressions exactly describe the response of a multi-binding system only at zero hormone concentration. However, they serve as useful approximations at concentrations that are low in relation to those of the higher-energy binding sites present in the system.

MCHUGH   That is what you are using at present?

EKINS   Yes, but only in arriving at optimal conditions for maximizing assay sensitivity.

SMITH   Why do you need so many points? Would not a mathematical formulation of the curve imply that only a few essential parameters are needed? Conceivably, three points would suffice to fit the model.

YALOW   If the reaction of antigen with antibody involved only one or two orders of antibody binding sites of known energy and concentration, and if the labeled antigen were identical from assay to assay, then it would be possible to draw a standard curve from mathematical formulations of the type I have described. In practice we often deal with a heterogeneous antibody system, so that an experimental approach is generally somewhat easier. For such hormones as insulin and growth hormone we have supplied large numbers of other investigators with antisera suitable for immunoassay and provided them with typical standard curves. If the specified conditions are followed, it is remarkable how reproducible the standard curves are both in our own laboratory and in those of the recipients. However, overiodination and other chemical manipulations of these hormones can change the immunoreactivity of the tracer and alter the standard curve. In addition, significant change in the concentration of the tracer also alters the shape of the standard curve. For hormones that do not have the stability of insulin, such as parathyroid hormone, or when the requirements for sensitivity demand maximal specific activity and minimal size of tracer (i.e., ACTH), the exact reproducibility of the standard curves depends critically on the nature of the labeled-hormone preparation and may not always be obtained. For this reason we feel it is best to run a standard curve with each assay, especially since the work of preparing it represents but a small fraction of the time involved in a several-hundred-specimen assay.

MEINERT   How do you choose the doses for determining the standard curve?

EKINS   We ordinarily take doubling dilutions of any initial concentration of hormone that will enable us to measure the desired concentrations.

YALOW   Our standard curve is a linear (not a logarithmic) plot of B/F versus hormone concentration. Except at the lowest hormone concentrations, where the slope of the curve is very sharp, we use standards much closer together than doubling dilutions. Thus, for most of our standard curves the hormone concentrations are 20 to 30% apart, to enable us to determine unknown hormone concentrations with better precision.

EKINS   I should perhaps add that occasionally we interpolate additional points between the doubling dilutions. However, in general, since plots of the free-to-bound ratio (F/B) frequently approach linearity, we find that quite a small number of standards suffices to define the response curve with adequate precision.

ALBERT   What is the error of a single determination of an unknown, say a sample of serum for an assay of growth hormone? And if one gave the same sample of serum and the same reactants to each of ten different laboratories with the same sensitivity and precision, what variation would one expect?

TASHJIAN   If one had not only the same reactants but also the same assay, what would the answer be?

YALOW   The answer depends on the hormone being assayed. For insulin and growth hormone we could probably determine hormone concentrations to $\pm 10\%$ in terms of given standards. In a routine assay, in which we assay only a single dilution of unknown and in which the hormone concentration corresponding to that dilution may not be in the optimal portion of the standard curve, the precision might not be this good. For these two hormones I probably could name at least ten laboratories that could duplicate each other's results within 20 to 30% or better, if they used the same hormone for standard. However, this degree of reproducibility for most of the other hormones is not being obtained. One may question whether such precision is required for those hormones for which there is a tenfold or greater change in plasma concentration within a matter of minutes. As I showed in the case of ACTH, there is an increase in hormone concentration from 25 to 280 $\mu\mu g/ml$ within 5 minutes after electric shock stimulation. Here the exact time of sampling has a greater effect on the measured hormone concentration than limitations on the precision of assay. Hormones such as human parathyroid hormone do not show the large variations in concentration in response to stimuli that are characteristic of insulin, ACTH, and growth hormone. For hormones of relatively constant concentration reproducibility would be more important. Since a suitable standard preparation of human parathyroid hormone is not available, inter-laboratory comparisons of parathyroid hormone concentrations are currently impossible.

TAIT   I would be grateful if the two speakers would expand their definitions of precision and sensitivity. Their sensitivity definitions are reciprocal, and Dr. Ekins' definition contains an error term. However, I find it rather difficult to reconcile their two definitions of precision.

EKINS   I feel very strongly that one should define precision in the terms that we have shown in our Figure 10. If one makes an error ΔR_h in the measurement of the ratio R_h, it implies an error Δh in the measurement of the hormone concentration h at that level, and the latter error is what we regard as the precision of the measurement.

In Figure 10 the error Δh corresponds to λ, the so-called index of precision of the assay. However, in bioassay work both the slope and the variance are usually treated as constant within a single assay, and therefore their ratio, the index of precision, is also constant. On the other hand, Δh, as defined here, is clearly a variable. The variance will alter as one moves up the response curve, and so also will the slope, since the response curve is not a straight line. Moreover, since bioassay response curves are customarily plotted in terms of log dose, the index of precision is a dimensionless quantity, whereas Δh has the dimensions of concentration. Nonetheless, Δh has a clear equivalence to the index of precision as invoked in bioassay.

In selecting assay conditions for optimizing the precision of measurement of any desired hormone concentration h, one is implicitly attempting to select concentrations of reagents that will minimize the associated error, Δh. However, we emphasize that an optimal assay incubation mixture relates to the maximal precision of measurement of only *one* hormone concentration; maximal precision of measurement of any other hormone concentration necessitates the use of different concentrations of reagents. In practice we optimize for an expected range of hormone concentrations, taking into account the relative importance of different portions of the anticipated range.

With regard to sensitivity, a definition solely in terms of the slope of the response curve has the difficulty of leading to the proposition that a balance with a pointer of infinite length has "infinite" sensitivity without any gain in the exactness of the indication. It is also readily demonstrated that in saturation assay techniques the conditions that lead to maximization of slope are not identical with those in which the "minimal hormone concentration detectable" is, in fact, an absolute minimum.

For these reasons we believe that our definition and mathematical formulation of "sensitivity," given in our Figure 9, is more meaningful than that of Yalow and Berson.

YALOW   A plot of the B/F ratio as a function of bound antigen concentration was the most useful form for studying the reactions of antigen with antibody, which are based on the law of mass action. Furthermore, measurement of the B/F ratio does not require precise sampling of the incubation mixture or certainty of the stability of the counting system. Therefore, we have chosen to plot the standard curve as B/F versus hormone concentration. However, it should be appreciated that large changes in B/F at very high B/F ratios may result from small changes in percent bound (b) and therefore be difficult to measure. For example, a change in percent bound from 99 to 98 reduces the B/F from 99/1, or 99, to 98/2, or 49, which is a large absolute drop but one not easily measured. Similarly, changes in low B/F ratios (<0.1) are not readily measured for a number of reasons, including limitation of statistical accuracy in counting the samples and variability of damage to labeled hormone. Therefore, it is more useful to define sensitivity and precision in terms of b. It can be shown from our Equation 8 (this volume) that

$$\text{sensitivity} = db/dH \approx -Kb(1-b)^2$$

when H approaches 0 or, that is, when the tracer is negligibly small. The sensitivity depends on the equilibrium constant for the reaction of antigen with antibody and on the fraction bound. This term has a maximum at $b = 1/3$. At that value it is

$$\text{maximal sensitivity} = \frac{db}{dH} = -\frac{4}{27}K$$

Precision and sensitivity are defined differently, and maximal precision and maximal sensitivity are not obtained under the same conditions. In the case of a single order of antibody binding sites reacting with the antigen the *maximal* precision is obtained when the antiserum is highly concentrated and the antibody binding sites are virtually all occupied by antigen; that is, when

$$\frac{B}{F} \ll K[\text{Ab}]_0$$

Then,

$$\text{maximal precision} \approx \frac{db}{dH/H} \approx -b$$

Under these conditions, if the hormone concentration changes by 10% (i.e., $dH/H = 0.1$), then db is about $0.1b$, and the change in the percent bound is 10% of the value of b. This relation is independent of K and holds for all antisera under the conditions specified.

Finally, I should like to return to what appears to be a difference in Dr. Ekins' and our approaches. Dr. Ekins has described situations in which a millionfold decrease in tracer concentration would not improve sensitivity. If we return to the theoretical reaction of antigen with a single order of antibody binding sites, we can appreciate the condition under which this situation obtains:

$$B/F = K([\text{Ab}]_0 - B) \qquad \text{and} \qquad \lim_{B \to 0} B/F = K[\text{Ab}]_0$$

Thus, when the tracer concentration is sufficiently low for it to occupy, say, less than 1% of the antibody binding sites ($B < 0.01[\text{Ab}]_0$), then any further decrease in tracer would have an undetectable effect on B/F, and no improvement in the sensitivity could be expected from such reduction. Even were B equal to $0.10[Ab]_0$, little improvement in sensitivity could be expected by a further decrease in the concentration of tracer. Under the conditions that we employ for the assay of ACTH the maximal binding capacity of our antiserum is 6 $\mu\mu g/ml$. Therefore, we consider that sensitivity would continue to improve as we reduced the tracer concentration to 1 $\mu\mu g/ml$ or below, were that possible. Furthermore, if the antiserum were to contain another order of antibody binding sites of low concentration but very high K, a dilution of antiserum and reduction of tracer concentration might unmask such a site. The existence of such a site would be undetected when too large a tracer was employed. I am sure Dr. Ekins does not mean to suggest that one should not reduce the amount of tracer until it can be shown experimentally that further reduction would bring no advantage.

EKINS   Though our mathematical approaches are entirely different, in practice the manner in which we perform our assays is likely to be very similar. This follows from the quantitative similarity in the precepts relating to the composition of optimal assay incubation mixtures which stem from the two analyses. As I understand her position, Dr. Yalow recommends that the experimenter minimize his concentration of tracer hormone so long as he retains sufficient counts. However, she does not specify exactly what she regards as adequate statistical accuracy of counting. Our own conclusion is that there will exist an optimal concentration of tracer hormone somewhere between zero and $4/K$. The exact point depends, among other things, on the "experimental" error arising in the determination of free-to-bound ratios. This optimal concentration of tracer may, in practice, be very small. Dr. Yalow has cited the example of the assay of ACTH. Referring to the assay for vitamin B_{12} shown in our Figure 18, it seems probable that the equilibrium constant for the B_{12} reaction is very similar to that governing the ACTH reaction. Our own analysis predicts that, assuming a 2% "experimental" error in the estimate of a free-to-bound ratio close to unity, one should use 4 $\mu\mu g/ml$ of binding site and 3 $\mu\mu g/ml$ of B_{12} tracer (taking realistic values for tracer specific activity and counting times). These concentrations were in fact used in the assay shown in Figure 18. In short, the optimal concentrations of reagents prescribed by our own analysis agree quite closely in order of magnitude with those actually employed by Dr. Yalow. But this does not mean that we agree with her theoretical precepts.

ALBERT   There is a point which has some overtones for bioassay. An unrelated substance displaced the labeled hormone in the same fashion as did the cold, or unlabeled, hormone. Hence, true parallelism was present; in fact, it was a complete superimposition. Does this mean that complete superimposition is not a test of the identity of substances? Conversely, when a substance displaces the label in a manner different from that of the unlabeled hormone, does this imply heterogeneity?

O'RIORDAN The problem is that it is extremely difficult to demonstrate that two substances are identical. Moreover, though standard and unknown may masquerade as identical, it is easy to miss differences. If one can detect differences, then there is no problem. The detection is probably easier when several species of binding sites are present, and when the relative affinities of the standard and unknown for these multiple species are not uniform. As you say, though, "parallelism" does not mean the standard and unknown are identical.

TASHJIAN What about the use of an independent determination of concentration? In other words, is it not possible to express the concentration on the abscissa in experimentally determined units rather than by merely sliding the curve along to see whether it can be "normalized"?

O'RIORDAN Yes, with an independent estimate of concentration, for example, in terms of micromicrograms of a pure protein or units of biological activity, one is in a favorable situation. On the other hand, if one is assaying plasma without any independent criterion of concentration and can assay it only over a limited range, one can be in considerable difficulty and not realize that differences do exist. One way out of this is use antisera from several animals, as we did in showing immunological differences between human and bovine parathyroid hormones (O'Riordan et al., in preparation).

YALOW It is possible for other hormonal substances and nonhormonal substances to interfere with the reaction of labeled antigen with antibody and thus to mimic the immunological behavior of the specific hormone that is being assayed. Generally, a simple dilution experiment will reveal the existence of nonspecific interference or nonidentity between standard and unknown hormone. But, as we have shown, on occasion dilution over a fiftyfold range of standard and unknown may result in a proportionate decrease in apparent hormone concentration, while a similar dilution experiment carried out with another antiserum will reveal differences. Thus, proper behavior on dilution is a necessary but not sufficient condition for immunologic identity of standard and unknown. It is the responsibility of the investigator to establish the validity of the specific immunoassay that he describes. It is quite important, too, to appreciate that plasma hormonal concentrations must agree with those obtained by bioassay or other means of estimating reasonable concentrations of hormone in plasma. When these results are markedly different, as in the first immunoassay for ACTH reported by Felber (1963), who found ACTH concentrations more than a hundred times higher than other workers had found by bioassay, it was the immunoassay results that were in error, presumably because proper attention had not been paid to interference by nonspecific factors. On the other hand, bioassay results may, on occasion, be suspect. Fat-pad assays for insulin in plasma show continued insulin-like activity long after pancreatectomy, when the pancreatectomized animals are markedly hyperglycemic. Immunoassay shows an appropriate decrease in plasma insulin after pancreatectomy. In this case it would appear that something other than insulin behaves like insulin in the fat-pad system and that the latter system is not specific for insulin. Specificity of the assay procedure cannot be taken for granted but must be demonstrated for each assay that is described.

REFETOFF   Do I understand that specific activity achieved after labeling is not crucial in attaining high assay sensitivity?

EKINS   The answer depends on the magnitude of the "experimental" errors (as distinct from counting errors) that arise in the assay; errors, that is, in the determination of the ratios of the free and bound fractions. We have distinguished between the statistical error of counting, which is directly dependent on the concentration and specific activity of the tracer used, the counting time available, and so on, and the "experimental" or "manipulation" error (ε) which is not thus dependent. If the latter is high, say of the order of 5 or 10%, an increase of specific activity (implying a decrease in the magnitude of the counting-error component of the overall error) may make little difference to the total error and thus have a negligible influence on sensitivity or precision. Conversely, if "experimental" errors are small, then an increase in specific activity may significantly increase the sensitivity of the assay (see our Figure 13). This is not to deny that high-specific-activity tracer has value; an increase clearly can lead to the use of shorter counting times or smaller incubation volumes without loss in sensitivity, as is also implicit in Figure 13. Nevertheless, sometimes the reward in terms of gain in assay sensitivity is negligible. It is important to realize that a hormone concentration of less than $2\varepsilon/K$ *cannot* be detected, whatever the specific activity of the tracer used (this contention applies only to assay systems in which the reagents are in equilibrium). The value of our analysis lies, we believe, in the guidance it gives regarding the circumstances in which it is useful to incur the technical difficulties associated with the synthesis and use of high-specific-activity materials. This is not to assert that they are never of value.

YALOW   We should decrease the concentration of the tracer until further decrease had no effect on the B/F ratio ($B < 0.1[\text{Ab}]_0$). If the antiserum had been diluted so the B/F were approximately 0.5, then one would have the maximal sensitivity possible with that antiserum. Obviously one must have a reasonably large total number of counts in order to obtain some degree of accuracy in determining the B/F ratio. Increasing the specific activity of the tracer, increasing the volume of incubation mixture assayed, and increasing the counting times are all ways of reducing the concentration of tracer without sacrificing too much statistical accuracy in the determination of B/F. I might add that the methods used at present in our laboratory permit the counting error in B and F to be reduced to 1% or less, so that statistical accuracy does not present a problem in our hands.

TASHJIAN   Dr. Ekins, would you care to comment on this?

EKINS   I can only comment by saying that I disagree completely with Dr. Yalow's definition of sensitivity, with the subsequent analysis, and with the conclusions drawn. I do not therefore agree that a reduction in tracer concentration is necessarily associated with the detection of a lower concentration of hormone. On the other hand, the premises on which our definition of sensitivity relies seem to be quite impeccable. The mathematical derivations that stem from this definition appear equally impeccable and lead to expressions for tracer and binding-site concentration and assay sensitivity that survive experimental test. All I can do is to invite the reader to compare our analysis with that of Dr. Yalow and come to some conclusion about which one represents the more legitimate approach.

REFETOFF   Concern was expressed earlier about a 5% experimental error. What about the error in calculating specific activity? I would think that the error in this estimation is of the order of 100% or more.

YALOW   Our recent concern has been with the determination of the specific activity of the iodine used for iodination. We have demonstrated that whereas ^{125}I is available with virtually no ^{127}I contamination, the ^{131}I content of presumably "carrier-free" ^{131}I from the Sterling Forest reactor may be as low as 5% and generally is no more than 20 or 25% of the total chemical iodine in the preparation.

However, the question relates to the determination of the specific activity of the labeled hormone. If one pipettes known amounts of the radionuclide and hormone into the iodination mixture, then one knows the maximal specific activity obtainable for 100% iodination with an accuracy that is limited only by the accuracy of pipetting. If immediately after iodination one samples the iodination mixture and applies an aliquot to paper for chromatoelectrophoresis, then from a scan of the chromatoelectrophoretogram one can determine the percentage of iodide that has not reacted. From this percentage and the maximal specific activity one can calculate the specific activity of the labeled preparation. There is another way to check the specific activity. If the hormone has been lightly iodinated and is of the same species as hormone used for standard, the labeled hormone should behave immunologically in the same fashion as the standard. If multiple tracers superimpose on the standard curve, one can use immunoassay to give the chemical concentration of the tracer. For hormones such as insulin and growth hormone estimates of specific activity determined by the two methods generally agree within 20 to 30%. From the point of view of the immunoassay procedure, it is not necessary to know the specific activity of the tracer. It is only necessary that the tracer concentration be small enough for variations in the tracer to be inappreciable compared with the minimal hormone concentrations to be assayed. As Dr. Ekins pointed out, one cannot use a tracer of 200 $\mu\mu$g/ml to assay an unknown with a concentration of 1 $\mu\mu$g/ml.

TASHJIAN   Dr. Ekins, how do you estimate your specific activity?

EKINS   As Dr. Yalow has pointed out, it's not very distressing if one does not know the value particularly accurately. However, by making the assumption that the equilibrium constant of the tracer is equal to that of the inactive hormone (a reasonable assumption with respect to many hormones), one can use the assay system to measure the tracer specific activity with a high degree of precision (see Ekins and Sgherzi, 1964).

TAIT   In the field of steroids, where practical saturation analysis methods are not yet equal to the sensitivity of the labeled reagent methods, this question of optimization of the assay methods and the difference in the conclusions between Dr. Ekins and Dr. Yalow is not an academic matter. I am sure that the mathematical derivations of both speakers are impeccable, but their starting definitions are quite different. There is an error term in the sensitivity expression of Dr. Ekins that Dr. Yalow does not have, and the dimensions of Dr. Yalow's expression for precision are different from those of Dr. Ekins. This must exert a fundamental effect on the conclusions. Furthermore, Dr. Ekins assumes that the error is dependent on counting time rather than constant total count conditions.

EKINS   As I have already indicated, there is a fundamental cleavage in our respective approaches, in that our analysis formally takes into account both counting and other experimental errors.

With regard to your latter point, we did, indeed, specify that the counting of the specimens be restricted by a time limit. In other words, we specify that each pair of specimens be counted for a total time T. This seems to us to be an appropriate approach in comparing assay systems. It would clearly be invalid to regard assay A as more sensitive than assay B (other things being equal) if, say, ten times more counting time were expended in A than in B. An analogous situation arises in the comparison of radioactive specimen counters. The best counter is the one that yields the highest precision of measurement of a given sample within a given overall (sample plus background) counting time. It is, of course, permissible to base the mathematical analysis on such postulates as that all samples are counted, without restriction on time, to any given statistical confidence level. As one might expect, however, this approach leads to the unrealistic conclusion that the optimal concentration of tracer is zero. As other experimental errors increase compared with the errors of counting, this particular element of the analysis becomes less important.

YALOW   I agree with Dr. Ekins that our theoretical analysis does not take into account counting errors. Obviously sensitivity depends both on the slope of the dose–response curve (a function of K) and the experimental error. The concept is really quite simple. If the slope of b versus H is 10% per mμg/ml, then 1 mμg/ml is detectable when the error is less than, but not greater than, 10%; if the slope is only 1% per mμg/ml, then 1 mμg/ml is not detectable until the error is made less than 1%. For any given error the sensitivity is greater according as the slope is greater — an obvious reason for evaluating the conditions of maximal slope regardless of the experimental error. We congratulate Dr. Ekins on the impeccability of his approach and would defend his right to program all sorts of errors into his analysis, but we reserve the right to keep our counting errors to 1% and to maximize the slope of the dose–response curve. This will ensure the best possible sensitivity for him and for us, whatever experimental errors he and we make, a conclusion that is undeniable.

If the maximal sensitivity for a particular antiserum is not sufficient to permit the detection of very low hormone concentrations, another antiserum must be sought. If the maximal sensitivity is barely adequate, then it must be fully exploited by reducing the tracer to such a low value that the high-energy antibody binding sites are not fully occupied by tracer alone. The counting accuracy is then improved as needed by increasing the counting time, when other methods (such as increasing the specific activity of the tracer, increasing the sensitivity of the counting system, and increasing the volume of incubation mixture) have been exploited fully. It is trite to note that, if the hormone concentrations to be measured are high, and maximal sensitivity is not required, one can increase the amount of tracer and thereby decrease the counting time.

In summary, the maximal sensitivity for an assay is dependent on the choice of antiserum; one can exploit that sensitivity, when necessary, as we have described. The investigator should choose his operating conditions while keeping in mind the question whether there exists a need for high sensitivity; but limiting sensitivity by unnecessary restriction of counting time is hardly prudent, especially when relatively long-lived isotopes, such as ^{125}I, are being used.

Dr. Tait is quite right in stating that the dimensions implicit in our definitions of sensitivity and precision are different. For sensitivity, we are concerned with the minimal hormone concentration we can detect, and the dimensions of the defining equation are percent change in b divided by the change in hormone concentration, db/dH. For precision, we are concerned with how great is the change in B/F ratio for a given fractional change in hormone concentration, $(db/dH)/H$. Precision, as we have defined it, is a dimensionless quantity. At present the problems of applying the specific reactor method to steroidal hormone assays seem to be more concerned with specificity than with sensitivity or precision. Unfortunately, the "specific" reactions are not always that "specific," and cross-reactivity with more than one steroid is the rule rather than the exception. Since the relative concentrations of the various competing steroids may be different in the plasmas of different subjects or even in the plasmas of the same subjects at different times, the problem is to find a binding protein of greater specificity for assay of the particular steroid. Alternatively, specificity may be improved by conjugating the steroid to a protein and developing an antiserum that will then react specifically with the uncomplexed steroid. No such assay has been reported, but the method has been considered (Hayashida, 1964).

*EKINS   So great is the confusion surrounding the concepts of assay "sensitivity" and "precision," particularly the former, that at least one worker (Jones, 1959) has recommended that the term "sensitivity" be discarded from scientific literature.

Two chief definitions of sensitivity either have been formally prescribed or are implicit in contemporary scientific usage (Morrison and Skogerboe, 1965). They are, briefly, the slope of the response curve (Finney, 1964; Macurdy et al., 1954) and the minimal quantity or concentration of the measured substance detectable within an assay system.

Confusion has arisen because this term is employed almost randomly in both senses, frequently in the same publication, with the implication that no conceptual distinction exists between the two. Thus, Drs. Yalow and Berson, in their presentations here and elsewhere, define sensitivity as db/dH (although b is not the measured response metameter in most of the assay systems they describe) and have emphasized that the dimen-

_____

* Comment submitted after termination of the Conference.

sions of their defining equation are "percent change per unit hormone concentration." Nonetheless, they often state explicitly that they are concerned with the measurement of small concentrations of hormone and imply that their procedures are designed to lower the detection limits of their assay systems.

These workers' failure to distinguish between the two extant definitions of sensitivity reflects, in our view, a logical fallacy, which is at the heart of the present controversy. The fallacy arises from the fact that the definitions are in no sense synonymous. Usually, moreover, they are not directly related: high "sensitivity" in the second sense given is not a logical consequence of high "sensitivity" in the first.

Thus, a balance is not necessarily capable of detecting smaller weights as the length of the pointer is increased — a truism which has led Mettler, the balance manufacturers, to abandon the word "sensitivity" in their descriptive literature. Likewise, a radioactive sample counter is not necessarily capable of detecting smaller amounts of radioactive material because of enhancement of its counting efficiency; nor is a radio receiver more capable of distinguishing a distant station because the amplifier gain is increased. In short, as is evident in each of these examples, a decrease in the detection limit is *not* a necessary consequence of an increase in the "response" of the system to a given stimulus. Rather, the detection limit depends both upon the response of the detector *and* upon the "noise," "blank," "zero," or "background" level observed in the absence of the stimulus.

This proposition can be clarified by rigorous definition of the detection limit of any analytical technique. Kaiser and Specker (1956), as quoted by Morrison and Skogerboe (1965), state that, if in an assay system the standard deviation of the blank reading is S_b and the mean value of this blank reading is $\bar{x}_b$, the minimal detectable difference between the average analytical reading $\bar{x}$ and the blank is defined by $\bar{x} - \bar{x}_b = k\sqrt{2}S_b$, where k is a constant determined by the degree of confidence specified by the experimenter. [Kaiser and Specker's expression may be approximately rewritten as $\bar{x} - \bar{x}_b = k\sqrt{2}S_b^1/(dy/dx)_b$, where S_b^1 represents the standard deviation of the blank value of the response metameter y, and $(d\bar{y}/dx)_b$ is the slope of the response curve at the zero, or blank, point. Note that this expression is identical in form with our own: $\Delta p = \Delta R_0/(dR/dp)_0$.]

Wilson (1961) has published a similar expression for the detection limit of a measurement system; likewise, Brodie and Tait (1969) have recognized the dependence of the detection limit on the standard deviation of the blank reading in the measurement of aldosterone.

Thus, an increase in the slope of the response curve yielded by the detector will lower the detection limit only if there is no concomitant increase in the standard deviation of the blank response. In certain systems, as exemplified by saturation assays, increasing the slope of the response curve (by alteration of the assay incubation mixtures) may occasion a disproportionate increase in the standard deviation of the blank readings, so that the minimal detectable concentration of hormone in the system likewise increases. In such circumstances the sensitivity of the assay is *increased* in the first sense but *decreased* in the second.

Recognizing this anomaly, we have consistently emphasized that in using the term sensitivity we are referring explicitly to the detection limit of the assay. In all illustrations intended to represent the variation of assay sensitivity with change in any specified parameter we have used the expression "minimal detectable hormone concentration." Regrettably, insofar as Kaiser and Specker's definition has been employed in scientific literature, there has been no agreement on a common value of k, which would facilitate comparison among the analytical methods reported by different workers. In our own theoretical studies we have implicitly set the value of k at $1/\sqrt{2}$. However, the choice of a particular value of k does not affect the optimal reagent concentrations required for minimizing the detection limit, nor are our conclusions regarding the effect on "sensitivity" of variation in tracer specific activity, equilibrium constant, etc., dependent on the magnitude of k.

In adopting this definition of sensitivity we recognize that the use of the term in scientific literature is essentially a semantic matter and would necessarily bow to a consensus of scientific opinion that favored its restriction to the first definition. Notwithstanding the pronouncements of the American Chemical Society (Macurdy et al., 1954) and statisticians such as Finney (1964), we would nonetheless argue that the first definition, which could lead to the statement that bathroom scales are more sensitive than microbalances, is intrinsically absurd.

Regardless of the resolution of this semantic problem, we contend that it is inadmissible to base a mathematical treatment of the optimization of assay "sensitivity" upon the first definition and subsequently to imply that the conclusions of the analysis are relevant to the optimization of assay "sensitivity" in the sense of the second definition. In our view the conclusions drawn by Drs. Yalow and Berson are both irrelevant and incorrect, in that they do not follow logically from their fundamental premises.

Essentially similar considerations underlie the use of the term "precision" and the contrasting conclusions that Drs. Yalow and Berson and ourselves have drawn regarding its optimization in saturation and radioimmunoassay techniques.

II
Statistical Aspects

CHAPTER TWENTY-ONE

Introduction

GRIFF T. ROSS

The statistician acquires a role in the design and analysis of radioimmunoassays, once the possibility of random variation is recognized. I should like to review briefly, as a prologue to the following three chapters, the requirements and procedure for a radioimmunoassay and to identify potential sources of error.

The equation of the reactions that take place in a radioimmunoassay are given by

$$Ab + Ag^* \rightleftharpoons AbAg^*$$
$$\text{addition of } Ag \rightarrow \downarrow AbAg^{**} \uparrow Ag^*$$

Labeled antigen reacts with antibody, and the addition of unlabeled antigen decreases the quantity of labeled antigen complexed with the antibody and similarly increases the proportion of the free, or unbound, labeled species.

The reagents and techniques required for developing a radioimmunoassay are summarized in Table 1. First, one obviously needs an antigen that is capable of stimulating the production of antibodies in a suitable species. Second, a suitable antiserum, specific for the antigen it is to measure, is required. It must be capable of reversible binding and,

TABLE 1   Requirements for Radioimmunoassay

A. Immunogenic antigen

B. Suitable antiserum
   1. Specific for antigen
   2. Capable of reversible binding:
        $Ag + Ab \rightleftharpoons AbAg$
   3. High titer

C. Highly purified antigen that can be labeled without loss of immunoreactivity

D. Method of separating antibody-bound tracer antigen from free tracer antigen

E. Suitable standard or reference preparation

therefore, be subject to the law of mass action. Although a high titer is not absolutely essential, it has some practical value, particularly when one wishes to perform a large number of assays with a single antiserum. The third requirement is a highly purified antigen that can be labeled without losing its immunoreactivity. It must be capable of reversible binding to the antibody, with affinities similar to those of the unlabeled antigen. Fourth, methods of separating the antibody-bound hormone from the free hormone and of measuring either or both are needed. Many techniques are available, including chromatoelectrophoresis (the bound and free forms have different mobilities in an electrical field), precipitation of antibody-bound hormone by a second antibody directed against the first (double-antibody method), and physical methods, such as molecular sieving on Sephadex gels or adsorption on silica, charcoal, Florisil, and polyethylene.

The last requirement is a suitable standard or reference preparation. Table 2 summarizes a general procedure for performing double-antibody radioimmunoassays. With minor variations this technique may be used for any of the protein and polypeptide hormones. The reaction is carried out in the presence both of a buffer with specified ionic strength and of some carrier protein that coprecipitates with the bound hormone.

The method of separating bound and free hormone requires the presence of some ethylenediaminetetraacetic acid. This inhibits the series of reactions that eventuate in the formation of complement, the presence of which may lead to spurious results. The volumes of the buffer and the EDTA added appear to constitute a negligible component of error.

The next ingredient added is a measured volume of standard or unknown containing the hormone to be assayed. Here the measurement of the quantity of added material is an unavoidable source of variation.

TABLE 2   Steps in Performing Double-Antibody
Radioimmunoassay

A. Addition of reagents
  1. Buffer containing carrier normal serum
  2. EDTA in final concentration of 0.1 M
  3. Varying volumes of solutions of standards or unknowns
  4. Constant volume of tracer of known specific activity
  5. Constant volume of antiserum

B. Addition of second antibody and incubation

C. Separation of Ag* from AbAg*

D. Determination of Ag*, AbAg*, or both

Volumes of solutions of reactants are measured with micropipettes. There is necessarily variation in the calibrated volumes of different pipettes and also in the volumes delivered by the repeated use of a single pipette. This is the first important source of error.

The next reagent to be added is the radioactively labeled tracer. It is necessary to measure the quantity of tracer accurately, in terms both of mass and of total counts. The assessment of tracer specific activity (mass) and the addition of constant quantities (total counts) to each tube constitute additional components of error.

The antiserum is the next reagent to be added. Its pipetting contributes further to error.

After all of the ingredients have been added, they are permitted to react for a constant period at a constant temperature. The conditions of incubation may give rise to between-laboratory variation. Some workers prefer to conduct so-called disequilibrium assays, in which equilibrium in the reaction of antigen and antibody has not been established. Others prefer to extend the period of incubation until equilibrium has been reached.

In the double-antibody assays a second antibody, directed against the gamma globulin of the species in which the first antibody was raised, is added. Since the proportions of antigen and antibody may influence the proportion of material precipitated, this is another potential source of error.

Finally, having converted the bound material into a precipitate, one can separate the bound and free fractions by centrifugation. The supernatant is aspirated and the precipitate counted. Besides minor variations in the volume of the remaining supernatant, lack of adequate separation and counting errors may contribute to variability.

If the plasma levels of all hormones exhibited the meteoric changes exemplified by adrenocorticotropic hormone, it might be that these errors could be ignored. When the magnitude and rate of change greatly exceed the error of the method, clearly the time of sampling becomes the more important determinant of variation. However, for other hormones, such as the gonadotropins and parathormone, the magnitude and rate of change of plasma levels are much smaller than those for adrenocorticotropin, and in their case the delineation of the sources and magnitude of error in radioimmunoassays would appear to be mandatory for obtaining maximal information.

CHAPTER TWENTY-TWO

A Theoretical Model for Statistical Inference in Isotope Displacement Immunoassay*

R. B. MCHUGH AND C. L. MEINERT

1. Introduction

Our interest in the biometric problems of hormone immunoassay was stimulated by the work of two colleagues, Goetz and Lazarow, at the University of Minnesota (Goetz et al., 1963; Morgan and Lazarow, 1963), and by the work of Yalow and Berson (1960b).

The methodological issue on which we have focused our attention is illustrated in Table 1 and Figure 1, which present experimental results of an actual insulin immunoassay. In such immunoassays the antigen Ag being assayed (which in Table 1 is insulin) and the appropriate antibody Ab, when brought together in the same system, lead to a reaction in which the antigen and antibody bind to form an antigen-antibody complex, AgAb. At equilibrium the proportion of bound antigen, AgAb, is observed (as illustrated in Figure 1) to be a *curvilinear* function of the initial concentration of antigen, $[Ag]_0$. Hence the problems of statistical inference include the following steps.

1. Choosing a calibration function, the "standard curve," with which specimens of unknown potency can be compared.

2. Fitting this curve to the data.

3. Estimating inversely the unknown ("test") antigen potency from the results of steps 1 and 2.

The major purpose of the assay is the completion of step 3.

As has been pointed out in Chapter 18, a complicating factor arises: the actual concentrations of bound antigen cannot be measured directly. However, they can be inferred if a part of the antigen in the system is labeled with a radioactive isotope, such as ^{131}I. A basis of indirect measurement is then provided by the displacement of unlabeled antigen $Ag_{\overline{L}}$ by the corresponding labeled antigen, Ag_L, in the antigen-antibody complex. Table 2 and Figure 2 illustrate didactically this essential point.

* This work was supported in part by National Institutes of Health Grant 5-SO1-FR-5448.

TABLE 1   An Example of Actual Data Generated
in an Insulin Immunoassay*

Concn. of unlabeled insulin of standards, mμg/ml	Observed proportion of labeled insulin bound
0	0.581
0.008	0.550
0.020	0.521
0.04	0.515
0.10	0.425
0.20	0.348
0.4	0.264
0.6	0.232
0.8	0.174
1.4	0.114

* Data of Yalow.

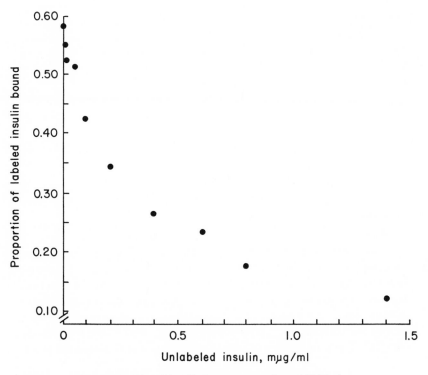

FIGURE 1   Plot of insulin immunoassay data of Table 1.

TABLE 2   Schematic Illustration of the Composition of Tubes in an Immunoassay with an Isotope-Labeled Antigen

Composition of tubes prior to incubation:

	Standards			Unknown ("test")
	20 $Ag_{\bar{L}}$ 10 Ag_L 40 Ab	40 $Ag_{\bar{L}}$ 10 Ag_L 40 Ab	60 $Ag_{\bar{L}}$ 10 Ag_L 40 Ab	? $Ag_{\bar{L}}$ 10 Ag_L 40 Ab
Unlabeled-insulin concn.:	A	$2A$	$3A$	$?A$

Assumed composition of tubes after incubation to equilibrium:

	Standards			Unknown ("test")
	16 $Ag_{\bar{L}}Ab$ 8 Ag_LAb 4 $Ag_{\bar{L}}$ 2 Ag_L 16 Ab	24 $Ag_{\bar{L}}Ab$ 6 Ag_LAb 16 $Ag_{\bar{L}}$ 4 Ag_L 10 Ab	30 $Ag_{\bar{L}}Ab$ 5 Ag_LAb 30 $Ag_{\bar{L}}$ 5 Ag_L 5 Ab	? $Ag_{\bar{L}}Ab$? Ag_LAb ? $Ag_{\bar{L}}$? Ag_L ? Ab
Concn. unlabeled insulin:	A	$2A$	$3A$	$?A$
Proportion of labeled insulin bound	8/10	6/10	5/10	0.68
Proportion of unlabeled insulin bound	16/20	24/40	30/60	
Proportion of total counts bound	0.8	0.6	0.5	

2. The statistical model

At the initial step of statistical analysis (the choice of a calibration curve to fit the curvilinear response data) we sought a function having a theoretical basis in immunochemistry instead of taking a strictly empirical approach (although we have also employed curves such as the logistic on an empirical basis). We arrived at the following equation, the "statistical model," as such a biomathematical basis for the immunoassay:

$$y_{ij} = \frac{\theta_1 + \theta_2^{-1} + A_L + X_i - [(\theta_1 + \theta_2^{-1} + A_L + X_i)^2 - 4\theta_1(A_L + X_i)]^{1/2}}{2(A_L + X_i)} + e_{ij}$$

(1)

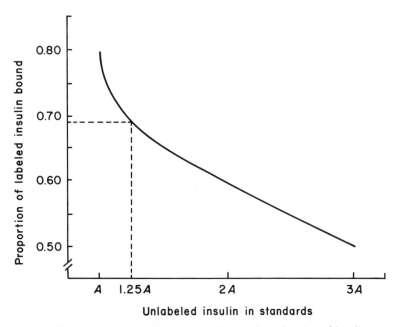

FIGURE 2   Standard curve and illustration of its use in estimation of insulin concentration, based on the data in Table 2.

Here y_{ij}, the observable random variable, is the proportion of counts associated with bound antigen in the jth tube ($j = 1, \ldots, n_i$) of the ith set of tubes ($i = 1, \ldots, s$). As illustrated in Table 2 and Figure 2, the y_{ij} provides indirect assessment of the theoretical quantity

$$\frac{[Ag_L Ab]_i + [Ag_{\overline{L}} Ab]_i}{[Ag_L] + [Ag_{\overline{L}}]}$$

which is the ratio of total concentration of labeled and unlabeled bound antigen in the ith tube to the total concentration of Ag, both labeled and unlabeled. The e_{ij} denotes the unobservable random error — a composite of experimental and counting errors — associated with observation in the jth tube of the ith set. Furthermore, in Equation 1 the parameters requiring estimation, θ_1 and θ_2, are not arbitrary but have specific physical meaning:

$$\theta_1 = [Ab]_0$$

is the true initial concentration of antibody combining sites in the system, and

$$\theta_2 = K = \frac{[AgAb]}{[Ag][Ab]}$$

is the corresponding equilibrium constant for the antigen-antibody reaction. The quantities A_L and X_i are known: A_L is the concentration $[Ag_L]$ of labeled antigen added to each tube, and X_i is the concentration $[Ag_{\bar{L}}]_i$ of unlabeled antigen added to the ith tube (thus the total concentration of the ith tube is $A_L + X_i$). The theoretical standard curve is Equation 1, assuming error-free measurement; that is, the deterministic model is

$$\eta_i = \frac{\theta_1 + \theta_2^{-1} + A_L + X_i - [(\theta_1 + \theta_2^{-1} + A_L + X_i)^2 - 4\theta_1(A_L + X_i)]^{1/2}}{2(A_L + X_i)}$$

(2)

where η_i is the theoretical average of the y_{ij}.

Four assumptions are involved in the derivation of Equation 1:

1. The antigen is univalent.
2. The antibody combining sites are of a single order.
3. The antigen-antibody reaction is reversible and follows the law of mass action.
4. The antibody-binding capacity of labeled antigen is the same as that of unlabeled antigen.

The actual details of this derivation (and others omitted here) are given by Meinert and McHugh (1968).

A further assumption made in practice, although not a part of the derivation of the model, is the adequacy of cross-reactive assay systems. Thus, in the experiment generating the data of Table 1 human plasma is assayed for human insulin by means of a pork or a beef system. That is, the labeled antigen and the assay antibody were prepared from insulin drawn, not from man, but from the pig or cow.

We should like to emphasize that the ability to provide this physical interpretation of the model parameters θ_1 and θ_2 is the primary characteristic distinguishing our biomathematical approach from the usual empirical method of curve-fitting applied to most biological assay problems. The fit to a given set of data that is obtained with an empirical function may be as good as that obtained with a theoretical model. However, the empirical "model" itself does not provide as stable a basis for the design of future experiments as does a model with an adequate theoretical basis.

3. The inverse of the theoretical standard curve

In principle the assay employs a function the inverse of the original model for the calibration of a preparation of unknown strength but known response. Let τ $(i = 1, \ldots, t)$ represent a test preparation that is to be assayed against the theoretical standard curve. The inverse relationship obtained from Equation 2 is

$$X_\tau = [\theta_1 \theta_2 - \eta_\tau(1 - \eta_\tau)^{-1}](\theta_2 \eta_\tau)^{-1} - A_L \tag{3}$$

where X_τ is the concentration of unlabeled antigen in the system, corresponding to the test preparation τ yielding the theoretical response η_τ. Equation 3 provides the theoretical solution to the immunoassay problem.

4. Estimation of the standard-curve inverse

In practice the theoretical quantity X_τ must be estimated. That is, Equation 3 is not immediately applicable, because the theoretical quantity η_τ is unknown and must be replaced with its observed value y_τ, and because the parameters θ_1 and θ_2 are also unknown and must be replaced with estimators $\hat{\theta}_1$ and $\hat{\theta}_2$, respectively, calculated from the data of the standards. The resulting point estimator of X_τ is obtained from Equation 3 by these substitutions:

$$\hat{X}_\tau = [\hat{\theta}_1 \hat{\theta}_2 - y_\tau(1 - y_\tau)^{-1}](\hat{\theta}_2 y_\tau)^{-1} - A_L \tag{4}$$

The least-squares estimation of θ_1 and θ_2 poses a problem, because the immunoassay model, Equation 1, is nonlinear in these parameters. Hence the least-squares estimators $\hat{\theta}_1$ and $\hat{\theta}_2$ must in general be approximated numerically. We have developed a FORTRAN program for the Gauss-Newton iterative solution of the desired estimators. The rate of convergence of the procedure to the desired least-squares estimates depends upon $\hat{\theta}_{1,0}$ and $\hat{\theta}_{2,0}$, the starting values used. Fortunately, the formulæ we have developed for starting values have, in our experience, assured rapid convergence. The "stopping rule" used is illustrated in Section 6.

5. Confidence limits for the standard-curve inverse X_τ

The calculation of an approximate $100(1 - \alpha)\%$ confidence interval estimate for X_τ, the expected concentration of unlabeled antigen in the τth set of tubes containing a test preparation, proceeds in two steps.

First, an approximate $100(1 - \alpha)\%$ confidence interval for η_τ is computed as

$$(\bar{y}_{\tau.})_L \le \eta_\tau \le (\bar{y}_{\tau.})_U$$

where

$$(\bar{y}_{\tau.})_L = \bar{y}_{\tau.} - t_{\alpha/2,\, n-2} \sqrt{\operatorname{var}(\bar{y}_{\tau.})}$$
$$(\bar{y}_{\tau.})_U = \bar{y}_{\tau.} + t_{\alpha/2,\, n-2} \sqrt{\operatorname{var}(\bar{y}_{\tau.})} \tag{5}$$

and the subscripts U and L denote "upper" and "lower." Here $\bar{y}_{\tau.}$ is the mean proportion of counts bound observed in the number of test tubes containing the τth unknown test preparation, and var $(\bar{y}_{\tau.})$ is the estimated variance function, readily obtained numerically as an output of the FORTRAN program for estimating θ_1 and θ_2. The true variance of $\bar{y}_{\tau.}$ is discussed in Section 7; see Equation 7. Finally, $t_{\alpha/2, \, n-2}$ is Student's t for $n-2$ DF (degrees of freedom) at the $100(1-\alpha/2)$ percentile point. The approximateness of Equation 4 arises partially from the use of probability assumptions concerning the distribution of errors, assumptions satisfied approximately in practice; see Section 7 below. In addition, owing to the nonlinearity of the model, Equation 1, the variance function var $(\bar{y}_{\tau.})$ is derived by the statistical approach to the propagation of error.

Second, the desired limits of $1-\alpha$ on X_τ are calculated from

$$(X_\tau)_{\mathrm{U}} = \{\hat{\theta}_1\hat{\theta}_2 - (\bar{y}_{\tau.})_{\mathrm{L}}[1 - (\bar{y}_{\tau.})_{\mathrm{L}}]^{-1}\}[\hat{\theta}_2(\bar{y}_{\tau.})_{\mathrm{L}}]^{-1} - A_{\mathrm{L}}$$
$$(X_\tau)_{\mathrm{L}} = \{\hat{\theta}_1\hat{\theta}_2 - (\bar{y}_{\tau.})_{\mathrm{U}}[1 - (\bar{y}_{\tau.})_{\mathrm{U}}]^{-1}\}[\hat{\theta}_2(\bar{y}_{\tau.})_{\mathrm{U}}]^{-1} - A_{\mathrm{L}} \qquad (6)$$

where $(\bar{y}_{\tau.})_{\mathrm{L}}$ and $(\bar{y}_{\tau.})_{\mathrm{U}}$ are obtained from Equation 5, $\hat{\theta}_1$ and $\hat{\theta}_2$ are obtained as described in Section 4, and A_{L} is known.

The two steps of the procedure are illustrated geometrically in Figure 3, where it is observed that the upper and lower limits for X_τ are given by the coordinates on the abscissa corresponding to the intersection of the line $y = \bar{y}_{\tau.}$ with the confidence interval about η_τ.

6. Application to the data of Yalow

The stated concentration of labeled antigen for the data furnished by Yalow was $A_{\mathrm{L}} = 0.1$ mμg/ml. The computer routine devised for fitting the model given by Equation 1 to data such as these yields starting values of

$$\hat{\theta}_{1,0} = 0.1795 \text{ m}\mu\text{g/ml}$$
$$\hat{\theta}_{2,0} = 9.6297 \text{ ml/m}\mu\text{g}$$

Three iterations were required to give the least-squares estimates:

$$\hat{\theta}_1 = \hat{\theta}_{1,3} = 0.1641 \text{ m}\mu\text{g/ml}$$
$$\hat{\theta}_2 = \hat{\theta}_{2,3} = 11.3125 \text{ ml/m}\mu\text{g}$$

These satisfied the "stopping rule":

$$(\hat{\theta}_{1,3} - \hat{\theta}_{1,2})^2 + (\hat{\theta}_{2,3}^{-1} - \hat{\theta}_{2,2}^{-1}) \leq 10^{-8}$$

where $\hat{\theta}_{1,2}$ and $\hat{\theta}_{2,2}$ are the results of the second iteration.

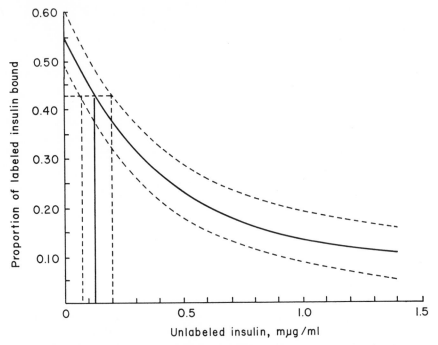

FIGURE 3   Illustration of inverse point and 95% confidence interval estimation. The standard curve is based on the data in Table 1.

Now, the equation of the estimated standard curve $\hat{\eta}$ can be obtained from Equation 2 by replacing the unknown θ_1 and θ_2 with their corresponding estimated values $\hat{\theta}_1$ and $\hat{\theta}_2$. This fitted calibration curve has been plotted in Figure 4 together with the original data of Table 1 for comparison. Table 3 gives the estimated values $\hat{\eta}_i$ and observed values y_i of the response for each level of standard considered. The last column in the table gives the difference between these two values for each standard. The sample mean square error $\hat{\sigma}^2$ for the fit is 0.000445.

Finally, to illustrate the principle of inverse estimation, suppose that one of the tubes of a test preparation that had been run with the standards of Table 1 yielded an observed proportion of counts of bound insulin of $y_\tau = 0.425$. Then the point estimate $\hat{X}_\tau$ of the true unknown insulin concentration X_τ is calculated from Equation 4. Using the value of A_L and the estimates $\hat{\theta}_1$ and $\hat{\theta}_2$ given above yields $\hat{X}_\tau = 0.133$ mμg/ml.

The corresponding 95% confidence limits for X_τ, given a point estimate of $\hat{X}_\tau$ of 0.133 mμg/ml, are

$$(X_\tau)_L = 0.075 \text{ m}\mu\text{g/ml}$$
$$(X_\tau)_U = 0.200 \text{ m}\mu\text{g/ml}$$

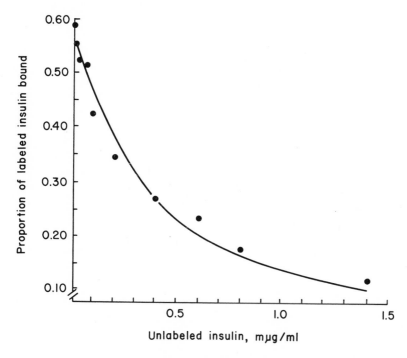

FIGURE 4   Plot of immunoassay data of Table 1, with corresponding least-squares fit for the model.

TABLE 3   Observed and Estimated Responses in the Insulin Immunoassay Data of Table 1

Observed proportion of labeled insulin bound	Estimated proportion of labeled insulin bound	Difference between observed and estimated
0.581	0.552	+0.029
0.550	0.544	+0.006
0.521	0.532	−0.011
0.515	0.512	+0.003
0.425	0.454	−0.029
0.348	0.372	−0.024
0.264	0.265	−0.001
0.232	0.202	+0.030
0.174	0.163	+0.011
0.114	0.103	+0.011

This interval estimate of X_τ is obtained from Equation 6 by using the values of $\hat{\theta}_1$, $\hat{\theta}_2$, and A_L given above for this example and

$$(y_\tau)_L = 0.372$$
$$(y_\tau)_U = 0.477$$

computed from Equation 5, where var $(y_\tau) = 0.0005185$.

7. Discussion

In Section 2 the four assumptions involved in the derivation of the theoretical model were stated. Assumption 1, univalency of the antigen, is supported with respect to insulin by the work of Yalow. The indications are that several other hormonal substances for which immunoassays are being developed may also be viewed as univalent. Likewise, the third assumption, that the antigen-antibody reaction follows the law of mass action, appears to be reasonable and generally acceptable with respect to most of the substances for which immunoassays are being developed.

On the other hand, the work of Berson and Yalow and others suggests that, in the insulin immunoassay assumption 2 — that there is a single order of antibody combining sites — is only an approximation. In this connection it is of interest to note that in principle an appropriate statistical model can be developed for any given number of orders of antibody combining sites and for a specific valence of the antigen by using the general approach employed in obtaining Equation 1. In fact, we have developed a model for univalent antigen and two orders of antibody combining sites. The usefulness in routine assay work of this substantially more complex model is under consideration.

Assumption 4, that the labeled and unlabeled antigen in all tubes of the assay have equal antibody-binding capacities, is frequently violated by intent, as noted at the end of Section 2. That is, pure preparations of the test antigen being assayed are difficult to obtain and, hence, the assay standards may be set up by using antigen taken from a species unlike the one from which the test preparations are drawn. For example, it is common practice to assay human insulin by using standards prepared with beef or pork insulin. The labeled antigen and antibody also are usually prepared from beef or pork insulin. Hence, the degree of similarity in reactivities between labeled and unlabeled antigen is likely to be different in tubes containing standards from that in tubes containing test preparations. However, at least at present the dissimilarities have not been viewed as a major contributor to errors in the results obtained from the immunoassay.

The assumptions underlying the derivation of confidence interval estimates for the test preparation (given in Section 5) appear to be well approximated in practice. The assumption of unbiased and independent errors can usually be satisfied by an application of appropriate randomization procedures in the preparation of the assay standards and unknowns. The assumption of normally distributed errors appears reasonable, particularly since a sizable contribution to the resulting error distribution is the Poisson variability associated with the counting process. The Poisson distribution for the level of radioactivity in most immunoassays is well approximated by a normal distribution. However, a large Poisson contribution to the variability, relative to the other types of variability in the assay, may vitiate the assumption of common variance and require a weighted least-squares approach similar to that referred to by Cornfield in another connection (Chapter 6). The estimation procedure discussed may thus be modified to take unequal variances into account.

Finally, some comments on experimental design may be of interest. We have not yet translated the conflicting concepts of sensitivity and precision presented by Yalow and Berson (Chapter 18) and Ekins et al. (Chapter 19) into terms that can be usefully applied in the statistical design of an immunoassay. However, with respect to the definition of assay precision we feel that a variant of the statistician's usual interpretation of this concept is worth considering. It seems reasonable to select that experimental design which for a particular type of assay gives a desired *precision* in the sense of a satisfactorily small inverse confidence estimator for the unknown X_τ of interest.

It is clear from the confidence interval given for X_τ (see Equations 6) that the length of the desired inverse interval depends upon the variance of $\bar{y}_{\tau.}$. The first approximation to this function is

$$\text{Var}\,(\bar{y}_{\tau.}) = \left[\frac{1}{q_\tau} + \sum_k^2 \sum_m^2 f_k(X'_\tau;\,\theta)f_m(X'_\tau;\,\theta)S^{km}\right]\sigma^2 \qquad (7)$$

where q_τ is the number of times the τth unknown is replicated, and where

$$f_1(X'_\tau;\,\theta) = (1/2X'_\tau)\{1 - (\theta_1 + \theta_2^{-1} - X'_\tau) \\ \times\,[(\theta_1 + \theta_2^{-1} + X'_\tau)^2 - 4\theta_1 X'_\tau]^{-1/2}\} \qquad (8)$$

$$f_2(X'_\tau;\,\theta) = (\theta_2^{-2}/2X'_\tau)\{(\theta_1 + \theta_2^{-1} + X'_\tau) \\ \times\,[(\theta_1 + \theta_2^{-1} + X'_\tau)^2 - 4\theta_1 X'_\tau]^{-1/2} - 1\} \qquad (9)$$

$$\hat{\sigma}^2 = \sum_i^s \sum_j^{n_i} \frac{(y_{ij} - \hat{\eta}_i)^2}{n-2} \qquad (10)$$

and S^{km} denotes the inverse element of the kth row ($k = 1, 2$) and mth column ($m = 1, 2$) of the matrix containing terms of the type

$$S_{km} = \sum_{i}^{s} \sum_{i}^{n_i} [f_k(X'_i; \theta) f_m(X'_i; \theta)] \qquad (11)$$

From inspection of the variance expression for $\bar{y}_{\tau.}$ given above it can be readily seen that any modification in design that reduces σ^2 will increase the precision of inverse confidence estimation; that is, such modifications will yield smaller confidence estimates for a given unknown.

From Equation 7 it is seen that the precision of the assay will be improved by increasing q_τ, the number of times the τth unknown is replicated, and also by increasing s, the number of standards, or n, the total number of tubes on which the calibration curve is based. Further, it will be improved by a judicious selection of standards over the range under consideration.

Finally, it follows from the role of Equations 8, 9, and 11 in the variance function given by Equation 7 that the values of θ_1, θ_2, and A_L will influence the assay precision. Of these quantities θ_1, the concentration of antibody combining sites, and A_L, the concentration of labeled antigen, are under the control of the investigator. Therefore Monte Carlo studies of the variance function for a variety of dose placements and numbers of standards may permit the determination of a set of optimal values of θ_1 and A_L for a given range over which inverse estimates are desired.

CHAPTER TWENTY-THREE

Statistical Quality Control of Radioimmunoassays

D. RODBARD, P. L. RAYFORD, AND
GRIFF T. ROSS

1. Introduction

Our experience with the statistical analysis of data from radio-immunoassays for human growth hormone, luteinizing hormone, chorionic gonadotropin, and follicle-stimulating hormone, and from a competitive protein-binding assay for progesterone provides the basis for this chapter. A pragmatic "quality control" system for data analysis is described and illustrated.

2. Data and dose–response curves

The data from ten assays for human luteinizing hormone are shown in Table 1. Odell et al. (1967) have reported the details of the "double antibody" radioimmunoassay, together with the automated procedure employed for counting the radioisotope. Since the data are materially affected by the magnitude and distribution of counting errors, the counting procedure is important.

A schematic form of the dose–response curve is shown in Figure 1, where the ordinate is in counts per minute, Y, of the radioactive tracer precipitated, or "bound," and the abscissa is in arbitrary units, X, of the dose (of the standard or unknown preparations).

The value T, the total number of counts, is the amount of tracer added to each incubation tube. This will be determined in part by the specific activity of the tracer. Ideally, T is a constant in all tubes; in practice, there is a small tube-to-tube variation. This variation presumably follows a normal distribution. We have found it adequate to determine T from a subsample of approximately 10% of the tubes in an assay.

The value N represents the number of counts that are nonspecifically precipitated, or "trapped." A similar blank or correction factor is encountered in radioimmunoassays that employ methods other than double-antibody precipitation for the separation of bound and free hormone and in competitive protein-binding assays. The blank has an

TABLE 1   Calibration Curves from Ten Assays for Human Luteinizing Hormone with Response Tabulated as B/B_0

Dose, mIU-IRP	Assay no. and date (1966)									
	1 10/4	2* 10/5	3 10/7	4* 10/7	5* 11/15	6 11/15	7 11/17	8* 11/17	9* 11/28	10 11/28
0.4	95.9	95.3	97.8	93.8	99.9	98.7	95.1	93.3	96.8	96.4
	98.6	96.6	95.9	93.8	96.4	97.7	96.7	96.3	96.6	90.0
	96.2	94.5	97.8	95.2	99.5	98.2	96.4	99.1	96.3	93.9
	99.9	96.2	96.0	93.9	98.1	99.9†	94.4	93.8	97.6	90.9
0.5	90.8	94.8	95.2	91.4	98.6	96.3	91.9	95.3	93.3	98.6
1.0	90.7	89.0	91.4	91.0	92.4	95.6	90.9	89.9	91.5	95.1
2.0	85.5	82.8	84.9	81.8	89.1	86.5	80.3	82.3	87.5	87.9
3.0	79.3	74.2	81.1	77.0	84.3	81.0	76.9	79.9	80.0	79.8
4.0	77.1	74.5	75.4	73.7	77.1	75.4	72.4	69.5	76.5	80.0
	76.7	74.1	76.6	72.7	78.1	76.8	67.6	70.7	74.7	77.4
	75.1	72.0	77.7	74.3	79.6	77.9	72.0	69.8	78.6	75.0
	76.1	73.6	76.5	72.9	78.6	79.4	72.3	73.2	77.4	78.7
5.0	72.8	70.6	74.1	69.2	75.8	72.1	66.8	70.9	75.9	76.6
10.0	59.7	58.4	63.2	59.0	62.2	59.0	54.5	56.0	60.0	64.8
20.0	41.6	40.7	45.9	39.1	44.0	44.1	40.4	40.2	46.7	46.9
30.0	33.0	30.7	38.5	30.6	31.7	35.0	30.2	29.2	34.2	33.2
40.0	24.6	24.4	32.0	23.2	27.2	24.3	23.2	23.7	29.9	28.0
	25.1	26.2	32.7	23.8	26.9	26.7	21.0	23.6	29.1	27.0
	25.4	24.2	34.3	24.0	28.4	26.0	23.4	29.5	28.3	30.1
	23.5	23.4	32.5	24.2	28.5	25.7	23.9	25.3	27.8	29.0
50.0	18.7	18.7	26.9	17.5	25.4	23.4	18.1	22.5	23.5	24.4
100.0	10.7	10.5	14.1	9.9	14.2	12.0	10.7	11.5	13.3	13.0
T	11382	11968	10696	10696	10570	10570	8640	8640	10288	10288
N	680	600	600	600	686	686	573	573	624	624
$B_0 - N$	8130	8610	5962	5962	4394	4394	2651	2651	5536	5536
B_0	8810	9210	6562	6562	5080	5080	3224	3224	6160	6160
$\frac{(B_0 - N)}{(T - N)}$	0.759	0.854	0.59	0.59	0.45	0.45	0.33	0.33	0.57	0.57

* New IRP–HMG standard used.   † Actual value was 100. Read as 99.9 to maintain finite logit.

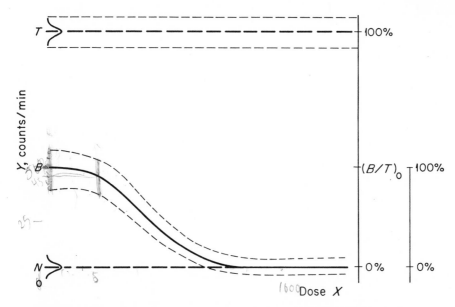

FIGURE 1   The general format of the dose–response curve for radioimmunoassay and competitive protein-binding assay data, where T is total counts, B is counts of bound, and N is nonspecific counts (blank). The areas within the light dashed lines indicate the residual variance. It is conventional to redefine N as 0%. Either T or $(B/T)_0$ may be designated 100%, depending on the type of analysis to be employed.

error which may likewise be assumed to be normally distributed, and upon which is superimposed a counting error following a Poisson distribution.

The value B represents the number of counts that are precipitated or bound. In theory, it is a monotonically decreasing function of dose. Again, there are errors from many sources, including variability in the pipetting of antibody, variation in the antigen-antibody reaction, failure to reach equilibrium, and counting errors. The variance of B is not uniform over the dose–response curve, nor does it exhibit any simple relationship with the magnitude of B (as would be true of the binomial and Poisson distributions).

It is customary to transform the dose–response curve and to work with derived variables. The value T is arbitrarily taken as 100% and N as 0%. This new scale corresponds to results expressed in terms of the ratio of bound-to-total, B/T, or of bound-to-free, B/F, counts. For B/T we are actually calculating $(B - N)/(T - N)$, and for B/F we calculate $(B - N)/(T - B)$. This distinction appears trivial. However, it changes the nature of the variables and prohibits the use of straightforward methods of handling inequality of variance. The heteroscedasticity

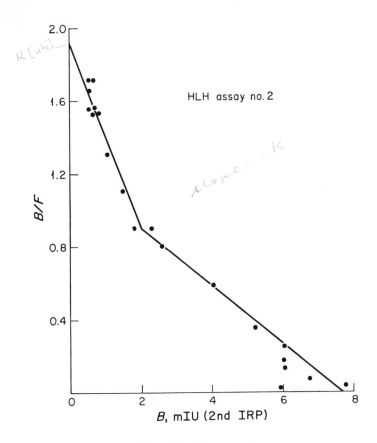

FIGURE 2   *B/F* versus *B*.

becomes greater as one approaches the upper and lower ends of the dose–response curve.

Alternatively, the value of B/T when $X = 0$, the so-called "initial B/T," written as $(B/T)_0$, may be arbitrarily defined as the 100% mark on a scale. The response is then expressed as $B/B_0 = (B - N)/(B_0 - N)$, where B_0 is the number of counts precipitated in the absence of an unknown or standard. Thus, each response B/T is divided by the initial B/T. This procedure, which can be accomplished automatically by the counter, standardizes the scale and, by forcing the dose–response curve to range from 0 to 100%, facilitates the use of such transformations as the logit and probit.

Many forms of presenting the dose–response curve have been employed, each having characteristic advantages and disadvantages. A number of these are illustrated in Figures 2 to 8, with the same data from one particular assay of luteinizing hormone.

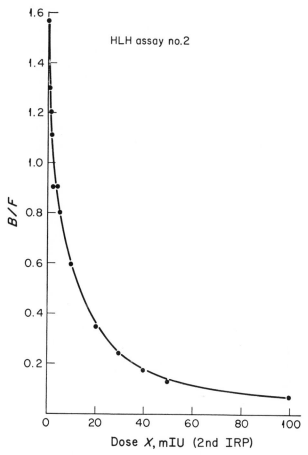

FIGURE 3 B/F versus X.

B/F versus B

The ratio of bound to free tracer versus bound tracer is sometimes referred to as a Scatchard plot (Scatchard, 1949) and was utilized by Berson and Yalow (1959b, 1964). For a univalent, homogeneous antibody this plot results in a straight line with a slope of $-K$ and intercepts $K[\text{Ab}^\circ]$ on the ordinate and B_0 on the abscissa, where K is the association constant for antigen-antibody complex (or steroid protein binding) and $[\text{Ab}^\circ]$ is the molar concentration of total antibody combining sites. Characteristic curves are also obtained for a heterogeneous mixture of univalent antibodies and for multivalent antibodies; see Figure 2. These have been analyzed and discussed by Berson and Yalow (1959b). Such plots are useful for examining the nature of the antigen-antibody (or steroid protein) reaction and permit the estimation of $[\text{Ab}^\circ]$ and K. However, the plot of B/F versus B is inconvenient for the estimation of potency.

B/F versus X

The form of dose–response curve given by *B/F* versus *X*, a natural extension of the Scatchard plot, yields a nonlinear, hyperbolic curve, which cannot be approximated by a linear segment except over a very narrow range; see Figure 3. This limits its usefulness for dose interpolation and for statistical analysis, although dose interpolation may be accomplished by graphical methods. A serious disadvantage is that the standard curve usually covers a hundredfold range of doses, which is not readily handled by a linear, arithmetic scale on the abscissa.

B/B₀ versus X

Although the *B/F* ratio arises in the derivation of the Scatchard plot, it is often more convenient to plot *B/B₀* as the response variable versus *X*; see Figure 4. This standardizes the scale (from 0 to 100%) and obviates the need to calculate *B/F*. Moreover, since the error in the denominator is small and uniform, the *B/B₀* percentage is more stable than the *B/F* ratio.

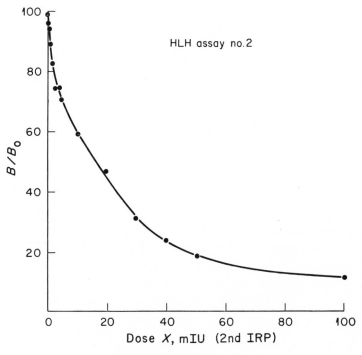

FIGURE 4   *B/B₀* versus *X*.

B/F versus $\log X$

By means of a logarithmic transformation of the dose the curve is partially linearized, and dose interpolation in the lower range is facilitated; see Figure 5. This is one of the most popular forms of the dose–response curve.

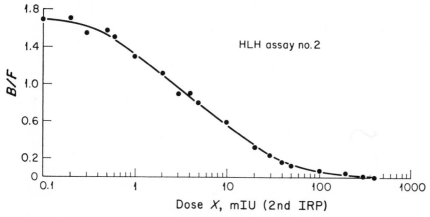

FIGURE 5 B/F versus $\log X$.

B/B_0 versus $\log X$

The plot of B/B_0 versus $\log X$ results in a sigmoidal curve, which can be approximated by a linear segment for at least a tenfold range of doses, thereby facilitating dose interpolation and potency estimation; see Figure 6. This form of the dose–response curve is still distinctly nonlinear.

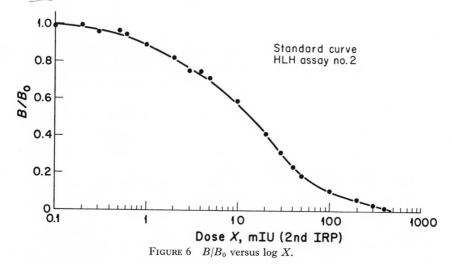

FIGURE 6 B/B_0 versus $\log X$.

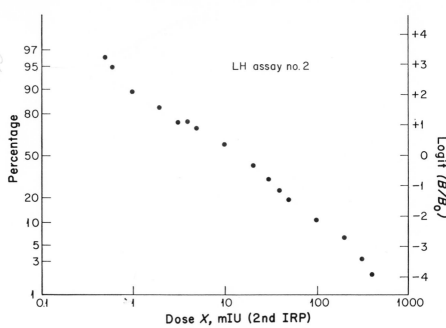

FIGURE 7   Logit (B/B_0) versus log X.

Logit (B/B_0) versus log X

When the logit transformation, logit $Y = \log_e [Y/(1 - Y)]$, is applied to B/B_0, the sigmoidal curve just described becomes almost linear; see Figure 7. The curve does not depart significantly from linearity between 10 and 90% or for logits between -2.2 and $+2.2$. Accurate estimation of slope and intercept, either by means of linear-regression analysis or graphical methods, is thereby permitted. We have found the graphical methods to be entirely satisfactory when the assay is "in control" (see the section on quality control below). Arc sine or probit transformations will also produce adequate linearization of the dose–response curve.

3. Statistical analysis

By employing the logit (B/B_0) versus log X adequate linearization of the dose–response curve is usually obtained. Results of conventional unweighted regression analysis for each of the ten assays in Table 1 are summarized in Table 2. In only one instance, in assay 10, did the subsequent analysis of variance indicate a statistically significant departure from linearity, $P < 0.05$, on the basis of 11 DF (degrees of freedom) for lack of linear fit.

unweighted

TABLE 2   Regression Analysis of the Data in Table 1 after Logit Transformation of Response and Log Transformation of Dose

Assay no.	Date	$\bar{y}$	s^2	b	λ	s^2 at dose: 0.4	4.0	40.0
1	10/4	1.01	1.029	−2.51	0.405	3.084	0.002	0.002
2	10/5	0.73	0.020	−2.12	0.066	0.052	0.003	0.004
3	10/7	1.02	0.045	−2.07	0.102	0.130	0.003	0.002
4	10/7	0.64	0.007	−2.01	0.041	0.018	0.001	0.001
5	11/15	1.32	0.857	−2.74	0.338	2.566	0.004	0.002
6	11/15	1.21	0.716	−2.70	0.313	2.135	0.009	0.003
7	11/17	0.66	0.029	−2.12	0.080	0.070	0.012	0.005
8	11/17	0.78	0.314	−2.17	0.258	0.915	0.007	0.020
9	11/28	0.95	0.016	−2.12	0.060	0.038	0.009	0.002
10	11/28	0.93	0.088	−2.01	0.148	0.247	0.014	0.004
	Pooled values:		0.312	−2.26	0.248	0.925	0.006	0.004

At each dose at which observations were replicated (that is, 0.4, 4.0, and 40.0 mIU of the Second International Reference Preparation for Human Menopausal Gonadotrophin) the variances of the four observations (after logistic transformation) were calculated, and they also are exhibited in Table 2. The results reveal the large degree of heteroscedasticity along this form of dose–response curve.

Table 3 and Figures 8 and 9 further illustrate these points. Table 3 gives the data for ten replications of an assay of luteinizing hormone. In

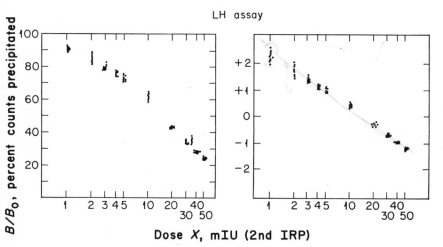

LH assay

FIGURE 8 B/B_0 versus log X and logit (B/B_0) versus log X for the data in Table 3.

Figure 8 log dose is plotted against the response before and after logistic transformation. The right-hand portion of the figure exhibits both the linearization of the curve obtained by employing the logistic transformation for response and the resultant heteroscedasticity along the curve. Further, Table 3 shows the variances of the ten replicates at each dose after logistic transformation of response. Figure 9 gives a plot of these variances (on a logarithmic scale) versus the response level (on a logistic scale). It would appear from these data that the logarithm of the residual variance of the logit (B/B_0) values is linearly related to the mean logit B/B_0. However, this is not generally true. The important point is that variance along the dose–response curve in this form cannot be assumed to be uniform.

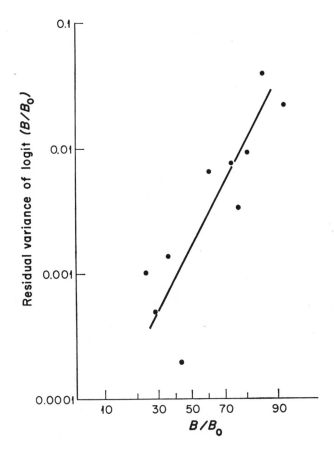

FIGURE 9   Residual variance of response variable logit (B/B_0) as a function of response level for the data in Table 3.

TABLE 3 Ten Replicates of a Standard Curve for Luteinizing Hormone with Response Tabulated as B/B_0

Dose, mIU-IRP	Assay no. (11/25/66)										After logit transform	
	1	2	3	4	5	6	7	8	9	10	Mean	Variance
1.0	91.6	88.6	90.5	93.0	92.1	90.2	91.4	88.7	90.9	90.7	2.30	0.0279
2.0	84.3	83.5	88.2	87.7	85.9	86.3	81.9	82.4	89.1	84.7	1.78	0.0404
3.0	79.1	78.1	78.5	79.5	80.4	80.6	81.5	78.3	79.8	83.0	1.38	0.0098
4.0	75.3	76.5	76.0	77.2	74.5	76.9	74.9	77.2	74.0	76.5	1.15	0.0040
5.0	72.2	74.7	72.8	71.3	72.5	70.7	71.1	72.2	74.7	75.9	0.99	0.0080
10.0	63.3	61.4	61.7	61.4	63.7	58.7	60.8	58.9	59.4	58.1	0.44	0.0066
20.0	43.3	42.9	43.0	42.8	43.2	43.4	42.8	42.2	43.2	43.2	−0.28	0.0002
30.0	33.7	33.5	33.3	34.7	33.8	35.7	34.2	35.1	32.9	33.7	−0.66	0.0015
40.0	28.2	28.8	28.2	29.0	27.8	28.0	29.0	28.1	28.2	27.8	−0.93	0.0004
50.0	23.9	23.5	25.0	23.7	22.8	23.4	24.2	24.0	24.2	24.1	−1.16	0.0011

In consequence of the heteroscedasticity the unweighted regression analysis as summarized in Table 2 is not appropriate. A weighted least-squares procedure is required, and a model for determining the shape and magnitude of the residual variance of logit (B/B_0) is currently being developed. As Cornfield has indicated in Chapter 6, heteroscedasticity also implies that the index of precision, λ, varies along the curve. Hence, each λ value calculated in Table 2 merely represents an average for the curve.

Comparison of the ten assays in Table 1 revealed statistically significant differences ($P < 0.01$) in the mean levels of response and in slope. Since different standards and differently labeled tracers are employed, and since minor, unnoticed differences in technique may affect assay results, this finding is to be anticipated. In consequence, the analysis of any one assay underestimates the total error. An important corollary is that comparisons of physiological interest should be made within the same assay.

4. Quality control

For quality control several parameters describing the assay are arbitrarily selected and displayed graphically, together with acceptable "tolerance ranges." Any departure from the "tolerance" limits signals that the assay is "out of control." Although the methods described below assume an underlying normal distribution, the results are insensitive to departures from this assumption.

The following parameters have been selected for the quality-control analysis. Note that the first three parameters are not mutually independent, since knowledge of any two determines the value of the third. However, we have found it convenient to maintain a check on each.

Specific activity of the tracer

Although a wide range of specific activities may be used (for example, 50 to 250 microcuries per microgram) and the method of Greenwood et al. (1963) yields reproducible results, the specific activity of the tracer reflects to some extent the nature of the iodination. There is evidence that damage to the tracer may increase with increasing specific activity or with overiodination (Berson and Yalow, 1964).

Amount of tracer

The amount of the tracer influences the performance of the assay. If present in an excessive amount, the tracer may shift the equilibrium between bound and free hormone, resulting in a decrease in initial B/T, or $(B - N)/(T - N)$, and in a loss of sensitivity.

Total counts T

The total counts T may be arbitrarily determined by the experimenter, since it is proportional both to the counting efficiency of the detector and to the amount of tracer present divided by the specific activity. The number of counts determines the counting error for T and indirectly influences the counting errors for B_0, B, and N. Since these errors are essentially additive, the overall error in B/T increases rapidly if T becomes too low.

Nonspecific, or background, counts

Nonspecific, or background, counts may be affected by the conditions of incubation (time, temperature, pH, damage, etc.) and by the efficiency of the separation technique, whether chromatoelectrophoresis, precipitation with second antibody, a Sephadex column, activated charcoal, or whatever be employed. A value greater than 5% of the total counts is indicative of trouble in the system.

We obtain an estimate of N with a small number of tubes, usually three. If there is wide variation, or if N exceeds 5% of the total counts, then the error in estimating N begins to contribute appreciably to the overall error in the B/B_0 response. To avoid introducing bias it is then advisable to increase the number of determinations of N so as to obtain a more precise estimate of mean N.

$(B/T)_0$

The "initial B/T" is the "100% control." This is the bound counts (minus the "blank," or nonspecific, counts N) divided by the total counts (minus the blank) when only tracer is present. In the assays for human growth, luteinizing, and follicle-stimulating hormones and for chorionic gonadotropin this quantity is obtained empirically from the three tubes containing antibody and a labeled tracer with no added unlabeled hormone.

The $(B/T)_0$ is one of the most important parameters describing the performance of an assay. It may be low for a variety of reasons, such as high nonspecific counts (N), low binding affinity (K) or titer [Ab°] of antibodies, incomplete separation of bound from free hormone, or failure to reach equilibrium. Whenever $(B/T)_0$ is low, the fractional error (standard error divided by the mean) will be unduly high, and assay precision will be decreased. It then becomes necessary to increase the number of determinations of B_0 in order to reduce the error of the estimate of $(B/T)_0$.

Slope

The slope of the dose–response curve is constant when the assay is under control. In fact, the slopes are remarkably similar in several assays (human follicle-stimulating, luteinizing, and growth hormones, and progesterone).

The slope may be calculated by conventional linear-regression methods, or it may be determined graphically by plotting the dose–response curve on logit-log paper. We have found that when the curve is in control, the graphically determined slope is virtually identical with that calculated by linear-regression methods. The standard error of the slope provides little additional information, since the heteroscedasticity of the data vitiates its applicability.

Abscissa intercept

Several parameters could be used to provide an estimate of the sensitivity of the assay. Since the dose–response curve is rarely reliable for interpolation above a 90% response, the 90% intercept may be used as one such measure. However, the 90% intercept is rather variable. We therefore prefer the 50% intercept as an index of sensitivity, since its value is estimated with greater precision.

Within-assay variability

Within-assay variation may be estimated by running a small number of samples in duplicate. For example, 5 duplicate samples provide an estimate of residual variance with 5 DF for each assay, 1 DF for each set of duplicates. Hence, n assays yield $5n$ DF for this estimate. Thus, after four or five assays one has a fairly reliable estimate of residual variance. Pooling the estimates over several assays, however, involves the assumption of homogeneity of variance. When all of the samples are within a tenfold range, we have found this assumption to be reasonable.

There are situations, however, where the results span a hundredfold range as, for example, in the case with growth hormone in hypophysectomized patients and acromegalics, gonadotropins in prepuberal or postmenopausal patients, and HCG titers in trophoblastic diseases. Under these circumstances one encounters heteroscedasticity along the dose–response curve besides errors in dilution that magnify the variances. The problem can be resolved by obtaining estimates of the variance from several different portions of the dose–response curve and then pooling the values from samples within a small range of dose. A variance that is proportional to the square of the dose level calls for logarithmic transformation of the dose to achieve homoscedasticity. However, near the minimal detectable quantity on the dose–response scale such an approach will not suffice, since the error becomes very large relative to the dose level.

Between-assay variability

Between-assay variability can be directly estimated by a repetition of the sample in successive assays. In our laboratory 300 µl aliquots from pooled plasma obtained from several subjects are frozen for incorporation into each assay.

The ratio of the between-assay to the within-assay variance provides an index of the stability of the system. For the ideal system the ratio should be unity; that is, there should be no greater variation from week to week than obtains between duplicates within a single assay.

Averages or totals

The averages or totals of several control samples that have been run in a series of assays can easily be obtained and plotted. If these values fluctuate by more than 5 or 10%, the assay is suspect.

To illustrate the monitoring of within-assay and between-assay variance, duplicate estimates of human luteinizing hormone in three subjects whose plasma was assayed ten times are set out in Table 4. For each assay the mean response of the six observations and the within-assay mean square (obtained from the duplicate determinations from each subject) are shown. These individual within-assay mean squares are also displayed in Figure 10, where it may be seen that assays 5 and 6 are out of control with respect to this parameter. The means of the six observations tend to rise until assay 6 and then to fall.

After each assay's results are available, an analysis of variance may be made on the cumulative data. After k assays (k in this case is between 2 and 10) this analysis of variance takes the following form:

Term	DF	
Between assays	$3(k-1)$	3 subjects
Between subjects	2	10 times
Within assays	$3k$	6 observation
Total:	$6k-1$	

Here the between-assay term $3(k-1)$ DF consists of a pooling of a between-different-assays term, $k-1$ DF, with the interaction-of-assays-and-subjects term, $2(k-1)$ DF.

For the data in Table 4 the resulting cumulative mean squares for between and within assays are indicated. When the cumulative mean

TABLE 4   Results of Samples Run in Duplicate for Each of Three Subjects in Ten Assays

Assay no.	Subject no. 1		Subject no. 2		Subject no. 3		Mean	Individual MS within assays (DF)	Cumulative MS within assays (DF)	Cumulative MS between assays (DF)	Individual MS between assays (DF)
1	24.4	24.4	32.3	29.7	33.0	32.3	29.4	1.21(3)	1.21 (3)	—	—
2	19.8	22.4	33.0	32.3	27.7	33.0	28.0	5.89(3)	3.55 (6)	6.30 (3)	6.30 (3)
3	29.7	29.7	39.6	39.6	39.6	39.6*	36.3	0 (3)	2.37 (9)	41.89 (6)	77.50 (3)
4	36.3	31.0	40.0	40.0	36.3	34.7	36.4	5.11(3)	3.05 (12)	45.69 (9)	53.27 (3)
5	33.0	33.0	56.1	49.5	49.5	49.5	45.1	7.26(3)	3.89 (15)	107.11 (12)	291.37 (3)
6	42.9	52.8	59.4	56.1	56.1	56.1	53.9	18.15(3)	6.27 (18)	204.40 (15)	593.57 (3)
7	36.3	33.0	47.9	46.2	46.2	44.6	42.4	2.73(3)	5.76 (21)	175.54 (18)	31.23 (3)
8	29.0	29.0	46.2	44.6	44.6	42.9	39.4	0.91(3)	5.16 (24)	152.22 (21)	12.35 (3)
9	29.0	28.3	38.0	38.0	36.3	36.3	34.3	0.08(3)	4.59 (27)	138.02 (24)	38.61 (3)
10	29.7	29.0	39.6	38.0	34.7	33.0	34.0	0.99(3)	4.23 (30)	127.38 (27)	42.28 (3)

* Estimated value of missing observation.

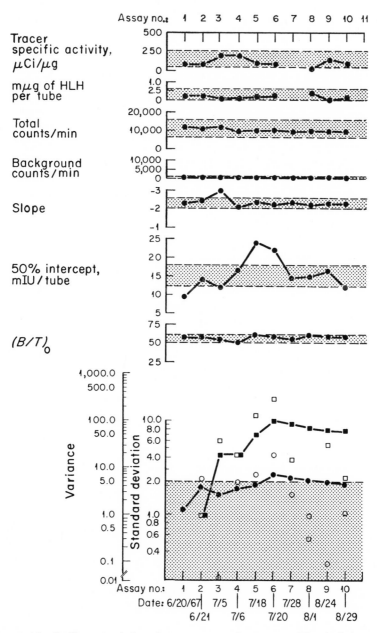

FIGURE 10 Quality-control chart for parameters of ten assays. The shaded areas indicate the tolerance limits.

squares for both are compared, it is clear that after the third assay the variability between assays becomes significantly larger than that within assays.

For an examination of the effect of the most recent assay on the between-assay variance the $3(k - 1)$ DF for between assays may be subdivided into a component, 3 DF, comparing the mean of the most recent assay (that is, the kth) with the means of the $k - 1$ preceding assays and a remainder term, $3(k - 2)$ DF. The former component, called the individual between-assay mean square, can be obtained by subtracting the between-assay sum of squares for the preceding $k - 1$ assays from the between-assay sum of squares including all k assays and dividing by the corresponding change in degrees of freedom. The results are shown in Table 4 and plotted in Figure 10 on the same scale as the individual within-assay mean squares.

Figure 10 displays the quality-control charts for the parameters listed above in ten assays for luteinizing hormone. The shaded areas define the tolerance limits, the determination of which is described by Bliss (1952), Grant (1952), and Duncan (1965). The departure of any point from the tolerance limits constitutes a warning that this aspect of the assay is "out of control." In our experience the four most informative parameters are the $(B/T)_0$, the 50% intercept, and the within-assay and between-assay variances. If the value for any of these parameters falls outside the tolerance limits, something is wrong (for example, tracer, antibody, standard, or technician) and the source of the error must be sought so that corrective action can be taken. The source of the difficulty may be apparent as, for example, excessively low specific activity or damaged tracer, but is more frequently obscure. We have therefore adopted the practice of including controls for the tracer, the antibody, and the standard. The tracer used on the previous assay is included as a check on the tracer, and a second batch of antibody is used as a check on the antibody. The control samples which are run on successive assays serve as a secondary standard. In addition, we insert a control to test for cross-reactivity (in the assay for luteinizing hormone, for example, we include a tube containing a known standard of follicle-stimulating hormone). Thus, in the event of a departure from the tolerance limits the source of the error can be detected and corrected before the next assay is run.

An additional quality-control parameter that is useful deals with pipetting error. If every tube received the same number of tracer molecules, the total count T in each tube would follow the Poisson distribution, in which the variance is equal to the mean. Denoting the mean of total counts among k tubes by $\bar{T}$ and their standard deviation by s_T, the agreement with Poisson variation can be tested by calculating

$$\chi^2 = (k - 1)s_T^2/\bar{T}$$

and using the chi-square distribution with $k - 1$ DF; see Snedecor and Cochran (1967, p. 232). In our laboratory we define the percentage error due to pipetting as

$$\% \text{ error} = 100\% \sqrt{s_T^2 - \bar{T}}/\bar{T}$$

In our experience this error is customarily of the order of 1%.

5. Discussion

A quality-control system such as that described is a convenience to the experimenter. The necessary data can be tabulated, calculated, and charted immediately upon completion of an assay. The graphical methods provide an immediate warning of poor correspondence between duplicates and of departures from linearity and parallelism. The use of repetitive control samples permits the direct determination of experimental error unburdened by assumptions of linearity, homoscedasticity, and normality of distribution. The price exacted is, of course, the necessity of running samples repetitively. However, the economy of the radioimmunoassay method is such that surveillance can be maintained with minimal effort.

CHAPTER TWENTY-FOUR

Dose–Response Curves for Radioimmunoassays*

C. I. BLISS

1. Introduction

An initial stage in developing a bioassay is determining the form of a practicable dose–response curve, its precision, and its stability. If some unit of response can be plotted as a straight line against a function of the dose over a sufficiently wide dose range, the potency of a test or unknown preparation can be estimated by standard techniques. To avoid weighting, the response should be equally variable or homoscedastic within this linear range.

More than one pair of variates may meet these conditions, depending upon both the hormone and the assay technique. A curve in which the response plots linearly against the log dose of hormone indicates a parallel-line assay. If, instead, the response is related linearly to the dose in arithmetic units, reciprocals, or powers, potency may be computed from the slopes for standard and unknown as a slope ratio assay. Both relations occur in radioimmunoassays. When an unknown preparation is tested at a single dose level, its potency may be estimated in either case from a concurrent standard curve, but there is then no test of qualitative equivalence.

The kinetic relations of enzyme chemistry, which have much in common with the antigen-antibody reaction, can often be reduced theoretically or empirically to rectangular hyperbolæ. It therefore seemed that the rectangular hyperbola might be particularly suitable for the fitting of radioimmunoassay data. In this chapter the fit of this curve to the measurements of human luteinizing hormone presented by Rodbard et al. in Chapter 23 is examined.

The rectangular hyperbola has three parameters, two asymptotes x'_0 and y'_0 and a constant c, as defined in the equation

$$(x' - x'_0)(y' - y'_0) = x'_0 y'_0 + c \qquad (1)$$

where x' is the independent variate, or dose, and y' is the dependent

* Material from *Statistics in Biology*, Vol. 3, copyrighted by the McGraw-Hill Book Co., New York.

variate, or response, in its initial form. In comparison with the response the dose may be considered free from random error. When the equation is solved in the same units y as the initial response y', so that y' equals y, the hyperbola may be converted to a straight line having the form

$$Y = y_0 + \frac{x_0' y_0 + c}{x' - x_0'} = a' + b\frac{1}{x' + d} = a' + bx \qquad (2)$$

where d is equal to $-x_0'$. Since this equation is nonlinear in its parameters, its solution is indirect or stepwise (Bliss and James, 1966).

2. Estimation from a single series

In Table 3 of Chapter 23 a dose–response curve was determined on 25 November 1966 with ten replicates at ten dose levels ranging from 1.0 to 50.0 mIU of the Second International Reference Preparation for Human Menopausal Gonadotrophin. The initial response in counts per minute above a nonspecific, or background, count N was transformed by the equipment at the National Cancer Institute directly to the ratio of counts of bound hormone to total counts, B/B_0, with a range of 0 to 100%. For direct analysis the responses have been transformed back to y, in counts per minute above the mean background count of $N = 632$, by multiplying each ratio B/B_0 by the counts of bound hormone in excess of N in the absence of antibody: $(B_0 - N)/100 = 57.388$. The means $\bar{y}$ of the ten replicate counts at each dose level ranged from 1,370 to 5,209 c/min, as listed in the second column of Table 1. If the counts in each mean differed

TABLE 1   Mean Responses to Ten Dosage Levels of Human Luteinizing Hormone from the Counts per Minute above the Background Count (from Table 3 of Chapter 23)

Dose x', mIU	$y = $ c/min			$z = \sqrt{c/min}$		
	$\bar{y}$	$\sum (y - \bar{y})^2/9$	Y	$\bar{z}$	$\sum (z - \bar{z})^2$	Z
1.0	5,209.1	6,298.9	5,154.6	72.172	2.7288	71.702
2.0	4,900.9	19,918.6	4,878.9	70.002	9.1416	69.843
3.0	4,584.2	7,857.9	4,631.3	67.703	3.8238	68.106
4.0	4,355.7	4,396.2	4,407.5	65.995	2.2885	66.480
5.0	4,178.4	9,980.4	4,204.4	64.638	5.3678	64.954
10.0	3,485.7	12,265.3	3,417.1	59.034	7.8780	58.555
20.0	2,467.7	402.2	2,486.0	49.676	0.3712	49.815
30.0	1,954.6	2,477.4	1,953.7	44.209	2.8465	44.125
40.0	1,624.7	693.2	1,609.1	40.303	0.9518	40.126
50.0	1,370.4	1,125.3	1,367.9	37.019	1.8651	37.162

$Y = 912.848 \times 100/(x' + 16.7)$; $Z = 17.2133 + 15.4204 \times 100/(x' + 27.3)$.

solely by random variation, they would be Poisson variates with an expected variance equal to the mean. This could be tested by computing χ^2 from the observed variances, $\sum (y - \bar{y})^2/9$, in Table 1. At seven of the ten doses the variation between replicates agreed satisfactorily with their Poisson expectations ($\chi^2 = 59.57$, 63 DF) but at doses of 2, 5, and 10 mIU the variation was excessive ($\chi^2 = 89.59$, 27 DF), an excess that could not be traced to any obvious outlier. On the assumption that the variation was predominantly Poisson, despite these discrepancies, two approaches may be considered.

Analysis in units of $z = \sqrt{c/min}$

One approach is to transform each reading to $z = \sqrt{c/min}$, which equalizes the variance of a Poisson or Poisson-type count, as is evident from the sums of squares in terms of z (column 6 in Table 1), with the three exceptions noted above. The three-parameter hyperbola in Equation 2 may then be computed without weighting. Its parameter d is estimated first; each observed dose x' is then transformed to

$$x = \frac{100}{x' + d}$$

and a linear regression of the mean responses $\bar{z}$ on x (column 5 in Table 1) is computed by least squares. The necessary equations from Bliss and James (1966) are summarized in the Appendix.

For a preliminary estimate of d the means $\bar{z}$ were plotted against the log dose of hormone and fitted by eye with a smooth curve (Figure 1), from which interpolated values (Table A1 of the Appendix) gave $d_0 = 20.7$. With trial values of d_i equal to 20, 24, 28, and 32 a provisional x was then computed for each dose (Table A2), and with the x's for each d_i a provisional regression equation of $\bar{z}$ on x was computed. The objective was to determine from the scatter of the $\bar{z}$'s about these four regressions the d_m which would minimize the scatter. For each regression the standard deviation $\bar{s}$, the square root of the scatter mean square, has been plotted against its d_i and fitted in Figure 2 (the upper curve) with a parabola from which d_i giving the minimal $\bar{s}$ could be estimated, in the present case at $d_m = 27.3$. The hyperbola in Equation 2 was the regression of $\bar{z}$ on $x = 100/(x' + d_m)$, with the estimated parameters a' and b in

$$Z = 17.2133 + 15.4204 \left(\frac{100}{x' + 27.3} \right) = 17.2133 + 15.4204x$$

as plotted with the mean responses $\bar{z}$ in the left side of Figure 3.

Agreement with the rectangular hyperbola in units of $z = \sqrt{c/min}$ may be measured by the ratio of the mean square for scatter to that

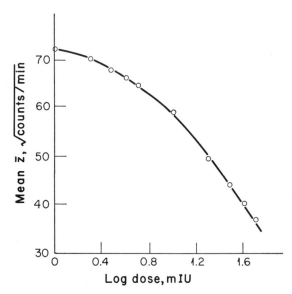

FIGURE 1   Freehand fit to the log dose of the mean square root of the counts per minute.

within doses. Even though the mean square between replicates within doses, 0.4140 with 90 DF, exceeded its Poisson expectation of 0.25, the mean square for scatter about the hyperbola with 7 DF was significantly larger, giving $F = 1.5091/0.4140 = 3.65$ ($P < 0.005$). Hence, this scatter mean square $\bar{s}^2$ would be the error variance for computing the standard error of each of the three statistics of the hyperbola.

Analysis in units of $y = $ c/min

Alternatively, a rectangular hyperbola may be fitted directly to the means $\bar{y}$ for counts per minute in column 2 of Table 1. In units of counts of bound hormone per minute a zero response would be expected when the dose x' of the unlabeled hormone under test was so large relative to the level of tracer that its reciprocal was effectively zero. If the true value of the intercept a' were zero, Equation 2 would reduce to a two-parameter hyperbola with a forced zero intercept:

$$Y = c\left(\frac{1}{x' - x_0'}\right) = b_0\left(\frac{1}{x' + d}\right) = b_0 x \tag{3}$$

When a hyperbola reduces to these two parameters, it can be solved directly for a provisional estimate d_0 of the parameter d. The original doses x' are plotted against $1/y$ and fitted by eye with the straight line

$$x' = -d_0 + b_0(1/y)$$

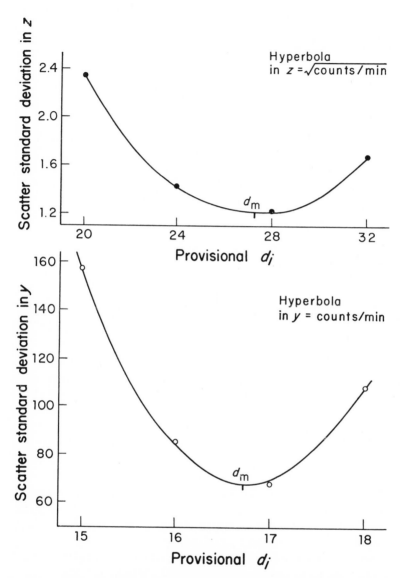

FIGURE 2 Estimation of the d_m giving a minimal standard deviation from parabolas relating the scatter standard deviation $\tilde{s}$ to d_i in hyperbolæ for y and z.

as in Figure 4 for the data in Table 1. Interpolating $10^4/\bar{y}$ equal to 1.85 and 7.25 from this line at an x' of 0 and 50 gives a d_0 of $1.85 \times 50/(7.25 - 1.85) = 17.13$. Each observed dose x' of hormone was then transformed as before (with trial values of d_i equal to 15, 16, 17, and 18) to the four trial series of the independent variate x (Table A3).

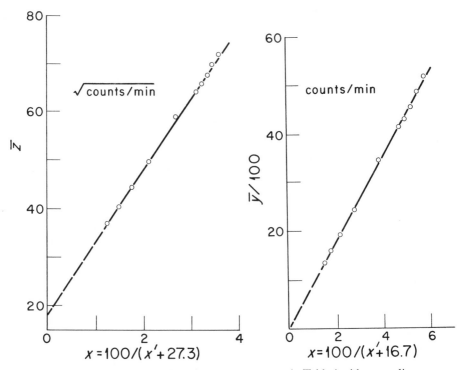

FIGURE 3   Two solutions of the dose–response curve in Table 1 with ten replicates at each dose.

Since the counts per minute were predominantly Poisson variates, fitting a regression of $\bar{y}$ upon each series of transformed doses x required weighting the $\bar{y}$'s by the inverse of their expected variances, $1/\sigma^2$, to adjust approximately for the increasing variability in $\bar{y}$ as x increased. With $\sigma^2 = \eta x$ at each x, the slope of a weighted least-squares regression with a zero intercept reduces to the ratio of the two totals, $\sum T_t$ and $f \sum x$ in Equation A10, the σ^2 and η canceling out (here f is the number of tubes at each dose level and is constant). A parallel weighting was required in Equation A12 for computing the scatter variance $\tilde{s}^2$ about each trial regression. The standard deviations $\tilde{s}$ have been plotted against the trial d_i's in the lower part of Figure 2 and fitted with a parabola, as in the upper curve. The estimate of d giving a minimal scatter standard deviation $\tilde{s}$ was $d_m = 16.7$. The resulting hyperbola with a zero intercept,

$$Y = 912.848 \left(\frac{100}{x' + 16.7} \right) = 912.848x$$

has been plotted with the observed means in the right side of Figure 3.

Estimates of its precision may be computed with the scatter variance $\tilde{s}^2 = 4{,}364.8$ with 8 DF.

3. Curves replicated in time

Table 1 in Chapter 23 gives the percentage response to thirteen different doses of the human luteinizing hormone from ten assays over an eight-week period. The dose levels ranged from 100 mIU in undiluted stock solution to 0.4 mIU, prepared with three 1:10 dilutions of stock to 40.0, 4.0, and 0.4 mIU. Before and after each dilution its accuracy was tested with duplicate tubes, giving four responses at each of these concentrations.

If each response were to be transformed from percentages to counts per minute, from u to y, it would be multiplied by $(B_0 - N)/100$, which ranged between assays from 26.51 to 86.10. In counts per minute the slopes of the computed hyperbolæ varied over an equivalent range. The initial transformation to a percentage scale has placed a ceiling of $u = 100\%$ upon the response for $x' = 0$ and $x = 100/d$ and a floor of $u = 0\%$ for $x' \approx \infty$ and $x = 0$, giving an anticipated slope of $\tilde{b}_0 = (100-0\%)/(100/d) = d$, as Rodbard et al. noted. For greater stability between curves the response in percentages may be retained, but each

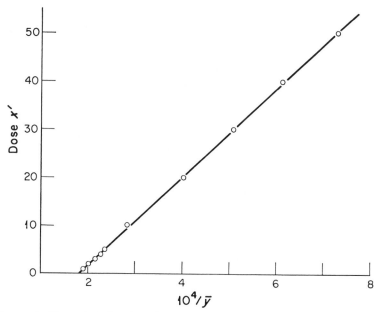

FIGURE 4   Dose plotted against the inverse of the mean response $\bar{y} = c/min$, for estimating d_0 in a rectangular hyperbola with a zero intercept.

curve is analyzed as a hyperbola with a zero intercept and weighted, as in the preceding section, for a Poisson-type response. The variance between the four replicate tubes within each assay at doses of 40.0, 4.0, and 0.4 mIU supported this approach, since over the ten assays their respective means of 26.5, 75.2, and 96.2 percent bound had increasing variances of $s^2 = 1.69$, 2.28, and 2.67 with 30 DF.

Like the replicate tubes of the preceding section, the duplicate counts before and after each dilution of stock have been tested in counts per minute for random variation, as defined by the Poisson distribution, giving $\chi^2 = 97.52$ (60 DF, $P = 0.001$). They still included an additional component when χ^2 was computed without the two most divergent pairs of tubes ($\chi^2 = 76.89$ for 58 DF, $P = 0.05$). The percentage readings from the two tubes before and after each dilution of test solution were then averaged and their means handled as single determinations, giving sixteen responses for each assay.

The doses x' and means $\bar{u}$ from the response totals T_t for the ten assays are listed in Table 2. For a starting point in estimating d the doses x' were plotted against $100/\bar{u}_i$ and fitted by eye with a straight line, from which interpolated values gave $d_0 = 14.54$. For an estimate of the d_m that would minimize the standard deviation $\tilde{s}$ for these means, and also

TABLE 2   Mean Dose–Response Curve in Terms of Mean Percent Response $\bar{u}_i$ from Ten Assays of Human Luteinizing Hormone (from Table 1 of Chapter 23)

Dose x', mIU	Mean resp. $\bar{u}_i = T_t/10$	$100/\bar{u}_i$	$x =$ $100/(x' + 14.9)$
0.4	96.08	1.04	6.54
	96.39	1.04	6.54
0.5	94.62	1.06	6.49
1.0	91.75	1.09	6.29
2.0	84.86	1.18	5.92
3.0	79.35	1.26	5.59
4.0	74.85	1.34	5.29
	75.54	1.32	5.29
5.0	72.48	1.38	5.03
10.0	59.68	1.68	4.02
20.0	42.96	2.33	2.87
30.0	32.63	3.06	2.23
40.0	26.13	3.83	1.82
	26.87	3.72	1.82
50.0	21.91	4.56	1.54
100.0	11.99	8.34	0.87
Total:	988.09		68.15

for each component assay, trial series of $x = 100/(x' + d_i)$ were computed with d_i from 10.5 to 21.0, spaced at intervals of $i_* = 1.5$. Starting with x for $d_i = 15.0$, the variance $\tilde{s}^2$ about the weighted regression of u upon x was determined with the responses u in each assay and with their means $\bar{u}$, continuing with additional trial values, until these bracketed a minimal $\tilde{s}^2$, and the d_m in Table 3 could be computed for each assay. The percentage responses in the assays with the largest and smallest d_m (assays 3 and 7) have been plotted in Figure 5 against their respective dose metameters x, together with the means for all ten assays as the center curve.

The estimated slopes b_0 of the percentage u of bound hormone upon the dose x transformed with the d_m for each assay have been calculated in Table 3 together with their standard errors. In addition, the variances $\tilde{s}^2$ are shown in Table 3. The assay in Table 1 recomputed in units of u and x has been added to the table. A plot of b_0 versus d_m in Figure 6 has been fitted with the regression $b_0 = 0.27846 + 0.95467 d_\mathrm{m}$, each estimate being weighted equally. The near-unity slope of this regression, with a squared correlation coefficient of 0.98, supports the suggestion of an obligatory relation between these two statistics when the response is in units u of the percentage bound. However, even if both d_m and b_0 were estimates of a single parameter, the difference of 0.40 between their means in these eleven assays indicates that, as calculated here, the relation is still a two-parameter hyperbola.

TABLE 3   Regressions of Percent Response u upon the Transformed Dose x for d_m in Each of Ten Assays for Human Luteinizing Hormone (from Table 1 of Chapter 23) and for the Assay in Table 1

Assay no.	Date, 1966	$\bar{u}$	$d_\mathrm{m} \pm \mathrm{SE}(d_\mathrm{m})$	$\bar{x}$ for d_m	$b_0 \pm \mathrm{SE}(b_0)$	$\tilde{s}^2$, 14 DF
1	10/4	61.25	13.59 ± 0.18	4.57	13.41 ± 0.12	1.05
2	10/5	59.87	13.37 ± 0.18	4.62	12.93 ± 0.11	0.96
3	10/7	64.24	19.17 ± 0.26	3.49	18.40 ± 0.15	1.24
4	10/7	59.33	13.03 ± 0.26	4.73	12.54 ± 0.11	0.91
5	11/15	64.18	15.59 ± 0.10	4.11	15.62 ± 0.09	0.58
6	11/15	63.03	14.59 ± 0.22	4.33	14.57 ± 0.10	0.72
7	11/17	58.74	12.70 ± 0.12	4.81	12.20 ± 0.11	0.85
8	11/17	60.10	13.82 ± 0.26	4.52	13.30 ± 0.12	1.11
9	11/28	63.17	16.47 ± 0.14	3.93	16.06 ± 0.10	0.61
10	11/28	63.66	16.54 ± 0.32	3.93	16.18 ± 0.15	1.35
Mean:		61.76	14.87 ± 0.08	4.26	14.50 ± 0.07	0.30
Table 1*:	11/25	59.48	16.72 ± 0.05	3.73	15.93 ± 0.06	0.13†

* From Table 1 recomputed in units of percent bound.   † 8 DF.

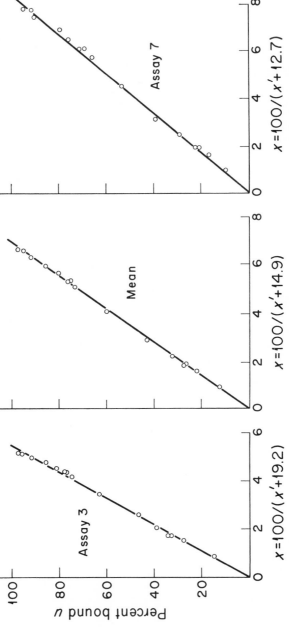

FIGURE 5 Rectangular hyperbolæ in units of percent bound u and the transformed dose x for the mean (Table 2) of ten assays and for the component assays with the largest and smallest d_m (Table 3).

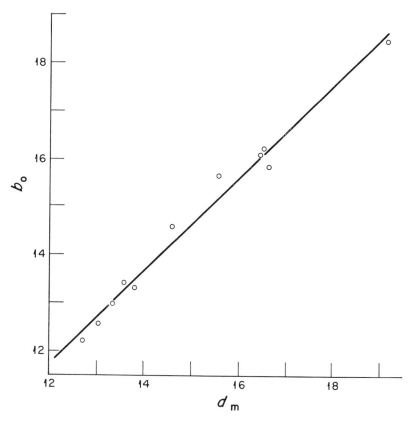

FIGURE 6   Relation between the statistics d_m and the slope b_0 of rectangular hyperbolæ with a zero intercept, in units of u from Table 3.

4. Estimation of relative potency

This analysis of assays for human luteinizing hormone shows that the two-parameter rectangular hyperbola with a zero intercept provides a relatively simple and effective description of its dose–response curve. When a test sample or unknown is to be assayed, and the dose is expressed in units of $1/(x' + d)$ or $100/(x' + d)$ with an intercept at $x = 0$, the assay is a slope-ratio one. The potency is computed from the ratio of two slopes b_0, one for the unknown (b_U) and the other for the standard (b_S) as

$$P = b_U/b_S \tag{4}$$

A slope factor may be computed for the standard curve as

$$C = b_S^2/(b_S^2 - \tilde{s}^2 t^2/f \textstyle\sum x) \tag{5}$$

With a single error variance $\tilde{s}^2$, applying to both the standard and the unknown, the confidence interval for a slope-ratio assay (Bliss and White, 1967) may be computed as

$$X'_L = CP \pm \sqrt{(C - 1)(CP^2 + N_S/N_U)} \tag{6}$$

where N_S and N_U are the number of observations on the standard and on the unknown, respectively.

Since the intercept is zero, and each slope is estimated, by Equation A10, from the simple ratio $b_0 = \sum u / \sum x$, then P and its precision may be determined by the same equations from a single dose level of the unknown ($N_U = 1$) and the standard curve.

If the three forms of the rectangular hyperbola that have been fitted to the present data are compared, it appears that the equation in terms of the percent bound (u) and a forced zero intercept is perhaps the simplest to compute and the most adaptable to methods of quality control.

APPENDIX

Fitting the three-parameter rectangular hyperbola with the response $z = \sqrt{c/min}$

Initial estimate of d   For an initial estimate of d the values of z or $\tilde{z}$ may be plotted against the k values of log x' and fitted graphically with a smooth curve as in Figure 1. At three equally and widely spaced levels of log x'_1, log x'_2, and log x'_3, the corresponding values of z_1, z_2, and z_3 are interpolated from the curve, and the three log doses are transformed to their antilogarithms x'. From the ratio

$$h = \frac{x'_3 - x'_2}{x'_2 - x'_1} \tag{A1}$$

an initial estimate of d may be computed as

$$d_0 = \frac{hx'_1 z_1 - (h + 1)x'_2 z_2 + x'_3 z_3}{(h + 1)z_2 - hz_1 - z_3} \tag{A2}$$

For the data in Table 1 two sets of overlapping values have been interpolated from this curve (see Table A1) for computing d_0 by means of Equations A1 and A2. The d_0 average, $\bar{d}_0$, is 20.70.

Improved estimate of d   The initial estimate of the statistic d, with which the doses are transformed to $x = 100/(x' + d)$, can be improved by a simple adjustment. For each of several values of d_i the slope of the response z upon the transformed dose x is computed by least squares and then the standard deviation $\tilde{s}$ for the scatter in z about each line. The required value of d is that for which $\tilde{s}$ is a minimum. For the data in

TABLE A1 Estimation of d_0 by Interpolation from the Curve in Figure 1 Fitted to the Means of $z = \sqrt{c/min}$

	$i = 1$	$i = 2$	$i = 3$	$i = 1$	$i = 2$	$i = 3$
Log x_i	0.2	0.8	1.4	0.3	0.9	1.5
x_i'	1.585	6.310	25.12	1.995	7.943	31.62
z_i	71.0	62.7	47.2	70.2	60.7	43.7
d_0, Eq. A2		19.21			22.20	

Here h is 3.981, Equation A1.

Table 1 the values of x have been computed in Table A2 with trial values of d_i equal to 20, 24, 28, and 32, spaced at equal intervals.

For each d_i the sum of squares with 2 DF for the slope of z upon k levels of x, with f constant at each x, is

$$B^2 = \frac{\{\sum x T_t - \sum x \sum T_t/k\}^2}{f\{\sum x^2 - (\sum x)^2/k\}} = \frac{[xT_t]^2}{f[x^2]} \tag{A3}$$

where T_t is the total response for each dose, and the terms in square brackets are sums of squares or products of the variates they enclose, measured from their respective means. The sum of squares of the treatment totals around their mean, in units of a single z,

$$[T_t^2] = \frac{\sum T_t^2}{f} - \frac{(\sum T_t)^2}{fk} \tag{A4}$$

is diminished by the sum of squares for slope, giving the variance, or mean square, for scatter as

$$\tilde{s}^2 = \frac{[T_t^2] - B^2}{k - 3} \tag{A5}$$

These estimates for each d_i are shown in the lower part of Table A2. From the square root of each $\tilde{s}^2$ the standard deviations $\tilde{s}$ in the last column bracketed the d_i giving a minimal scatter.[1]

The value of d_i at which $\tilde{s}$ is a minimum is an improved estimate of the statistic d. From the parabola relating $\tilde{s}$ to d_i,

$$\tilde{s} = a' + b_1 d_i + b_2 d_i^2 \tag{A6}$$

the minimal $\tilde{s}$ occurs at $d_m = -b_1/2b_2$. From four trial values of d_i, averaging $\bar{d}_i$ and spaced at equal intervals of length i_*, the d_m can be calculated more directly by replacing b_1 and b_2 with their numerators

[1] Suggested by Professor D. V. Lindley.

TABLE A2 Dose–Response Curve in $z = \sqrt{c/min}$ for Human Luteinizing Hormone as a Rectangular Hyperbola (from Table 3, Chapter 23)

Dose x', mIU	Total resp. T_t	$x = 100/(x' + d_i)$ for d_i equal to:				
		20.0	24.0	28.0	32.0	27.3
1.0	721.72	4.76	4.00	3.45	3.03	3.53
2.0	700.02	4.55	3.85	3.33	2.94	3.41
3.0	677.03	4.35	3.70	3.23	2.86	3.30
4.0	659.95	4.17	3.57	3.12	2.78	3.19
5.0	646.38	4.00	3.45	3.03	2.70	3.10
10.0	590.34	3.33	2.94	2.63	2.38	2.68
20.0	496.76	2.50	2.27	2.08	1.92	2.11
30.0	442.09	2.00	1.85	1.72	1.61	1.75
40.0	403.03	1.67	1.56	1.47	1.39	1.49
50.0	370.19	1.43	1.35	1.28	1.22	1.29
Total:	5,707.51	32.76	28.54	25.34	22.83	25.85

$[T_t^2] = 15,524.0645$ (9 DF), $f = 10$, $k = 10$.

d_i	$[x^2]$	$[xT_t]$	B^2, 2 DF	Scatter SS	$\tilde{s}^2$, 7 DF	$\tilde{s}$
20	14.52244	1,499.61144	15,485.2385	38.8260	5.5466	2.3551
24	9.18184	1,193.36156	15,510.0918	13.9727	1.9961	1.4128
28	6.12904	975.09966	15,513.3487	10.7158	1.5308	1.2373
32	4.26501	813.21467	15,505.6635	18.4010	2.6287	1.6213
27.3	6.52405	1,006.03605	15,513.5006	10.5639	1.5091	1.2285

$d_m = 26 - 4(- 2.3769)/(5 \times 1.3263) = 27.3$, Equation A7;
$b = 1,006.03605/(10 \times 6.52405) = 15.4204$; $a' = 57.0751 - 2.5850b = 17.2134$.

computed with the orthogonal coefficients x_1 equal to -3, -1, 1, and 3, and x_2 equal to 1, -1, -1, and 1, giving

$$d_m = \bar{d}_i - \frac{i_* \sum (x_1 \tilde{s})}{5 \sum (x_2 \tilde{s})} \tag{A7}$$

If the minimal standard deviation $\tilde{s}$ is bracketed more or less symmetrically with only three trial values of d_i, the orthogonal coefficients are x_1 equal to -1, 0, and 1, and x_2 equal to 1, -2, and 1, giving

$$d_m = \bar{d}_i - \frac{i_* \sum (x_1 \tilde{s})}{2 \sum (x_2 \tilde{s})} \tag{A8}$$

If five trial values of d_i are required, the orthogonal coefficients are x_1 equal to -2, -1, 0, 1, and 2, and x_2 equal to 2, -1, -2, -1, and 2, giving

$$d_m = \bar{d}_i - \frac{7i_* \sum (x_1 \tilde{s})}{10 \sum (x_2 \tilde{s})} \tag{A9}$$

As shown at the foot of Table A2, a d_m of 27.3 is the improved estimate in the present example for fitting a rectangular hyperbola with the variate $z = \sqrt{c/min}$, giving the values of x in the last column of that table.

Fitting a two-parameter rectangular hyperbola with the response $y = c/min$

Fitting the regression of $y = c/min$ on x as if the counts per minute were Poisson variates would adjust approximately for unequal variability at the different dosage levels. With a nearly fourfold range in the $\bar{y}$'s in Table A3 and, accordingly, in the expected variance of the mean at each dose, each mean response would be weighted by the reciprocal of its expected variance σ^2 in computation of the regression. When $\bar{y}$ increases linearly with the independent variate x, its expected variance as a Poisson type of variable is $\sigma^2 = \eta x$ at any given x. The slope b_0 of a

TABLE A3 Dose–Response Curve in $y = c/min$ for Human Luteinizing Hormone as a Rectangular Hyperbola with a Zero Intercept (from Table 3, Chapter 23)

Dose x', mIU	Total response T_t	$10^4/\bar{y}_i$	$x = 100/(x' + d_i)$ for d_i equal to:				
			15.0	16.0	17.0	18.0	16.7
1.0	52,091	1.92	6.25	5.88	5.56	5.26	5.65
2.0	49,009	2.04	5.88	5.56	5.26	5.00	5.35
3.0	45,842	2.18	5.56	5.26	5.00	4.76	5.08
4.0	43,557	2.30	5.26	5.00	4.76	4.55	4.83
5.0	41,784	2.39	5.00	4.76	4.55	4.35	4.61
10.0	34,857	2.87	4.00	3.85	3.70	3.57	3.75
20.0	24,677	4.05	2.86	2.78	2.70	2.63	2.72
30.0	19,546	5.12	2.22	2.17	2.13	2.08	2.14
40.0	16,247	6.15	1.82	1.79	1.75	1.72	1.76
50.0	13,704	7.30	1.54	1.52	1.49	1.47	1.50
Total:	341,314	36.32	40.39	38.57	36.90	35.39	37.39

d_i	$\sum (T_t^2/fx)$, 10 DF	B_0^2, 2 DF	Scatter SS	$\tilde{s}^2$, 8 DF	$\tilde{s}$
15.0	288,622,189.69	288,425,963.35	196,226.34	24,528.29	156.615
16.0	302,093,182.84	302,035,899.91	57,282.93	7,160.37	84.619
17.0	315,741,419.67	315,705,275.33	36,144.34	4,518.04	67.216
18.0	329,284,112.47	329,175,604.96	108,507.51	13,563.44	116.462
16.7	311,599,688.87	311,567,923.50	31,765.37	3,970.67	63.013

$d_m = 16.5 - (-137.862)/(5 \times 121.242) = 16.727;$ $b_0 = 341,314/(10 \times 37.39)$
$= 912.848.$

weighted least-squares regression with a zero intercept then reduces to the ratio

$$b_0 = \frac{\sum y}{\sum x} = \frac{\sum T_t}{f \sum x} \tag{A10}$$

when the number of tubes, f, at each dose level is constant. The sum of squares due to this regression with 2 DF, which is due to the estimated d in $x = 100/(x' + d_i)$, is

$$B_0^2 = \frac{(\sum y)^2}{\sum x} = \frac{(\sum T_t)^2}{f \sum x} \tag{A11}$$

The variance of the scatter of the k means about the regression computed with x for a given d_i is

$$\tilde{s}^2 = \frac{\sum (y^2/x) - B_0^2}{k - 2} = \frac{\sum (T_t^2/fx) - B_0^2}{k - 2} \tag{A12}$$

from which the variance of the slope b_0 is

$$V(b_0) = \frac{\tilde{s}^2}{\sum x} \quad \text{or} \quad \frac{\tilde{s}^2}{f \sum x} \tag{A13}$$

Improved estimates of the rectangular hyperbola

Two possible improvements in estimating the rectangular hyperbola may be noted, both minor. One would fit a weighted three-parameter hyperbola to the counts per minute and with its intercept adjust the background count based upon the negative control tubes with the additional evidence from known concentrations of hormone. For the data in Table 1 the background count would be adjusted to $\bar{N} = 632 + 39.3 = 671.3$. The two-parameter hyperbola with this adjustment in $\bar{N}$ would be

$$Y = 886.919[100/(x' + 16.3)]$$

As a second adjustment, the hyperbola in terms either of $z = \sqrt{c/min}$ or of $y = c/min$ can be corrected by means of maximum likelihood. Maximum-likelihood corrections in the present series changed none of the estimated parameters by more than a small fraction of their standard errors.

The variance of d_m in the two-parameter hyperbola

In the computations of d_m for each assay in Table 3 the d_i ranged from 10.5 to 15.0 for assay 7 and from 16.5 to 21.0 for assay 3, both requiring four sets of doses for computing d_m as the minimum of a parabola with Equation A7. In the remaining assays d_m was estimated similarly by means of Equation A8 from three successive values of d_i. The error variances for d_m from these equations may be approximated with $\bar{s}^2$ for each assay, Equation A5, as

$$V(d_m) = \frac{\bar{s}^2[(d_m - \bar{d_i})^2 + 0.1875]}{19\,[\sum (x_2\bar{s})]^2} \quad \text{for } k = 3 \tag{A14}$$

$$V(d_m) = \frac{\bar{s}^2[(d_m - \bar{d_i})^2 + 0.45]}{28.5\,[\sum (x_2\bar{s})]^2} \quad \text{for } k = 4 \tag{A15}$$

The standard errors of the separate assays were somewhat larger for d_m than for the slope b_0.

CHAPTER TWENTY-FIVE

Discussion

EKINS It seems to me that a great deal of unnecessary trouble is incurred by statisticians attempting to cope with data expressed in terms of the bound-to-free ratio. As we pointed out in 1963 (Ekins and Samols, 1963), one frequently observes curves that approach or, indeed, sometimes achieve linearity if the results are plotted in terms of the free-to-bound ratio (see Figure 18, Chapter 19).

I should also like to ask whether the fitting of a rectangular hyperbola to bound-to-free ratios is the same as the fitting of a straight line to free-to-bound ratios.

MCHUGH I agree with the utility of empirical curve-fitting for certain problems. However, there are two main considerations that motivated us to use y as the proportion of total counts of bound hormone. First, statistically one is interested in examining a random variable with properties that behave in some way that can be modeled probabilistically. The bound-to-free ratio is a ratio of random variables. Both the numerator and denominator have a Poisson variation (at least in part), and there may be certain statistical difficulties in dealing with such ratios. Second, there are various criteria for deciding upon the most useful response measure. If, beyond curve-fitting, one asks about a calibration curve relationship that has both a theoretical deterministic basis (that is, it can be deduced from the mass-action phenomenon of immunochemistry) and stochastic variability (that is, the experimental error and Poisson variability of counting), then one would attack the problem somewhat as we have. The statistician would first try to identify those quantities which are random variables, observable or unobservable (which I have denoted by y and e), then those which are under the direct control of the experimenter (which I have denoted by x), and finally those which need to be estimated (the parameters θ). There is no intent on our part to "hunt sparrows with an elephant gun." However, the advantage of our approach is that eventually a rational basis for experimental design can be developed. That is, if one is able to say, for example, that the variance is an explicit function of certain parameters, such as the equilibrium constant θ_2, then it should be possible to examine the behavior of the variance as one varies these parameters.

RODBARD In Dr. Bliss's model we would expect that the y intercept would be zero, because the bound-to-free or bound-to-total ratio approaches zero asymptotically as the transformed variable $x = 100/(x' + d)$ approaches zero, corresponding to there being an infinite amount of unlabeled hormone, x', present. In theory this would apply, irrespective of the nature of the antibody, even in the case of multivalency and/or heterogeneity. In practice the intercept may not be zero, owing to random errors in the estimate of the value of N, the nonspecific background counts per minute, which has been defined as our zero level for the ordinate. If we overestimate or underestimate N, then the best fit will have an intercept that is slightly different from zero. A large error in N could result in a significant departure from the rectangular hyperbola model.

When the intercept is zero, then Dr. Bliss's model becomes similar to (but not identical with) the use of linear regression for a plot of the total-to-bound ratio versus the arithmetic dose. The former is the case of $y = B/T = k_1/(x + k_2)$; the latter, of $1/y = T/B = c_1 x + c_2$. These are algebraically interconvertible. However, in practice the results from the two models may differ considerably, owing to an error in the estimation of N with a nonzero intercept or to the two models' making different implicit assumptions about the nature of the distributions of the variables and assigning different weights to different portions of the curve, or to both.

SMITH   With respect to the fitted function on p. 407, Dr. Ekins' point is well taken, because the fit is not very good. If one is interested in fitting that set of data, the inverse relationship fits almost perfectly. However, I understand that your concern is not solely with prediction.

MCHUGH   I agree that either a free-hand or empirical fitting of an observed dose–response curve for an estimate of potency is warranted in a routine laboratory situation. However, if one is concerned with a mathematical approach to the design problem in immunoassay, then the method we have employed may be superior. Dr. Frederick Goetz at the University of Minnesota approached us because of his interest in design and in the sources of variability. Moreover, the concepts of sensitivity and precision enunciated by Dr. Ekins and Dr. O'Riordan are both oriented around experimental design.

Consider an empirical fit such as the logistic one. It involves two parameters that may have little relevance to experimental design. A formulation in which the parameters have meaning in immunochemical terms is of interest to the endocrinologist. Even if the fitting of our model to experimental data provides poor or only fair results, the underlying mass-action aspect is fundamental. Our model corresponds to a univalent antigen with a single order of antibody combining sites.

Since the assumption of a single order of antibody combining sites is reasonable only in certain situations and it is thought that two orders may be more reasonable, we have extended our approach to a more complicated model. When one considers univalent antigen and two orders of antibody combining site, things get fairly complicated. At present we have not developed this model into a usable form, nor have we explored its implications for design.

MEINERT   We were interested in the derivation of a model that has a theoretical basis and also provides a satisfactory fit of the observed data. The parameters of our model have specific physical interpretations and, hence, provide a basis for the design of subsequent assays. The model can be used by the investigator for selecting the labeled antigen and antibody concentrations that are optimal for the range of standards employed. While it may be possible to fit the data given here equally well with some empirical curve, such an approach is not as useful from a design point of view.

COX   Do Dr. McHugh and Dr. Meinert have any replicate observations at the various concentrations? The agreement between such observations with what Dr. Bliss calls "scatter" is a good criterion for examining the effectiveness of the fit. A relatively poor fit with good biological explanation may be better than a close empirical fit which merely describes (I prefer to think of "description" rather than "prediction" in this context) the data in the local regions of the investigation but is weak when it comes to extrapolation outside that region. The well-known dangers of extrapolation from polynomial fits illustrate this point.

I should like to ask Dr. Bliss about his lack-of-fit tests. If I were testing for lack of fit, I would divide the mean square for scatter by the mean square for within replicates.

Finally, Dr. Bliss stated that if these lines have zero intercepts, a slope-ratio assay is obtained. It should be noted that taking logs gives a parallel-line assay and, further, if the intercept is zero, the parallel lines have unit slope.

BLISS   With respect to the mean square for replicates and for scatter, I looked upon the scatter as being the relevant term for estimating the error of these particular lines. It seemed to me that replicates of the same dose have less chance of variation than those in which dilution errors may arise.

The rectangular hyperbola is theoretically the correct curve in the Michaelis-Menten relation. The biochemists at the Connecticut Agricultural Experiment Station have found this procedure to constitute an improvement over other methods of fitting the Michaelis-Menten constant and related mass-action laws. In applying the same form of the rectangular hyperbola here, we are not becoming entirely empirical. As to the implication that unless one fits the relation as a curve that contains all of the theoretical inferences, the estimate is not satisfactory, I disagree.

ROSS   It appears to me that the approaches of Drs. McHugh, Meinert, Ekins, and O'Riordan, while neither simplifying the estimation of the error of a potency estimate nor facilitating interpolation from a dose–response curve, have two advantages: they permit examination of the effects of variation in the several components that enter into immuno-assay procedure, and they provide a secure framework for further research, being grounded not in the vagaries of particular experiments but in the rational constructs of immunochemistry.

References

Albert, A., D. Bennett, G. Carl, E. Rosemberg, P. Keller, and W. B. Lewis, 1965, "Assay characteristics of tannate complexes of human chorionic gonadotropin," *Endocrinology*, **76**:499.

Albert, A., and J. Berkson, 1951, "A clinical bio-assay for chorionic gonadotropin," *J. Clin. Endocr.*, **11**:805.

Althabe, O., Jr., I. C. Arnt, L. A. Branda, and R. Caldeyro-Barcia, 1966, "Comparison of the milk-ejecting potencies of oxytocin and deaminooxytocin in lactating women," *J. Endocr.*, **36**:7.

Anscombe, F. J., 1954, "Comments on 'The analysis of variance with various binomial transformations' by Sir Ronald Fisher," *Biometrics*, **10**:141.

Anscombe, F. J., 1960, "Rejection of outliers," *Technometrics*, **2**:123.

Anscombe, F. J., 1963, "Sequential medical trials," *J. Amer. Statist. Ass.*, **58**:365.

Anscombe, F. J., and J. W. Tukey, 1963, "The examination and analysis of residuals," *Technometrics*, **5**:141.

Armitage, P., 1960, *Sequential Medical Trials*, Blackwell Scientific Publications, Oxford, England, and Charles C. Thomas, Springfield, Illinois.

Armitage, P., and I. Allen, 1950, "Methods of estimating the L.D.50 in quantal response data," *J. Hyg.* (Cambridge), **48**:298.

Baird, D., R. Horton, C. Longcope, and J. F. Tait, 1968, "Steroid prehormones," *Perspect. Biol. Med.*, **11**:384.

Bangham, D. R., M. V. Mussett, and M. P. Stack-Dunne, 1962, "The third international standard for corticotrophin," *Bull. Wld. Hlth. Org.*, **27**:395.

Barakat, R. M., and R. P. Ekins, 1961, "Assay of vitamin B-12 in blood: a simple method," *Lancet*, **2**:25.

Bartee, T. C., 1966, *Digital Computer Fundamentals*, 2nd ed., McGraw-Hill, New York.

Bennett, C. A., and N. L. Franklin, 1954, *Statistical Analysis in Chemistry and the Chemical Industry*, Wiley, New York.

Berkson, J., 1955, "Maximum likelihood and minimum χ^2 estimates of the logistic function," *J. Amer. Statist. Ass.*, **50**:130.

Bernstein, J., 1963, *The Analytical Engine: Computers — Past, Present and Future*, Random House, New York.

Berson, S. A., 1957, in *Conference on Insulin Activity in Blood and Tissue Fluids: Résumé*, by R. Levine, and E. Anderson. National Institute of Arthritis and Metabolic Diseases, National Institutes of Health, Public Health Service, Department of Health, Education, and Welfare, Bethesda, Maryland, 1958.

Berson, S. A., and R. S. Yalow, 1957, "Kinetics of reaction between insulin and insulin-binding antibody," *J. Clin. Invest.*, **36**:873.

Berson, S. A., and R. S. Yalow, 1958, "Isotopic tracers in the study of diabetes," *Advances Biol. Med. Phys.*, **6**:349.

Berson, S. A., and R. S. Yalow, 1959a, "Recent studies on insulin-binding antibodies," *Ann. N.Y. Acad. Sci.*, **82**:338.

Berson, S. A., and R. S. Yalow, 1959b, "Quantitative aspects of the reaction between insulin and insulin-binding antibody," *J. Clin. Invest.*, **38**:1996.

Berson, S. A., and R. S. Yalow, 1959c, "Species-specificity of human anti-beef, pork insulin serum," *J. Clin. Invest.*, **38**:2017.

Berson, S. A., and R. S. Yalow, 1964, "Immunoassay of protein hormones," in *The Hormones*, vol. IV (G. Pincus, K. V. Thimann, and E. B. Astwood, Eds.), Academic Press, New York, ch. 11, p. 557.

Berson, S. A., and R. S. Yalow, 1966, "Insulin in blood and insulin antibodies," *Amer. J. Med.*, **40**:676.

Berson, S. A., and R. S. Yalow, 1968, "Principles of peptide hormones in plasma," in *Clinical Endocrinology II* (E. B. Astwood, and C. E. Cassidy, Eds.), Grune & Stratton, New York, p. 699.

Berson, S. A., and R. S. Yalow, 1969, "Recent advances in immunoassay of peptide hormones in plasma," in *Suppl. Proc. Int. Diabetes Fed. 6th Congr.* (J. Ostman, Ed.), Excerpta Medica Foundation, Amsterdam, p. 47.

Berson, S. A., R. S. Yalow, A. Bauman, M. A. Rothschild, and K. Newerly, 1956, "Insulin-I^{131} metabolism in human subjects: demonstration of insulin binding globulin in the circulation of insulin-treated subjects," *J. Clin. Invest.*, **35**:170.

Biggers, J. D., 1950, "Observations on the intravaginal assay of natural oestrogens using aqueous egg albumin as the vehicle of administration," *J. Endocr.*, **7**:163.

Bindon, B. M., and D. R. Lamond, 1966, "Diurnal component in the response by the mouse to gonadotrophin," *J. Reprod. Fertil.*, **12**:249.

Bliss, C. I., 1940, "Factorial design and covariance in the biological assay of vitamin D," *J. Amer. Statist. Ass.*, **35**:498.

Bliss, C. I., 1944, "The U.S.P. collaborative cat assays for digitalis," *J. Amer. Pharm. Ass.*, **33**:225.

Bliss, C. I., 1952, *The Statistics of Bioassay*, Academic Press, New York.

Bliss, C. I., 1956, "Analysis of the biological assays in USP XV," *Drug Stand.*, **24**:33.

Bliss, C. I., 1967, *Statistics in Biology*, vol. 1, McGraw-Hill, New York.

Bliss, C. I., and McK. Cattell, 1943, "Biological assay," *Ann. Rev. Physiol.*, **5**:479.

Bliss, C. I., and R. A. Fisher, 1953, "Fitting the negative binomial distribution to biological data" and "Note on the efficient fitting of the negative binomial," *Biometrics*, **9**:176.

Bliss, C. I., and A. T. James, 1966, "Fitting the rectangular hyperbola," *Biometrics*, **22**:573.

Bliss, C. I., and H. P. Marks, 1939, "The biological assay of insulin. I. Some general considerations directed to increasing the precision of the curve relating dosage and graded response," *Quart. J. Pharm.*, **12**:82.

Bliss, C. I., and A. R. G. Owen, 1958, "Negative binomial distributions with a common k," *Biometrika*, **45**:37.

Bliss, C. I., and C. L. Rose, 1940, "The assay of parathyroid extract from the serum calcium of dogs," *Amer. J. Hyg.*, **31**:A79.

Bliss, C. I., and C. White, 1967, "Statistical methods in biological assay of the vitamins," in *The Vitamins*, vol. VI (P. Gyorgy, and W. N. Pearson, Eds.), Academic Press, New York, ch. 2, p. 21.

Borth, R., B. Lunenfeld, and H. de Watteville, 1957, "Effect of serum used as a vehicle on the quantal assay of human chorionic gonadotrophin by the ovarian hyperaemia response in rats," *Acta Endocr.* (Kobenhavn), **24**:119.

Bradley, R., 1967, "Topics in rank-order statistics," in *Proc. 5th Berkeley Symp. Math. Statist. Prob.*, vol. 1 (L. M. Le Cam, and J. Neyman, Eds.), University of California Press, Berkeley, California, p. 593.

Bradley, T. R., and P. M. Clarke, 1956, "The response of rabbit mammary glands to locally administered prolactin," *J. Endocr.*, **14**:28.

British Pharmacopoeia, 1963, "Biological assay of heparin," Pharmaceutical Press, London, p. 1136.

Brodie, A. H., and J. F. Tait, 1969, "Assay of aldosterone and related compounds," in *Methods in Hormone Research*, 2nd ed., vol. 1 (R. Dorfman, Ed.), Academic Press, New York, p. 323.

Brodish, A., 1964, "Delayed secretion of ACTH in rats with hypothalamic lesions," *Endocrinology*, **74**:28.

Bross, I., 1950, "Estimates of the LD-50: a critique," *Biometrics*, **6**:413.

Brown, B. W., Jr., 1961, "Some properties of the Spearman estimator in bioassay," *Biometrika*, **48**:293.

Brown, B. W., Jr., 1966, "Planning a quantal assay of potency," *Biometrics*, **22**:322.

Brownlee, K. A., J. L. Hodges, Jr., and M. Rosenblatt, 1953, "The up-and-down method with small samples," *J. Amer. Statist. Ass.*, **48**:262.

Carlson, A., and G. Hannauer, 1964, *Handbook of Analog Computation*, Electronic Association, Princeton, New Jersey, p. 225.

Claringbold, P. J., 1955a, "Demonstration of a competition between bovine plasma albumin and the cells of the vaginal epithelium for oestrone," *J. Endocr.*, **12**:93.

Claringbold, P. J., 1955b, "A study of the individual median effective dose of oestrone in the ovariectomized mouse," *J. Endocr.*, **13**:11.

Claringbold, P. J., 1955c, "Use of the simplex design in the study of joint action of related hormones," *Biometrics*, **11**:174.

Claringbold, P. J., 1956, "The within-animal bioassay with quantal responses," *J. Roy. Statist. Soc. Ser. B*, **18**:133.

Claringbold, P. J., 1959, "Orthogonal contrasts in slope-ratio investigations," *Biometrics*, **15**:307.

Claringbold, P. J., J. D. Biggers, and C. W. Emmens, 1953, "The angular transformation in quantal analysis," *Biometrics*, **9**:467.

Claringbold, P. J., and D. R. Lamond, 1957, "Optimum conditions for the biological assay of gonadotrophins," *J. Endocr.*, **16**:86.

Clarke, P. M., 1955, "Nomograms for multiple slope-ratio assays arranged in blocks, and improved nomograms for assays without blocks," *Brit. J. Pharmacol.*, **10**:296.

Clarke, P. M., and Z. D. Hosking, 1953, "The graphical evaluation of simple and multiple slope-ratio assays," *J. Pharm. Pharmacol.*, **5**:586.

Cochran, W. G., 1940, "The analysis of variance when experimental errors follow the Poisson or binomial laws," *Ann. Math. Statist.*, **11**:335.

Cochran, W. G., 1941, "The distribution of the largest of a set of estimated variances as a fraction of their total," *Ann. Eugenics*, **11**:47.

Cochran, W. G., 1954, "Some methods for strengthening the common χ^2 tests," *Biometrics*, **10**:417.

Cochran, W. G., and G. M. Cox, 1957, *Experimental Designs*, 2nd ed., Wiley, New York, and Chapman and Hall, London.

Cochran, W., and M. Davis, 1965, "The Robbins-Monro method for estimating the median lethal dose," *J. Roy. Statist. Soc. Ser. B*, **27**:28.

Colton, T., 1963, "A model for selecting one of two medical treatments," *J. Amer. Statist. Ass.*, **58**:388.

Cornfield, J., 1964, "Comparative bioassays and the role of parallelism," *J. Pharmacol. Exp. Ther.*, **144**:143.

Cornfield, J., and J. W. Tukey, 1956, "Average values of mean squares in factorials," *Ann. Math. Statist.*, **27**:907.

Cox, C. P., 1967, "Statistical analysis of log-dose response bioassay experiments with unequal dose ratios for the standard and unknown preparations," *J. Pharm. Sci.*, **56**:359.

Cox, C. P., and P. E. Leaverton, 1966, "Statistical procedures for bioassays when the condition of similarity does not obtain," *J. Pharm. Sci.*, **55**:716.

Cox, C. P., and D. J. Ruhl, 1966, "Simplified computation of confidence intervals for relative potencies using Fieller's theorem," *J. Pharm. Sci.*, **55**:368.

Cox, D. R., 1958, *Planning of Experiments*, Wiley, New York, and Chapman and Hall, London.

Cramer, E. M., 1964, "Some comparisons of methods of fitting the dosage response curve for small samples," *J. Amer. Statist. Ass.*, **59**:779.

Daniel, C., 1959, "Use of half-normal plots in interpreting factorial two-level experiments," *Technometrics*, **1**:311.

Das, M. N., and G. A. Kulkarni, 1966, "Incomplete block designs for bioassays," *Biometrics*, **22**:706.

David, H. A., 1952, "Upper 5 and 1% points of the maximum F-ratio," *Biometrika*, **39**:422.

Diczfalusy, E., and J. A. Loraine, 1955, "Sources of error in clinical bioassays of serum chorionic gonadotropin," *J. Clin. Endocr.*, **15**:424.

Dixon, W. J., 1965, "The up-and-down method for small samples," *J. Amer. Statist. Ass.*, **60**:967.

Dixon, W. J., and A. M. Mood, 1948, "A method for obtaining and analyzing sensitivity data," *J. Amer. Statist. Ass.*, **43**:109.

Dixon, W. J., and J. W. Tukey, 1968, "Approximate behavior of the distribution of Winsorized t (Trimming/Winsorization 2)," *Technometrics*, **10**:83.

Dorfman, R. I., and A. S. Dorfman, 1948, "Studies on the bioassay of hormones — the comparative oviduct response of various breeds of chicks to stilbestrol," *Endocrinology*, **42**:102.

Drucker, W. D., M. S. Roginsky, and N. P. Christy, 1965, "Persistence of abnormal pituitary-adrenal relationship in patients with Cushing's disease partially corrected by bilateral subtotal adrenalectomy," *Amer. J. Med.*, **38**:522.

Duncan, A. J., 1965, *Quality Control and Industrial Statistics*, 3rd ed., Richard D. Irwin, Homewood, Illinois.

Duncan, D. B., 1955, "Multiple range and multiple F tests," *Biometrics*, **11**:1.

Dunn, O. J., and F. J. Massey, Jr., 1965, "Estimation of multiple contrasts using t-distributions," *J. Amer. Statist. Ass.*, **60**:573.

Dunnett, C. W., 1964, "New tables for multiple comparisons with a control," *Biometrics*, **20**:482.

Edwards, W., H. Lindman, and L. J. Savage, 1963, "Bayesian statistical inference for psychological research," *Psychol. Rev.*, **70**:193.

Ekins, R. P., 1960, "The estimation of thyroxine in human plasma by an electrophoretic technique," *Clin. Chim. Acta*, **5**:453.

Ekins, R., 1962, "Saturation analysis: a microanalytical technique for assaying some compounds of biological importance," in *Radioaktive Isotope in Klinik und Forschung*, vol. 5 (Vortrage am Gasteiner Internationalen Symposion), Urban & Schwarzenberg, Munich, 1963, p. 211.

Ekins, R. P., G. B. Newman, and J. L. H. O'Riordan, 1968, "Theoretical aspects of 'saturation' and radioimmunoassay," in *Radioisotopes in medicine: In vitro studies* (R. L. Hayes, F. A. Goswitz, and B. E. P. Murphy, Eds.), U.S. Atomic Energy Commission, Oak Ridge, Tennessee.

Ekins, R. P., and E. Samols, 1963, "Immunoassay of insulin with insulin-antibody precipitate," *Lancet*, **2**:202.

Ekins, R. P., and A. M. Sgherzi, 1964, "The microassay of vitamin B-12 in human plasma by the saturation assay technique," in *Radiochemical Methods of Analysis II, Proc. Symp. Radiochem. Methods Analysis*, Salzburg, I.A.E.C., Vienna, 1965.

Ellis, F., J. Parker, and M. Hills, 1964, "Experimental electrical stimulation of the bladder," *Brit. J. Surg.*, **51**:857.

Emmens, C. W., 1939a, "Analysis of the assays carried out in various laboratories on the contributions offered towards the International Standard preparation of the gonadotrophic substance of urine of pregnancy," *Bull. Hlth. Org. L.O.N.*, **8**:862.

Emmens, C. W., 1939b, "Reports on Biological Standards. 5. Variables affecting the estimation of androgenic and oestrogenic activity," *Med. Res. Counc. Spec. Rep. Ser.*, No. 234, Privy Council, Medical Research Council, Great Britain.

Emmens, C. W., 1948, *Principles of Biological Assay*, Chapman and Hall, London.

Emmens, C. W., 1950, "Statistical methods," in *Hormone Assay* (C. W. Emmens, Ed.), Academic Press, New York, p. 1.

Emmens, C. W., 1957, "Some properties of methylethylstilboestrol," *J. Endocr.*, **16**:148.

Emmens, C. W., 1960, "The role of statistics in physiological research," *Biometrics*, **16**:161.

Emmens, C. W., 1962, "Statistical methods," in *Methods in Hormone Research*, vol. II: *Bioassay* (R. I. Dorfman, Ed.), Academic Press, New York, p. 3.

Emmens, C. W., and L. Martin, 1963, "Intravaginal assay of oestrogens in mice," *Steroids*, **2**:221.

Federer, W. T., 1955, *Experimental Design*, Macmillan, New York.

Felber, J. P., 1963, "ACTH antibodies and their use for a radioimmunoassay for ACTH," *Experientia* (Basel), **19**:227.

Feuer, G., and P. L. Broadhurst, 1962, "Thyroid function in rats selectively bred for emotional elimination. III. Behavioural and physiological changes after treatment with drugs acting on the thyroid," *J. Endocr.*, **24**:385.

Fieller, E. C., 1940, "The biological standardization of insulin," *J. Roy. Statist. Soc.*, **Suppl. 7**:1.

Fieller, E. C., J. O. Irwin, H. P. Marks, and E. A. G. Shrimpton, 1939, "The dosage–response relation in the cross-over rabbit test for insulin. Part II," *Quart. J. Pharm.*, **12**:724.

Finney, D. J., 1950, "The estimation of the mean of a normal tolerance distribution," *Sankhya*, **10**:341.

Finney, D. J., 1952, *Probit Analysis*, 2nd ed., Cambridge University Press, Cambridge, England.

Finney, D. J., 1953, "The estimation of the ED_{50} for a logistic response curve," *Sankhya*, **12**:121.

Finney, D. J., 1955, *Experimental Design and Its Statistical Basis*, University of Chicago Press, Chicago, Illinois.

Finney, D. J., 1960, *An Introduction to the Theory of Experimental Design*, University of Chicago Press, Chicago, Illinois.

Finney, D. J., 1964, *Statistical Method in Biological Assay*, 2nd ed., Charles Griffin, London.

Fisher, R. A., 1935, *The Design of Experiments*, Oliver and Boyd, Edinburgh and London (1966, 8th ed., paperback).

Fisher, R. A., 1949, "A biological assay of tuberculins," *Biometrics*, **5**:300.

Fisher, R. A., and W. A. Mackenzie, 1923, "Studies in crop variation. II. The manurial response of different potato varieties," *J. Agric. Sci.* (Cambridge), **13**:311.

Fisher, R. A., and F. Yates, 1963, *Statistical Tables for Biological, Agricultural and Medical Research*, 6th ed., Oliver and Boyd, Edinburgh.

Forsham, P. H., A. E. Renold, and T. F. Frawley, 1951, "The nature of ACTH resistance," *J. Clin. Endocr.*, **11**:757.

Gaddum, J. H., 1950, "Hormone assay: introduction," *Analyst*, **75**:530.

Galicich, J. H., F. Halberg, and L. A. French, 1963, "Circadian adrenal cycle in C mice kept without food and water for a day and a half," *Nature* (London), **197**:811.

Gilbert, J. P., 1967, *Conversational Algebraic Language Student's Manual*, Harvard Computing Center, Cambridge, Massachusetts.

Glick, S. M., J. Roth, and E. T. Lonergan, 1964, "Survival of endogenous human growth hormone in plasma," *J. Clin. Endocr.*, **24**:501.

Glover, T. D., 1956, "The effect of scrotal insulation and the influence of the breeding season upon fructose concentration in the semen of the ram," *J. Endocr.*, **13**:235.

Goetz, F. C., B. Z. Greenberg, J. Ells, and C. L. Meinert, 1963, "A simple immunoassay for insulin: application to human and dog plasma," *J. Clin. Endocr.*, **23**:1237.

Gold, H., N. T. Kivit, and McK. Cattell, 1940, "Studies on purified digitalis glucosides. I. Potency and dosage of 'Digitaline Nativelle' by oral administration in man," *J. Pharmacol. Exp. Ther.*, **69**:177.

Goldin, A., J. M. Venditti, S. R. Humphreys, and N. Mantel, 1956, "Modification of treatment schedules in the management of advanced mouse leukemia with amethopterin," *J. Nat. Cancer Inst.*, **17**:203.

Good, B. F., and N. S. Stenhouse, 1966, "An improved bioassay for TSH by modification of the method of McKenzie," *Endocrinology*, **78**:429.

Goodman, L. A., and W. H. Kruskal, 1954, "Measures of association for cross-classifications," *J. Amer. Statist. Ass.*, **49**:732.

Goodman, L. A., and W. H. Kruskal, 1959, "Measures of association for cross-classifications: II. Further discussion and references," *J. Amer. Statist. Ass.*, **54**:123.

Goodman, L. A., and W. H. Kruskal, 1963, "Measures of association for cross-classifications: III. Approximate sampling theory," *J. Amer. Statist. Ass.*, **58**:310.

Grant, E. L., 1952, *Statistical Quality Control*, 2nd ed., McGraw-Hill, New York.

Greenwood, F. C., W. M. Hunter, and J. S. Glover, 1963, "The preparation of ^{131}I-labelled human growth hormone of high specific radioactivity," *Biochem. J.*, **89**:114.

Greep, R. O., H. B. Van Dyke, and B. F. Chow, 1941, "Use of anterior lobe of prostate gland in the assay of metakentrin," *Proc. Soc. Exp. Biol. Med.*, **46**:644.

Guillemin, R., and E. Sakiz, 1963, "Quantitative study of the response to LH after hypophysectomy in the ovarian ascorbic acid depletion test: effect of prolactin," *Endocrinology*, **72**:813.

Gurpide, E., and J. Mann, 1965, "Estimation of secretory rates of hormones from the specific activities of metabolites which have multiple secreted precursors," *Bull. Math. Biophys.*, **27**:389.

Harter, H. L., D. S. Clemm, and E. H. Guthrie, 1959, "Probability integral and percentage points of the Studentized range: critical values for Duncan's new multiple range test," *WADC Tech. Rep.*, vol. II, Wright Air Development Center, Ohio, p. 58.

Hawkins, D. F., 1964, "Observations on the application of the Robbins-Monro process to sequential toxicity assays," *Brit. J. Pharmacol.*, **22**:392.

Hayashida, T., 1964, "Frontiers in immunoendocrinology," *Proc. 2nd Int. Congr. Endocr.*, London (S. Taylor, Ed.), International Congress Series No. 83, Excerpta Medica Foundation, Amsterdam, Part II, p. 1356.

Hearon, J. Z., 1963, "Theorems on linear systems," *Ann. N.Y. Acad. Sci.*, **108**:36.

Hill, A. B., 1962, *Statistical Methods in Clinical and Preventive Medicine*, Oxford University Press, New York, and E. and S. Livingstone, Edinburgh.

Hill, W. J., and W. G. Hunter, 1966, "A review of response surface methodology: a literature survey," *Technometrics*, **8**:571.

Horton, R., and J. F. Tait, 1966, "Androstenedione production and interconversion rates measured in peripheral blood and studies on the possible site of its conversion to testosterone," *J. Clin. Invest.*, **45**:301.

James, G., and R. C. James, 1959, *Mathematics Dictionary*, 2nd ed., D. Van Nostrand, Princeton, New Jersey.

Jones, R. C., 1959, "Phenomenological description of the response and detecting ability of radiation detectors," *Proc. Inst. Radio Engineers*, **47**:1495.

Kaiser, H., and H. Specker, 1956, "Bewertung und Vergleich von Analysenverfahren," *Z. Anal. Chem.*, **149**:46.

Kaneto, A., K. Kosaka, and K. Nakao, 1967, "Effects of stimulation of the vagus nerve on insulin secretion," *Endocrinology*, **80**:530.

Kendall, J. W., Jr., G. W. Liddle, C. F. Federspiel, and J. Cornfield, 1963, "Dissociation of corticotropin-suppressing activity from the eosinopenic and hyperglycemic activities of corticosteroid analogues," *J. Clin. Invest.*, **42**:396.

Kendall, J. W., Jr., K. Matsuda, C. Duyck, and M. A. Greer, 1964, "Studies of the location of the receptor site for negative feedback control of ACTH release," *Endocrinology*, **74**:279.

Kennedy, T. J., Jr., M. Eden, and R. W. Berliner, 1957, "Interpretation of urine CO_2 tension," *Fed. Proc.*, **16**:72.

Keuls, M., 1952, "The use of the Studentized range in connection with an analysis of variance," *Euphytica*, **1**:112.

Kodlin, D., 1951, "An application of the analysis of covariance in pharmacology," *Arch. Int. Pharamcodyn.*, **87**:207.

Kotter, K., 1960, "General properties of oscillating systems," *Cold Spring Harbor Symposia on Quantitative Biology*, vol. 25, The Biological Laboratory, Long Island Biological Association, New York, 1961, p. 185.

Kruskal, W. H., 1958, "Ordinal measures of association," *J. Amer. Statist. Ass.*, **53**:814.

Krutchkoff, R. G., 1967, "Classical and inverse regression methods of calibration," *Technometrics*, **9**:425.

Labrie, N., J. G. Pacquet, J. C. Gille, and C. Fortier, 1966, "Dynamique de la sécrétion de corticosterone chez le rat," *Proc. 4th Int. Congr. Cybernetic Med.*, Nice, p. 345.

Labrie, F., J. P. Raynaud, P. Ducommun, and C. Fortier, 1965, "Physiological significance of corticosteroid binding by transcortin," *Proc. 47th Meeting Endocrine Soc.*, Abstract No. 85, New York, p. 63.

Lamond, D. R., and B. M. Bindon, 1966, "The biological assay of follicle-stimulating hormone in hypophysectomized immature mice," *J. Endocr.*, **34**:365.

Lamond, D. R., and C. W. Emmens, 1959, "The effect of hypophysectomy on the mouse uterine response to gonadotrophins," *J. Endocr.*, **18**:251.

Laumas, K. R., J. F. Tait, and S. A. S. Tait, 1961a, "The validity of the calculation of secretion rates from the specific activity of a urinary metabolite," *Acta Endocr.* (Kobenhavn), **36**:265.

Laumas, K. R., J. F. Tait, and S. A. S. Tait, 1961b, "Further considerations on the calculations of secretion rates. A correction," *Acta Endocr.* (Kobenhavn), **38**:469.

Lee, H. M., E. B. Robbins, and K. K. Chen, 1942, "The potency of stilbestrol in the immature female rat," *Endocrinology*, **30**:469.

Leech, F. B., and A. B. Paterson, 1952, "The effects of thyroxine and thiouracil on the tuberculin reactions of guinea pigs," *J. Endocr.*, **8**:96.

Liddle, G. W., D. Island, and C. K. Meador, 1962, "Normal and abnormal regulation of corticotropin secretion in man," in *Recent Progress in Hormone Research*, vol. 18 (G. Pincus, Ed.), Academic Press, New York, p. 125.

Lipscomb, H. S., and D. H. Nelson, 1960, "Dynamic changes in ascorbic acid and corticosteroids in adrenal vein blood after ACTH," *Endocrinology*, **66**:144.

Loraine, J. A., 1957, "Some general principles in the bioassay of anterior and placental hormones in blood with special reference to clinical problems," in *CIBA Foundation Colloquium on Endocrinology, No. 11, Hormones in Blood*, Churchill, London, p. 19.

Loraine, J. A., and E. T. Bell, 1966, *Hormone Assays and Their Clinical Application*, 2nd ed., Williams and Wilkins, Baltimore.

Lunenfeld, B., E. Rabau, A. Harell-Steinberg, and A. Szejnberg, 1957, "Effect of injection medium on quantal assay of chorionic gonadotrophin in male toads," *Acta Endocr.* (Kobenhavn), **24**:113.

McCracken, D. D., 1961, *A Guide to Fortran Programming*, Wiley, New York.

McKerns, K. W., and E. Nordstrand, 1955, "The *in vitro* adrenal response to corticotrophin subtypes: an improved assay design," *Canad. J. Biochem.*, **33**:681.

Mackinnon, P. C. B., M. E. Monk-Jones, and K. Fotherby, 1963, "A study of various indices of adrenocortical activity during 23 days at high altitude," *J. Endocr.*, **26**:555.

Macurdy, L. B., H. K. Alber, A. A. Benedetti-Pichler, H. Carmichael, A. H. Corwin, R. M. Fowler, E. W. D. Huffman, P. L. Kirk, and T. W. Lashof, 1954, "Terminology for describing the performance of analytical and other precise balances. Report and recommendations of the Committee on Balances and Weights," *Anal. Chem.*, **26**:1190.

Mandl, A. M., and S. Zuckerman, 1950, "The numbers of normal and atretic ova in the mature rat," *J. Endocr.*, **6**:426.

Martin, L., 1960, "The use of 2-3-5-triphenyltetrazolium chloride in the biological assay of oestrogens," *J. Endocr.*, **20**:187.

Martin, L., and P. J. Claringbold, 1960, "The mitogenic action of œstrogens in the vaginal epithelium of the ovariectomized mouse," *J. Endocr.*, **20**:173.

Meckler, R. J., and R. L. Collins, 1965, "Histology and weight of the mouse adrenal: a diallel genetic study," *J. Endocr.*, **31**:95.

Meinert, C. L., and R. B. McHugh, 1968, "The biometry of an isotope displacement immunologic microassay," *Math. Biosci.*, **2**:319.

Miller, L. C., 1944, "The U.S.P. collaborative digitalis study using frogs (1939–1941)," *J. Amer. Pharm. Ass.*, **33**:245.

Miller, R. P., Jr., 1966, *Simultaneous Statistical Inference*, McGraw-Hill, New York.

Morgan, C. R., and A. Lazarow, 1963, "Immunoassay of insulin: two antibody system," *Diabetes*, **12**:115.

Morrison, G. H., and R. K. Skogerboe, 1965, "General aspects of trace analysis," in *Trace Analysis: Physical Methods* (G. H. Morrison, Ed.), Interscience, New York, p. 1.

Mosteller, F., and J. W. Tukey, 1968, "Data analysis, including statistics," in *Revised Handbook of Social Psychology* (G. Lindsey, and E. Aronson, Eds.), Addison-Wesley, Reading, Massachusetts.

Munford, R. E., 1963, "Changes in the mammary glands of rats and mice during pregnancy, lactation and involution. 1. Histological structure," *J. Endocr.*, **28**:1.

Murphy, B. E. P., W. Engelberg, and C. J. Pattee, 1963, "Simple method for the determination of plasma corticoids," *J. Clin. Endocr.*, **23**:293.

Murphy, B. E. P., and C. J. Pattee, 1964, "Determination of thyroxine utilizing the property of protein-binding," *J. Clin. Endocr.*, **24**:187.

Mussett, M. V., and W. L. M. Perry, 1955, "The International Standard for thyrotrophin," *Bull. Wld. Hlth. Org.*, **13**:917.

Mussett, M. V., and W. L. M. Perry, 1956, "The Second International Standard for corticotrophin," *Bull. Wld. Hlth. Org.*, **14**:543.

Nicol, D. S. H. W., and L. F. Smith, 1960, "Amino-acid sequence of human insulin," *Nature* (London), **187**:483.

Normand, M., F. Labrie, J.–G. Paquet, J.–C. Gille, and C. Fortier, 1966, "Dynamique de la sécrétion de corticosterone chez le rat," *Proc. 4th Int. Congr. Cybernetic Med.*, Nice, p. 345.

Nugent, C. A., K. Eik-Nes, and F. H. Tyler, 1961, "The disposal of plasma 17-hydroxycorticosteroids. I. Exponential disposal from a single compartment," *J. Clin. Endocr.*, **21**:1106.

Odell, W. D., G. T. Ross, and P. L. Rayford, 1967, "Radioimmunoassay for luteinizing hormone in human plasma or serum: physiological studies," *J. Clin. Invest.*, **46**:248.

Parker, J. L., R. D. Utiger, and W. H. Daughaday, 1962, "Studies on human growth hormone. II. The physiological disposition and metabolic rate of human growth hormone in man," *J. Clin. Invest.*, **41**:262.

Parlow, A. F., 1961, "Bio-assay of pituitary luteinizing hormone by depletion of ovarian ascorbic acid," in *Human Pituitary Gonadotropins* (A. Albert, Ed.), Charles C. Thomas, Springfield, Illinois, p. 300.

Pearce, S. C., 1965, *Biological Statistics: an Introduction*, McGraw-Hill, New York.

Pearlman, W. H., 1957, "Circulating steroid hormone levels in relation to steroid hormone production," in *CIBA Foundation Colloquium on Endocrinology, No. 11, Hormones in Blood*, Churchill, London, p. 233.

Pearson, E. S., and H. O. Hartley, 1958, *Biometrika Tables for Statisticians*, vol. I, 2nd ed., Cambridge University Press, Cambridge, England, pp. 46 and 164.

Perry, W. L. M., 1950, "Biometrical aspects of biological assay: 2. The analysis of a collaborative assay of the Third International Digitalis Standard Preparation," *Biometrics*, **6**:322.

Piel, G., editor, 1966, papers concerning computers, *Sci. Amer.*, **215**:65–260.

Pillai, K. C. S., and K. V. Ramachandran, 1954, "On the distribution of the ratio of the i-th observation in an ordered sample from a normal population to an independent estimate of the standard deviation," *Ann. Math. Statist.*, **25**:565.

Pollard, I., and L. Martin, 1967, "The rate of uptake of locally applied oestradiol and oestrone by the vaginal epithelium of the ovariectomized mouse," *J. Endocr.*, **38**:71.

Pugsley, L. I., and C. A. Morrell, 1943, "Variables affecting the biological assay of estrogens," *Endocrinology*, **33**:48.

Robbins, H., and S. Monro, 1951, "A stochastic approximation method," *Ann. Math. Statist.*, **22**:400.

Rosemberg, E., J. Cornfield, R. W. Bates, and E. Anderson, 1954, "Bioassay of adrenal steroids in blood and urine based on eosinophil response: a statistical analysis," *Endocrinology*, **54**:363.

Rothenberg, S. P., 1961, "Assay of serum vitamin B-12 concentration using Co^{57}–B_{12} and intrinsic factor," *Proc. Soc. Exp. Biol. Med.*, **108**:45.

Rothenberg, S. P., 1965, "A radio-enzymatic assay for folic acid," *Nature* (London), **206**:1154.

Roughton, F. J. W., 1935, "Recent work on carbon dioxide transport by the blood," *Physiol. Rev.*, **15**:241.

Rümke, C. L., 1959, "The influence of atropine on the toxicity of thialbarbitone, thiopentone and pentobarbital (with an appendix on sequential toxicity testing)," *Arch. Int. Pharmocodyn.*, **119**:10.

Salassa, R. M., T. P. Kearns, J. W. Kernohan, R. G. Sprague, and C. S. McCarty, 1959, "Pituitary tumors in patients with Cushing's syndrome," *J. Clin. Endocr.*, **19**:1523.

Salvatierra, V., and A. Torres, 1952, "Acción inhibidora del suero sanguineo sobre la respuesta del mocho de 'R. esculenta' in la inyección de gonadotropina corionica," *Acta Ginec.* (Madrid), **3**:435

Samuels, L. T., H. Brown, K. Eik-Nes, F. H. Tyler, and O. V. Dominguez, 1957, "Extra-adrenal factors affecting the levels of 17-hydroxycorticosteroids in plasma," in *CIBA Foundation Colloquium on Endocrinology, No. 11, Hormones in Blood*, Churchill, London, p. 208.

Satterthwaite, F., 1946, "An approximate distribution of estimates of variance components," *Biometrics Bull.*, **2**:110.

Savage, I. R., 1957, "Nonparametric statistics," *J. Amer. Statist. Ass.*, **52**:331.

Savage, I. R., 1968, "Nonparametric statistics: the field," in *International Encyclopedia of the Social Sciences*, Macmillan, Free Press, New York, p. 175.

Scatchard, G., 1949, "The attractions of proteins for small molecules and ions," *Ann. N.Y. Acad. Sci.*, **51**:660.

Scheffé, H., 1953, "A method for judging all contrasts in the analysis of variance," *Biometrika*, **40**:87.

Scheffé, H., 1959, *The Analysis of Variance*, Wiley, New York.

Seeger, P., 1966, *Variance Analysis of Complete Designs — Some Practical Aspects*, Almqvist and Wiksells, Uppsala, Sweden.

Sharney, L., L. R. Wasserman, and N. R. Gewirtz, 1964, "Representation of certain mammillary *N*-pool systems by two-pool models," *Amer. J. Med. Electronics*, **3**:249.

Sheps, M. C., and P. L. Munson, 1957, "The error of replicated potency estimates in a biological assay method of the parallel line type," *Biometrics*, **13**:131.

Shizume, K., A. B. Lerner, and T. B. Fitzpatrick, 1954, "*In vitro* bioassay for the melanocyte stimulating hormone," *Endocrinology*, **54**:553.

Siegel, S., 1956, *Nonparametric Statistics for the Behavioral Sciences*, McGraw-Hill, New York.

Snedecor, G. W., and W. G. Cochran, 1967, *Statistical Methods*, 6th ed., Iowa State University Press, Ames, Iowa.

Steelman, S. L., and F. M. Pohley, 1953, "Assay of the follicle stimulating hormone based on the augmentation with human chorionic gonadotropin," *Endocrinology*, **53**:604.

Tait, J. F., and S. Burstein, 1964, "*In vivo* studies of steroid dynamics in man," in *The Hormones*, vol. 5 (G. Pincus, K. V. Thimann, and E. B. Astwood, Eds.), Academic Press, New York.

Tait, S. A. S., J. F. Tait, M. Okamoto, and C. Flood, 1967, "Production of steroids by *in vitro* superfusion of endocrine tissue. I. Apparatus and a suitable analytical method for adrenal steroid output," *Endocrinology*, **81**:1213.

Thompson, W. R., 1948, "On the use of parallel or non-parallel systems of transformed curves in bioassay: illustration in the quantitative complement-fixation test," *Biometrics*, **4**:197.

Tukey, J. W., 1949, "One degree of freedom for non-additivity," *Biometrics*, **5**:232.

Tukey, J. W., 1953, "The problem of multiple comparisons," unpublished.

Ungar, F., 1964, "*In vitro* studies of adrenal-pituitary circadian rhythms in the mouse," *Ann. N.Y. Acad. Sci.*, **117**:374.

Ungar, F., and F. Halberg, 1963, "*In vitro* exploration of a circadian rhythm in adrenocorticotropic activity of C mouse hypophysis," *Experientia* (Basel), **19**:158.

United States Pharmacopeia, XVII Revision, "Insulin injection," 1965, Mack Publishing, Easton, Pennsylvania, p. 306.

Utiger, R. D., M. L. Parker, and W. H. Daughaday, 1962, "Studies on human growth hormone. I. A radioimmunoassay for human growth hormone," *J. Clin. Invest.*, **41**:254.

Vande Wiele, R. L., P. C. MacDonald, E. Gurpide, and S. Lieberman, 1963, "Studies on the secretion and interconversion of the androgens," *Recent Progr. Hormone Res.*, **19**:275.

van Strik, R., 1961, "A method of estimating relative potency and its precision in the case of semi-quantitative responses," in *Quantitative Methods in Pharmacology* (H. De Jonge, Ed.), North Holland Publishing, Amsterdam, and Interscience Publishers, New York, p. 88.

Wajchenberg, B. L., A. A. Pupo, and C. M. Laves, 1964, "Adrenocorticotropic potency of a synthetic 24 amino acid polypeptide," *J. Clin. Endocr.*, **24**:1083.

Wales, R. G., and I. G. White, 1958, "The interaction of pH tonicity and electrolyte concentration on the motility of fowl spermatozoa," *Aust. J. Biol. Sci.*, **11**:177.

Watkinson, G., 1958, "Treatment of ulcerative colitis with topical hydrocortisone hemisuccinate sodium: a controlled trial employing restricted sequential analysis," *Brit. Med. J.*, **2**:1077.

Wetherill, G. B., 1963, "Sequential estimation of quantal response curves," *J. Roy. Statist. Soc. Ser. B*, **25**:1.

Williams, E. J., 1949, "Experimental designs balanced for the estimation of residual effects of treatments," *Aust. J. Sci. Res.*, **2**:149.

Wilson, A. L., 1961, "The precision and limit of detection of analytical methods," *Analyst*, **86**:72.

Yalow, R. S., and S. A. Berson, 1959, "Assay of plasma insulin in human subjects by immunological methods," *Nature* (London), **184**:1648.

Yalow, R. S., and S. A. Berson, 1960a, "Editorial: Plasma insulin in man," *Amer. J. Med.*, **29**:1.

Yalow, R. S., and S. A. Berson, 1960b, "Immunoassay of endogenous plasma insulin in man," *J. Clin. Invest.*, **39**:1157.

Yalow, R. S., and S. A. Berson, 1961a, "Immunological specificity of human insulin: application to immunoassay of insulin," *J. Clin. Invest.*, **40**:2190.

Yalow, R. S., and S. A. Berson, 1961b, "Immunoassay of plasma insulin in man," *Diabetes*, **10**:339.

Yalow, R. S., and S. A. Berson, 1968a, "General principles of radioimmunoassay," in *Radioisotopes in Medicine: in vitro Studies* (R. L. Hayes, F. A. Goswitz, and B. E. P. Murphy, Eds.), U.S. Atomic Energy Commission, Oak Ridge, Tennessee, p. 7.

Yalow, R. S., and S. A. Berson, 1968b, "Special problems in the radioimmunoassay of small polypeptides," in *Protein and Polypeptide Hormones, Part I*, International Congress Series No. 161 (M. Margoulies, Ed.), Excerpta Medica Foundation, Amsterdam, p. 71.

Yalow, R. S., S. M. Glick, J. Roth, and S. A. Berson, 1964, "Radio-immunoassay of human plasma ACTH," *J. Clin. Endocr.*, **24**:1219.

Yates, F. E., 1967, "The liver and the adrenal cortex," *Gastroenterology*, **53**:477.

Yates, F. E., and R. D. Brennan, 1967, "Study of the mammalian adrenal glucocorticoid system by computer simulation," Palo Alto Scientific Center, IBM Data Processing Division, *IBM Tech. Rep. No. 320–3228*, p. 51.

Yates, F. E., and J. Urquhart, 1962, "Control of plasma concentrations of adrenocortical hormones," *Physiol. Rev.*, **42**:359.

Young, D. M., and R. G. Romans, 1948, "Assay of insulin with one blood sample per rabbit per test day," *Biometrics*, **4**:122.

Index to Discussion Participants

Subject Index